As unprecedented numbers of women reach midlife, "menopause management" has become a major public healthcare issue. The North American Menopause Society (NAMS) is uniquely qualified to provide menopause-related information.

With the founding of NAMS in 1989, a forum was created to enhance the exchange of knowledge and experience among specialists from multiple disciplines. Physicians (including gynecologists, internists, psychiatrists, and cardiologists), physician assistants, nurse practitioners, nurses, pharmacists, psychotherapists, nutritionists, and other specialists, including those involved in research, have contributed to the better understanding of key issues — resulting in improved quality of life for women at midlife and beyond.

In mid-2000, NAMS published the first edition of the *Menopause Core Curriculum Study Guide*. It was designed to serve as a resource for healthcare professionals who are charged with providing care for women during these years. The study guide presents a comprehensive overview of the key issues in the field. With this second edition, NAMS has expanded the information to cover a wider range of menopause issues. NAMS hopes that this resource will play a role in standardizing practices — thereby eliminating confusion among peri- and postmenopausal women and resulting in their optimal health and well-being.

Every effort has been made to ensure that the contents are scientifically valid, current, and unbiased. NAMS recognizes, however, that a considerable amount of scientific research is ongoing and will undoubtedly render some material contained here out-of-date. There also are many unanswered questions about menopause.

This study guide is also designed to assist those who are preparing for the NAMS Menopause Practitioner competency examination, although studying this guide in preparation for the examination will not guarantee a passing score. For more information about the examination, contact the NAMS Central Office (440-442-7550).

This text is not designed to be a complete review. Healthcare providers must identify their own area(s) of weakness, seek out additional information from other sources, and develop an individualized plan that will meet their unique needs.

The development of this *Menopause Core Curriculum Study Guide* has been entirely through The North American Menopause Society. Special thanks are owed to the Society members and other experts mentioned on the following pages, who contributed their time, knowledge, and energy.

Wulf H. Utian, MD, PhD
Executive Director
The North American Menopause Society

Acknowledgments

The North American Menopause Society wishes to acknowledge the efforts of the following individuals who contributed editorial content and/or reviewed the text. Members of the NAMS 2001-2002 Board of Trustees are marked with an asterisk. The Society is also grateful to **Philip K. Lammers,** NAMS Medical Editor, and **Pamela P. Boggs, MBA,** NAMS Director of Education and Development, whose editorial skills were invaluable.

George I. Gorodeski, MD, PhD*
Professor of Reproductive Biology, Case Western
    Reserve University School of Medicine
Department of Obstetrics and Gynecology,
    University Hospitals of Cleveland
Cleveland, OH

Gail A. Greendale, MD*
Associate Professor of Medicine and Obstetrics
    and Gynecology
University of California, Los Angeles
Los Angeles, CA

Kathryn K. Havens, MD
Internist
Associate Professor of Family Medicine,
    University of Wisconsin Medical School
Milwaukee, WI

Victor W. Henderson, MD, MS
Center on Aging
University of Arkansas for Medical Sciences
Little Rock, AR

David M. Herrington, MD, MHS
Professor of Internal Medicine – Cardiology
Wake Forest University School of Medicine
Winston-Salem, NC

Andrew G. Herzog, MD
Director, Neuroendocrine Unit
Beth Israel Deaconess Medical Center
Boston, MA

Susan R. Johnson, MD
Professor of Obstetrics and Gynecology,
    and Epidemiology
University of Iowa
Iowa City, IA

Elaine E. Jolly, OC, MD, FRCS(C)
Associate Professor, Obstetrics and
    Gynecology, University of Ottawa
Director, Women's Health Centre, Ottawa
    Hospital
Ottawa, ON, Canada

Risa Kagan, MD
Associate Clinical Professor
Department of Obstetric and Gynecology
    and Reproductive Sciences
University of California, San Francisco
Co-Medical Director, Foundation for
    Osteoporosis Research and Education
Oakland, CA

Brinda M. Kalro, MD
Assistant Professor
Division of Reproductive Endocrinology
    and Infertility
Department of Obstetrics and Gynecology,
    and Reproductive Sciences
Magee-Womens Hospital
Pittsburgh, PA

Andrew M. Kaunitz, MD
Professor and Assistant Chair
Director, Menopause and Bone Density Services
University of Florida Health Science Center
Jacksonville, FL

Bruce Kessel, MD*
Associate Professor
Department of Obstetrics and Gynecology,
    and Women's Health
John A. Burns School of Medicine
University of Hawaii
Honolulu, HI

Rebecca S. Kightlinger, DO
Presque Isle Gynecology Center for
    Menopausal Health
Erie, PA

Sheryl A. Kingsberg, PhD
Assistant Professor
Departments of Reproductive Biology
    and Psychiatry
Case Western Reserve University School
    of Medicine
Department of Obstetrics and Gynecology,
    University Hospitals of Cleveland
Cleveland, OH

Nancy Lane, MD
Associate Professor of Medicine, Division
    of Rheumatology
University of California San Francisco
San Francisco, CA

Gretchen M. Lentz, MD
Associate Professor, Departments of Obstetrics
    and Gynecology, and Urogynecology
Associate Director, Women's Health Care Center
University of Washington
Seattle, WA

Sandra J. Lewis, MD, FACC
Portland Cardiovascular Institute
Portland, OR

Marian C. Limacher, MD
Professor of Medicine, Division of
    Cardiovascular Medicine
University of Florida
Gainesville, FL

Betsy Love McClung, RN, MN*
Associate Director
Oregon Osteoporosis Center
Portland, OR

Michael R. McClung, MD
Director
Oregon Osteoporosis Center
Portland, OR

Margaret F. Moloney, RN-C, PhD, ANP
Associate Professor, Clinical
Nell Hodgson Woodruff School of Nursing
Emory University
Atlanta, GA

Valerie C. Montgomery Rice, MD
Associate Professor, Department of Obstetrics
    and Gynecology
University of Kansas Medical Center
Kansas City, KS

Laura Mueller, MD
Park Nicollet Medical Center
Shakopee, MN

Lila E. Nachtigall, MD*
Professor of Obstetrics and Gynecology
New York University School of Medicine
New York, NY

Katherine M. Newton, PhD
Associate Investigator, Center for Health Studies
Group Health Cooperative
Affiliate Assistant Professor, Department of
    Epidemiology
Affiliate Assistant Professor, Department of
    Biobehavioral Nursing and Health Systems
University of Washington
Seattle, WA

Annette M. Cormier O'Connor, RN, PhD*
Professor, University of Ottawa
Faculty of Health Sciences, School of Nursing
Faculty of Medicine, Department of
    Epidemiology and Community Medicine
Senior Scientist, Ottawa Health Research
    Institute, Ottawa Hospital
Ottawa, ON, Canada

(continued)

Joan Otomo-Corgel, DDS, MPH
UCLA School of Dentistry
Department of Periodontics
Los Angeles, CA

Diane T. Pace, PhD, APRN, BC
Family Nurse Practitioner/Researcher
Regional Medical Center at Memphis
Memphis, TN

JoAnn V. Pinkerton, MD
Director, Midlife Health Center
Associate Professor, Department of Obstetrics
    and Gynecology
University of Virginia Health System
Charlottesville, VA

Jennifer L. Prouty, MSN, RNC
Women's Health Nurse Practitioner and
    Psychiatric Clinical Nurse Specialist
Perinatal and Reproductive Psychiatry Program
Massachusetts General Hospital
Boston, MA
Midlife Health Connections
Mattapoisett, MA

Natalie L. Rasgon, MD, PhD
Director, UCLA Menopause-Related Mood
    Disorder Program
Assistant Professor of Psychiatry, UCLA School
    of Medicine
Los Angeles, CA

Veronica A. Ravnikar, MD
Chairperson, Department of Obstetrics
    and Gynecology
St. Barnabas Medical Center
Livingston, NJ
Lecturer, Harvard Medical School
Associate Clinical Gynecologist, Massachusetts
    General Hospital
Boston, MA

Nancy E. Reame, MSN, PhD, FAAN
Professor of Nursing and Research Scientist
Reproductive Sciences Program
University of Michigan
Ann Arbor, MI

Marcie K. Richardson, MD*
Assistant Director of Obstetrics and
    Gynecology for Clinical Quality
The Copley Center
Harvard Vanguard Medical Associates
Boston, MA

Marilyn Rothert, PhD, RN, FAAN
Dean and Professor
College of Nursing
Michigan State University
East Lansing, MI

Andrew L. Rubman, ND
Adjunct Associate Professor of Clinical Medicine
University of Bridgeport, College of
    Naturopathic Medicine
Bridgeport, CT
Director, Southbury Clinic for Traditional
    Medicines
Southbury, CT

Ronald J. Ruggiero, PharmD
Clinical Professor, Department of Clinical
    Pharmacy and Obstetrics, Gynecology
    and Reproductive Sciences
University of California, San Francisco
San Francisco, CA

Nanette F. Santoro, MD
Professor of Obstetrics and Gynecology
Director, Division of Reproductive
    Endocrinology and Infertility
Albert Einstein College of Medicine
Bronx, NY

Isaac Schiff, MD*
Joe Vincent Meigs Professor of Gynecology
Harvard Medical School
Chief, Vincent Memorial Ob/Gyn Service
Massachusetts General Hospital, Women's
    Care Division
Boston, MA

Peter E. Schwartz, MD
John Slade Ely Professor of Obstetrics
    and Gynecology
Yale School of Medicine
New Haven, CT

Joan L.F. Shaver, PhD, RN, FAAN
Professor and Dean
College of Nursing
University of Illinois at Chicago
Chicago, IL

Jan L. Shifren, MD
Director, Menopause Program, Vincent
    Memorial Ob/Gyn Service
Massachusetts General Hospital
Assistant Professor of Obstetrics, Gynecology,
    and Reproductive Biology
Harvard Medical School
Boston, MA

James A. Simon, MD*
Clinical Professor of Obstetrics and Gynecology
George Washington University School
    of Medicine
Washington, DC

Janine A. Smith, MD
Deputy Clinical Director
Division of Epidemiology and Clinical Research
National Eye Institute
Bethesda, MD

Cynthia A. Stuenkel, MD
Clinical Professor of Medicine
Division of Endocrine/Metabolism
University of California, San Diego
La Jolla, CA

Eliza Sutton, MD
Women's Health Care Center
University of Washington
Seattle, WA

Maida B. Taylor, MD, MPH, FACOG
Associate Clinical Professor
Department of Obstetrics and Gynecology,
    and Reproductive Science
University of California, San Francisco
San Francisco, CA

Wulf H. Utian, MD, PhD*
Arthur H. Bill Professor Emeritus of Reproductive
    Biology, and Obstetrics and Gynecology
Case Western Reserve School of Medicine
Consultant in Women's Health, Cleveland
    Clinic Foundation
President, Rapid Medical Research
Executive Director, The North American
    Menopause Society
Cleveland, OH

Robert A. Wild, MD, MPH
Professor and Chief
Section of Reproductive
    Endocrinology/Infertility
Oklahoma University Health Science Center
Oklahoma City, OK

Nancy Fugate Woods, PhD, RN, FAAN*
Dean, School of Nursing
Professor, Family and Child Nursing
University of Washington
Seattle, WA

Sue A. Woodson, RNC, MSN, CNM
Nurse Midwife/Practitioner
The Women's Place – Midlife Health Center
University of Virginia Health Sciences Center
Charlottesville, VA

Contents

Section	Page
A. Introduction	9
A.01. Terminology	9
A.01.a. Menopause	9
A.01.b. Premenopause	10
A.01.c. Perimenopause	10
A.01.d. Menopausal/menopause transition	10
A.01.e. Postmenopause	10
A.01.f. Climacteric	11
A.01.g. Premature menopause	11
A.01.h. Induced menopause	11
A.01.i. Temporary menopause	11
A.02. Demographics	11
A.01.a. United States	11
A.01.b. Canada	12
A.01.c. Worldwide	12
A.03. Evaluating the literature	13
A.03.a. Types of studies	13
A.03.b. Analyses	14
Bibliography for A.	14
B. Normal physiology	15
B.01. Stages of reproductive aging	15
B.01.a. Reproductive interval	15
B.01.b. Menopause transition	16
B.01.c. Postmenopause stages	17
Bibliography for B.01.	18
B.02. Hypothalamic-pituitary-ovarian axis	18
Bibliography for B.02.	19
B.03. Receptor activity	19
Bibliography for B.03.	20
C. Perimenopause/menopause transition	21
C.01. Decline in fertility	21
Bibliography for C.01.	22
C.02. Irregular uterine bleeding	22
Bibliography for C.02.	22
C.03. Vasomotor symptoms	23
Bibliography for C.03.	24
C.04. Sleep disturbances	24
Bibliography for C.04.	25
C.05. Urogenital changes	25
C.05.a. Vulvovaginal changes	26
C.05.b. Urinary complaints	27
Bibliography for C.05.	28
C.06. Central nervous system changes	28
C.06.a. Headache	28
C.06.b. Mood swings	29
C.06.c. Depression and anxiety	30
C.06.d. Cognition	31
Bibliography for C.06.	32
C.07. Sexual function effects	33
Bibliography for C.07.	36

Section	Page
C.08. Skeletal system effects	36
C.08.a. Relationship with menopause	37
C.08.b. Pathophysiology	37
Bibliography for C.08.	38
C.09. Cardiovascular system effects	39
C.09.a. Relationship with menopause	39
Bibliography for C.09.	40
C.10. Other changes/complaints	40
C.10.a. Weight gain	40
C.10.b. Palpitations	41
C.10.c. Joint pain	41
C.10.d. Skin changes	41
C.10.e. Ocular changes	42
C.10.f. Hair changes	42
C.10.g. Dental/oral cavity changes	43
Bibliography for C.10.	43
D. Pathology	45
D.01. Premature menopause	45
D.01.a. Signs and symptoms	45
D.01.b. Etiology	45
D.01.c. Diagnosis	46
Bibliography for D.01.	46
D.02. Induced menopause	47
D.02.a. Effect on fertility	47
D.02.b. Effect on menopause symptoms	48
D.02.c. Effect on sexual function	48
D.02.d. Effect on mental health	49
D.02.e. Effect on long-term health	50
Bibliography for D.02.	50
D.03. Temporary menopause	51
Bibliography for D.03.	51
D.04. Pelvic pathology/abnormal uterine bleeding	51
Bibliography for D.04.	53
D.05. Dementia	53
Bibliography for D.05.	54
E. Clinical evaluation	55
E.01. Primary evaluation	55
E.01.a. History	55
E.01.b. Height	56
E.01.c. Weight	56
Bibliography for E.01.	57
E.02. Ovarian/adrenal function	57
Bibliography for E.02.	59
E.03. Thyroid function	59
Bibliography for E.03.	60
E.04. Diabetes risk	60
Bibliography for E.04.	60

(continued)

Contents continued

Section			Page

E.05. Cardiovascular risk 60
    E.05.a. Blood pressure 60
    E.05.b. Lipid tests 61
    E.05.c. Other tests 62
    Bibliography for E.05. 62

E.06. Osteoporosis risk 63
    E.06.a. History/physical examination . . . 64
    E.06.b. Evaluation 65
    E.06.c. Bone mineral density
          measurement 65
    E.06.d. Defining osteoporosis 66
    E.06.e. Biochemical bone markers 67
    E.06.f. Tests for secondary causes
          of osteoporosis 69
    Bibliography for E.06. 69

E.07. Abnormal uterine bleeding 70
    Bibliography for E.07. 72

E.08. Cancer risk 72
    E.08.a. Breast cancer 73
    E.08.b. Endometrial cancer 75
    E.08.c. Cervical cancer 76
    E.08.d. Ovarian cancer 77
    E.08.e. Colorectal cancer 78
    E.08.f. Pancreatic cancer 79
    E.08.g. Skin cancer 79
    Bibliography for E.08. 79

E.09. Vulvovaginal health 83
    Bibliography for E.09. 83

E.10. Sexual function 84
    Bibliography for E.10. 84

E.11. Urinary incontinence 85
    Bibliography for E.11. 86

E.12. Psychological health 86
    Bibliography for E.12. 87

E.13. Domestic abuse risk 88
    Bibliography for E.13. 88

E.14. Sexually transmitted infections 88
    Bibliography for E.14. 89

F. **Therapeutic options: Lifestyle modification** 91
F.01. Substance use 91
    F.01.a. Smoking 91
    F.01.b. Alcohol 92
    F.01.c. Caffeine 93

F.02. Exercise 93
F.03. Stress reduction 94
F.04. Nutrition 94
    F.04.a. Heart disease and diet 95
    F.04.b. Osteoporosis and diet 96
    F.04.c. Cancer and diet 96

F.05. Weight management 97
Bibliography for F. 99

G. **Therapeutic options: Nonprescription therapies** . . 103
G.01. Government regulations for
    dietary supplements 103
    Bibliography for G.01. 103

G.02. Vitamins and minerals 104
    G.02.a. Calcium 104
    G.02.b. Vitamin D 107
    G.02.c. Vitamin E 107
    G.02.d. B vitamins 108
    G.02.e. Vitamin A 109
    G.02.f. Vitamin C 109
    G.02.g. Chromium 109
    G.02.h. Iron 109
    G.02.i. Magnesium 110
    G.02.j. Others 110
    Bibliography for G.02. 110

G.03. OTC hormones 113
    G.03.a. Topical progesterone 113
    G.03.b. DHEA 114
    G.03.c. Melatonin 115
    Bibliography for G.03. 116

G.04. Aspirin 118
    Bibliography for G.04. 118

G.05. Vaginal lubricants/moisturizers 119
    Bibliography for G.05. 119

G.06. Nonhormonal contraceptives 120
    Bibliography for G.06. 120

H. **Therapeutic options: Prescription therapies** 121
H.01. Contraceptives 121
    H.01.a. Combination (estrogen-
          progestin) contraceptives 121
    H.01.b. Progestin-only contraceptives . . 122
    H.01.c. Emergency contraception 122
    H.01.d. Intrauterine devices 122
    H.01.e. Noncontraceptive use
          during perimenopause 123
    Bibliography for H.01. 123

H.02. ERT and HRT 124
    H.02.a. Estrogens and ERT 124
    H.02.b. Progestogens and HRT 128
    H.02.c. Custom-compounded
          formulations 133
    H.02.d. ERT/HRT safety issues 134
    H.02.e. Transition from hormonal
          contraception to HRT 136
    Bibliography for H.02. 136

H.03. Androgen 140
    Bibliography for H.03. 142

H.04. Osteoporosis agents 143
    H.04.a. Bisphosphonates 143
    H.04.b. SERMs 144
    H.04.c. Calcitonin 145
    H.04.d. Others 145
    H.04.e. Combining therapies 147
    Bibliography for H.04. 147

Section	Page

I. **Therapeutic options: Complementary and alternative medicine (CAM)** 151
    I.01. Alternative medical systems 151
        I.01.a. Traditional Chinese Medicine .. 152
        I.01.b. Other cultural systems 152
        I.01.c. Homeopathic medicine 152
        I.01.d. Naturopathic medicine 153
        Bibliography for I.01. 153
    I.02. Mind-body interventions 154
        Bibliography for I.02. 154
    I.03. Manipulative and body-based methods ... 154
        Bibliography for I.03. 154
    I.04. Energy therapies 154
        Bibliography for I.04. 154
    I.05. Biologically based treatment 154
        I.05.a. Government regulation of dietary supplements 155
          Bibliography for I.05.a. 155
        I.05.b. Botanical therapies 156
          I.05.b.1. General precautions 156
          I.05.b.2. Phytoestrogens 157
            Bibliography for I.05.b.2. 159
          I.05.b.3. Herbs 161
            Bibliography for I.05.b.3. 166
    I.06. Other biologically based therapies 167
        I.06.a. SAM-e 167
          Bibliography for I.06.a. 167
        I.06.b. Glucosamine/chondroitin 168
          Bibliography for I.06.b. 168

J. **Management strategies: Menopause symptoms** .. 169
    J.01. Vasomotor symptoms 169
        Bibliography for J.01. 171
    J.02. Sleep disturbances 172
        Bibliography for J.02. 173
    J.03. Headache 174
        Bibliography for J.03. 175
    J.04. Psychological symptoms 175
        Bibliography for J.04. 176
    J.05. Vulvovaginal changes 177
        Bibliography for J.05. 178
    J.06. Sexual dysfunction 178
        Bibliography for J.06. 180
    J.07. Incontinence 181
        Bibliography for J.07. 183
    J.08. Urinary tract infection 183
        Bibliography for J.08. 184
    J.09. Cognitive function 184
        Bibliography for J.09. 185

    J.10. Skin changes 186
        Bibliography for J.10. 187
    J.11. Ocular changes 188
        Bibliography for J.11. 189
    J.12. Hair changes 190
        Bibliography for J.12. 191
    J.13. Oral/dental changes 191
        Bibliography for J.13. 191

K. **Management strategies: Osteoporosis** 193
    K.01. Nutrition 193
    K.02. Exercise 194
    K.03. Smoking cessation 195
    K.04. Fall prevention 195
    K.05. Pharmacologic interventions 196
    K.06. Management of osteoporotic fractures ... 196
    Bibliography for K. 197

L. **Management strategies: Cardiovascular disease** .. 199
    L.01. Lifestyle modification 199
    L.02. Pharmacologic therapy 200
        L.02.a. Primary prevention 200
        L.02.b. Secondary prevention 202
    Bibliography for L. 202

M. **Management strategies: Abnormal uterine bleeding** 205
    M.01. Medical treatments 205
    M.02. Surgical management 207
    Bibliography for M. 207

N. **Management strategies: Cancer** 209
    N.01. Endometrial cancer 209
        Bibliography for N.01. 210
    N.02. Breast cancer 210
        N.02.a. Management of breast cancer survivors 211
        N.02.b. Management of women with benign breast disease 214
        Bibliography for N.02. 214
    N.03. Cervical/ovarian cancer 216
        Bibliography for N.03. 216
    N.04. Colorectal cancer 217
        Bibliography for N.04. 217

O. **Management strategies: Premature/induced menopause** 219
    Bibliography for O. 219

(continued)

Contents continued

Section	Page
P.	**Management strategies: Concomitant conditions** . 221
P.01.	Diabetes . 221
	Bibliography for P.01. . 223
P.02.	Thyroid disease . 225
	Bibliography for P.02. . 225
P.03.	Arthritis . 226
	Bibliography for P.03. . 227
P.04.	Lupus . 228
	Bibliography for P.04. . 228
P.05.	Epilepsy . 229
	Bibliography for P.05. . 229
P.06.	Pancreatitis . 230
	Bibliography for P.06. . 230
P.07.	Gallbladder disease . 230
	Bibliography for P.07. . 231
P.08.	Asthma . 231
	Bibliography for P.08. . 232
P.09.	Raynaud's syndrome . 232
	Bibliography for P.09. . 232

Section	Page
Q.	**Counseling issues** . 233
Q.01.	View of menopause/aging . 233
	Bibliography for Q.01. . 234
Q.02.	Social and cultural aspects of care . 234
	Bibliography for Q.02. . 236
Q.03.	Behavior modification . 237
	Bibliography for Q.03. . 238
Q.04.	Lifestyle modification . 238
	Bibliography for Q.04. . 238
Q.05.	Treatment counseling . 239
	Q.05.a. HEDIS requirements . 240
	Bibliography for Q.05. . 241
Q.06.	Improving medication continuance . 242
	Bibliography for Q.06. . 243
Q.07.	Importance of listening and building trust . . 245
	Bibliography for Q.07. . 246
Q.08.	Lesbian health . 246
	Bibliography for Q.08. . 248
Q.09.	Sexual function . 249
	Bibliography for Q.09. . 250
Q.10.	Preventing STIs . 250
	Bibliography for Q.10. . 251
Q.11.	Domestic violence . 251
	Bibliography for Q.11. . 252
Q.12.	Alcohol/drug abuse . 252
	Bibliography for Q.12. . 253

Menopause is a natural biologic process, not an estrogen deficiency disease. Menopause represents the permanent cessation of menses resulting from loss of ovarian follicular function. Menopause can occur spontaneously (ie, "naturally") or be induced through a medical intervention (ie, surgery, chemotherapy, or pelvic radiation therapy).

Aging is the natural progression of changes in structure and function that occur with the passage of time in the absence of known disease. Aging of the female reproductive system begins at birth and proceeds as a continuum. It consists of a steady loss of oocytes from atresia or ovulation, which does not necessarily occur at a constant rate, as evidenced by the relatively wide age range (42 to 58 years) for spontaneous menopause. Chronologic age is a very poor indicator of the beginning or the end of the menopause transition.

A.01. Terminology

Clinicians and researchers involved in the field of menopause have long recognized the need for universally accepted menopause terminology as well as a staging system to logically divide the last 10 to 15 years of reproductive aging. In 2001, the Stages of Reproductive Aging Workshop (STRAW) sponsored by The North American Menopause Society (NAMS), the National Institutes of Health, the American Society for Reproductive Medicine, and the National Institute of Child Health and Human Development, addressed nomenclature

and a staging system. Previously, the Council of Affiliated Menopause Societies (CAMS), an international policy organ of the International Menopause Society (IMS), had developed standardized definitions for menopause-related events. Although STRAW redefined some terms, other CAMS terms remain in use.

The reproductive aging continuum created by STRAW was divided into seven stages; five precede and two follow the final menstrual period (Fig 1). STRAW pointed out, however, that not all healthy women will follow this pattern; some will "seesaw" back and forth between stages or skip a stage altogether.

A.01.a. Menopause

The term *menopause* (ie, spontaneous or natural menopause), as described by STRAW, is the anchor point that is defined after 12 months of amenorrhea following the final menstrual period (FMP), which reflects a near complete but natural diminution of ovarian hormone secretion. Menopause means the end of natural childbearing (without assisted reproductive techniques). There is no adequate independent biological marker for menopause.

In the Western world, menopause occurs at an average age of 51.4 years, with a Gaussian distribution ranging from 40 to 58 years. Some women reach menopause in their 30s and a few in their 60s. Although there has been an increase in

---

Figure 1. Stages/nomenclature of normal reproductive aging in women

Final Menstrual Period (FMP)

Stages:	-5	-4	-3	-2	-1	0	+1	+2
Terminology:	Reproductive			Menopausal Transition			Postmenopause	
	Early	Peak	Late	Early	Late*		Early*	Late*
				Perimenopause				
Duration of Stage:	variable			variable		ⓐ 1 yr	ⓑ 4 yrs	until demise
Menstrual Cycles:	variable to regular	regular		variable cycle length (>7 days different from normal)	≥2 skipped cycles and an interval of amenorrhea (≥60 days)	Amen. x 12 mos	none	
Endocrine:	normal FSH		↑ FSH	↑ FSH			↑ FSH	

*Stages most likely to be characterized by vasomotor symptoms.

Source: Stages of Reproductive Aging Workshop (STRAW), *Menopause* 2001.

life expectancy over the years, the age of menopause has not changed during the past few centuries, unaffected by improving nutrition and reduction of disease. In previous centuries, fewer women lived beyond menopause because lifespans were shorter; today, most women spend at least one-third of their lives postmenopause.

Two factors have been identified as influencing when menopause occurs:

- Current smoking has been identified as a cause of earlier menopause, producing a shift of approximately 1.5 years. There is a dose-response relationship between the number of cigarettes smoked, the duration of smoking, and age at menopause.

- Familial factors as well as genetic polymorphisms of the estrogen receptor influence the age of onset of the menopause transition (as well as influencing the risk for surgical menopause).

Limited data support the association of the timing of menopause with the following:

- Multiparity (ie, more than one pregnancy) and increased body mass index are associated with menopause occurring later than average.

- Higher cognitive scores in childhood are associated with a later menopause.

- Nulliparity (ie, history of no pregnancy), medically treated depression, toxic chemical exposure, and treatment of childhood cancer with pelvic radiation and alkylating agents are associated with menopause occurring earlier than average.

- Epilepsy appears to be associated with menopause occurring earlier than average, especially in women with a high lifetime seizure frequency.

No link has been found between age at menopause and use of oral contraceptives, socioeconomic or marital status, race, or age at menarche.

Menopause is one point in time. The misnomers "in menopause" and "going through menopause" accurately describe perimenopause or the menopause transition. It is appropriate to say that one "reaches" menopause.

A.01.b. Premenopause

The term *premenopause,* according to CAMS, is often used ambiguously, either to refer to the 1 or 2 years immediately before menopause or to the whole of the reproductive period prior to menopause. CAMS recommends that this term should be used consistently in the latter sense, and should encompass the entire reproductive period up to the FMP. However, CAMS has also indicated that this term can be confusing and, preferably, should be abandoned.

A.01.c. Perimenopause

The term *perimenopause,* according to STRAW, is defined as about or around menopause. It begins with Stage -2 and ends 12 months after the FMP. STRAW suggests that the term *climacteric* be used synonymously with perimenopause. However, STRAW recommends that the terms *perimenopause* and *climacteric* only be used with patients or in the lay press. Nonetheless, NAMS will use the term *perimenopause* interchangeably with *menopause transition* in this study guide.

A.01.d. Menopausal/menopause transition

According to STRAW, the term *menopausal transition* (or *menopause transition*) is defined as stage -2 (early) and stage -1 (late) and it exhibits menstrual cycle and endocrine changes. The menopausal transition begins with variation in menstrual cycle length in a woman who has monotropic FSH rise and ends with the FMP (not able to be recognized until after 12 months of amenorrhea).

The median age for the onset of the menopause transition is 47.5 years. For most women, the transition lasts approximately 4 years. Only about 10% of women cease menstruating abruptly, experiencing no menstrual irregularity.

A.01.e. Postmenopause

The term *postmenopause* is the span of time dating from the FMP, regardless of whether menopause was spontaneous or induced. It is defined by STRAW as stage +1 (early) and stage +2 (late). STRAW further clarified that the early postmenopause is defined as within 5 years of the FMP. The participants agreed this time period is relevant, as it encompasses a further dampening of ovarian hormone function to a permanent level as well as the period of accelerated bone loss. Stage +1 was further subdivided into segment "a" (ie, the first 12 months after the FMP) and "b" (ie, the next 4 years). Stage +2 has a definite beginning, but the duration is variable because it ends with the woman's death. STRAW concluded that further divisions may be warranted as women live longer and more information is accumulated.

A.01.f. Climacteric

According to CAMS, the term *climacteric* describes the phase during the aging of women marking the transition from the reproductive phase to the nonreproductive state. This phase incorporates perimenopause by extending for a longer, variable period before and after perimenopause. Thus, the climacteric is a process, rather than a specific point in time. According to CAMS, the climacteric is sometimes, but not necessarily always, associated with symptomatology. When this occurs, it may be termed the *climacteric syndrome*.

However, as mentioned above, STRAW has suggested that the term climacteric be used synonymously with perimenopause, and that both terms — *perimenopause* and *climacteric* — should not be used in scientific papers. The global consensus on this terminology has not been achieved. The term *climacteric* is still widely used outside North America, where it often describes the reproductive transition for both women and men.

A.01.g. Premature menopause

According to CAMS, *premature menopause* should be defined as menopause that occurs at an age less than 2 standard deviations below the mean estimated age for the reference population. In practice, CAMS states, the age of 40 is frequently used as an arbitrary cutoff point, below which menopause is said to be premature.

Premature menopause and *premature ovarian failure* (POF) can be synonymous. Strictly speaking, however, menopause is by definition the very last menses. POF (ie, hypergonadotropic amenorrhea), while having all the characteristics of menopause, may not be permanent.

A.01.h. Induced menopause

According to CAMS, the term *induced menopause* is defined as the cessation of menstruation that follows either surgical removal of both ovaries (bilateral oophorectomy, with or without hysterectomy) or iatrogenic ablation of ovarian function (eg, by chemotherapy or pelvic radiation therapy). Bilateral oophorectomy is the most common cause of induced menopause.

In women who experience surgically induced menopause (*surgical menopause*), fertility ends immediately. With other types of induced menopause, fertility may end immediately or over several months.

A.01.i. Temporary menopause

The term *temporary menopause* describes a span of time when normal ovarian function is interrupted and temporary amenorrhea results.

A.02. Demographics

Menopause is a significant public health issue because of three factors: (1) menopause affects every woman, (2) an unprecedented number of women are reaching midlife, and (3) more women are living beyond age 65, with the elderly population also reaching unprecedented numbers. Therefore, treating this population gives clinicians an excellent opportunity to make a significant impact on public health.

A.02.a. United States

In the United States in 2000, there were an estimated 42.19 million women over age 50 (see Table 1). About 33.21 million women are over 55 years of age (compared with 28.7 million in 1990). By the year 2020, the number of US women over 55 is expected to be 45.9 million

Table 1. Numbers of US women				
	July 1, 1999	*July 1, 2000*	*% Change*	*Postmenopausal*
Age 50+	41,000,000	42,189,280	+2.9%	39,944,824
Age groups:				
Age 40-44	11,188,000	11,312,761	+1.1%	1,134,000
Age 45-49	9,832,000	10,202,898	+3.8%	2,017,600
Age 50-54	8,439,000	8,977,824	+6.4%	6,733,368

Source: US Census Bureau, 2000 Census.

A woman's life expectancy is estimated at 79.7 years. Today, a woman who reaches 54 can expect to reach the age of 84.3 years. About two-thirds of the total US population will survive to age 85 or longer.

NAMS is often asked (1) how many US women are postmenopausal and (2) how many women will reach menopause this year. No hard data exist. NAMS provides the following rough estimates, as well as the assumptions used to make these estimates.

1. *Spontaneous menopause.* The average age of spontaneous (natural) menopause in the Western world is approximately 51 years. US Census Bureau estimates of the population are made in 5-year age groups (see Table 1); the Census Bureau does not provide the exact number of women over age 51. The year 2000 report estimated that 8.98 million women would be aged 50 to 55 on July 1, 2000. One can assume that 50% of 51-year-olds have reached menopause and that percentage would increase to 90% at 55 years of age, allowing the overall percentage over the 5-year span to be

approximately 75%. Thus, 75% of 8.98 million is 6.73 million — the number of women who have reached menopause in this age group. This number is added to 33.21 million, the number of women aged 55-plus. Therefore, 39.94 million US women had experienced spontaneous menopause as of 2000. For a rough estimate of the number of women reaching spontaneous menopause during 2000, 6.73 million is divided by 5, for a total of 1.35 million.

2. *Premature (spontaneous) menopause.* Clinical trial data suggest that the incidence of premature ovarian failure (POF) in US women is about 0.3%, or approximately 146,000 cases in 2000. Although POF is not always synonymous with premature menopause, this figure could be used as a rough estimate for premature spontaneous menopause cases. However, this is the total number of US cases; the annual figure is not known.

3. *Surgical menopause.* To estimate this figure, the rates of hysterectomy with concomitant bilateral oophorectomy per 1,000 women from a 1993 surveillance study were applied to population data from the 2000 US Census.

4. *Induced menopause from other causes (eg, chemotherapy, pelvic radiation therapy).* There are no hard data from which to calculate estimates, so these women are not included.

Because of the limitations, these figures can only be used to provide a rough estimate of the number of US women reaching menopause — either naturally or induced — in the year 2000:

1. Spontaneous (natural) menopause	1,346,000
2. Premature spontaneous menopause	?
3. Surgical menopause	207,000
4. Other medically induced menopause	?
	1,553,000+ (or over 4,255 per day)

A.02.b. Canada

Canadian statistics also show an increase in life expectancy for midlife women. In 1922, a 50-year-old woman lived, on average, until age 75. Today, a woman the same age can expect to live until her mid-80s. Canadian women are, therefore, living at least one-third of their lives after menopause. Approximately 4.78 million women (15.4% of the Canadian population) were aged 50 and older in 2001. By 2021, that number is projected to increase to 7.4 million (21% of the Canadian population).

A.02.c. Worldwide

In 1998, there were more than 477 million postmenopausal women in the world, with approximately 9% expected to live to age 80. By 2025, the number of postmenopausal women is expected to rise to 1.1 billion. Life expectancy for women worldwide was 65 years in 1998 (79 in more developed countries). Women's lifespan is expected to rise to 72 years worldwide by 2025 (82 in more developed countries).

Bibliography

Clinical challenges of perimenopause: consensus opinion of The North American Menopause Society. *Menopause* 2000;7:5-13.

Cramer DW, Harlow BL, Xu H, et al. Cross-sectional and case-controlled analyses of the association between smoking and early menopause. *Maturitas* 1995;22:79-87.

Cramer DW, Xu H, Harlow BL. Family history as a predictor of early menopause. *Fertil Steril* 1995;64:740-745.

Executive summary: Stages of Reproductive Aging Workshop (STRAW) Park City, Utah, July 2001. *Menopause* 2001;8:402-407.

Harden CL, Nikolov BG, Koppel BS, et al. Seizure frequency and age of menopause in women with epilepsy. *Epilepsia* 2001; 42(suppl 7):291.

Hardy R, Kuh D. Reproductive characteristics and the age at inception of the perimenopause in a British National Cohort. *Am J Epidemiol* 1999;149:612-620.

Kato I, Toniolo P, Akmedkhanov A, et al. Prospective study of factors influencing the onset of natural menopause. *J Clin Epidemiol* 1998;51:1271-1276.

Lepine LA, Hillis SD, Marchbanks PA, et al. Hysterectomy surveillance: United States, 1980-1993. *Mor Mortal Wkly Rep CDC Surveill Summ* 1997;46:1-15.

McKinlay SM, Brambilla PJ, Posner JG. The normal menopause transition. *Maturitas* 1992;14:103-15.

Richards M, Kuh D, Hardy R, Wadsworth M. Lifetime cognitive function and timing of the natural menopause. *Neurology* 1999;53:308-314.

Smith T, Contestabile E. Executive summary: Canadian consensus on menopause and osteoporosis. *J SOGC* 2001;23:829-835.

Statistics Canada. CANSIM II. Ottawa, ON, Canada: Statistics Canada; 2000. Accessible at http://www.statcan.ca.

Torgerson DJ, Thomas RE, Reid DM. Mothers' and daughters' menopausal ages: is there a link? *Eur J Obstet Gynecol Reprod Biol* 1997;74:63-66.

United States Bureau of the Census. Current population reports. Accessible at http://www.census.gov/population/projections/nation/nas/npas9600.txt.

Utian WH. The International Menopause Society menopause-related terminology definitions. *Climacteric* 1999;2:284-286.

Weel AE, Uitterlinden AG, Westendorp IC. Estrogen receptor polymorphism predicts the onset of natural and surgical menopause. *J Clin Endocrinol Metab* 1999;84:3146-3150.

WHO Scientific Group on Research on the Menopause in the 1990s. Geneva, Switzerland: *WHO Technical Report Series* 866; 1994.

A.03. Evaluating the literature

The evidence base on which practitioners rely when informing women about the risks and benefits of treatment options is constantly changing. Reports of studies in the lay press can be both confusing and misleading to women, and frequently must be placed into a broader context. A basic understanding of the types of studies, and the meaning of the analyses, will help healthcare providers evaluate the evidence and its implication on clinical practice.

A.03.a. Types of studies

The two categories of studies that are most frequently reported are *experimental* and *observational* (sometimes called descriptive). In experimental studies, the interventions and conditions are strictly defined and controlled. Observational studies describe outcomes in relation to variables of interest but without intervention on the part of the investigator.

Some of the most common types of studies are listed here, ordered by the strength of evidence they provide.

Experimental studies
Two types of experimental studies are randomized controlled trials and crossover trials:

Randomized controlled trials are the gold standard of scientific inquiry. In these studies, a group of subjects with similar characteristics is identified and then randomly assigned to intervention or control groups. In this way, the biases of observational studies are avoided because participants have an equal and unbiased chance of being assigned to each treatment under study. Depending on the intervention, both participants and investigators may be blinded (ie, double-blinded) as to which treatment a participant is receiving, usually through the use of placebo medications. Blinding controls for potential placebo effects and the effects of a participant's expectation of benefit. Randomized controlled trials assess the efficacy of the treatment in a controlled setting, which may not reflect its actual effectiveness in a real-world, clinical-practice setting. Often, the trials use a highly defined patient population, so it may not be accurate to extrapolate the results to other patient populations. The Women's Health Initiative is an example of a randomized controlled trial.

Crossover trials allow subjects to serve as their own controls. Participants are randomly assigned to one treatment arm and later switched to the other treatment arm.

Observational studies
Types of observational studies include longitudinal cohort studies, case-control studies, case reports, and case series:

Longitudinal cohort studies begin with a defined group of subjects (eg, individuals of a certain age, or people who work in a certain industry) called the cohort. This cohort is then followed over time for a variety of outcomes. Most commonly, data are collected in a similar manner on all participating subjects at the beginning of the study (ie, baseline) and at set intervals during follow-up. The Nurses' Health Study and the Framingham Study are examples of large observational cohort studies. Cohort studies are usually prospective, but they may be retrospective. The evidence from prospective cohort studies is considered stronger because data on exposures are collected before outcomes occur.

Case-control studies most commonly begin with an outcome of interest (eg, hot flashes, breast cancer) and then compare the characteristics of individuals with the outcome (cases) and without the outcome (controls). Data are analyzed using a snapshot approach to determine at a single point in time the differences that may account for the outcome. Matching subjects for specific characteristics and defining strict eligibility criteria lessens, but cannot eliminate, the possibility that the results are caused by bias. For example, women who use ERT are known to smoke less and be generally healthier, and this biases any observation of ERT and health outcomes. Despite these limitations, case-control studies have many advantages. Because they begin with an outcome of interest, they can be performed efficiently and at less cost than cohort studies. They are important in situations in which it would be unethical to assign individuals to an exposure (eg, asbestos) or when an outcome is relatively rare so that the number of identified cases in any given cohort would be too small to analyze (eg, birth defects).

In *case reports* and *case series*, the experience of a single patient or series of patients is described. Such reports are useful in bringing new diseases or phenomena to the attention of the clinical and scientific community and for generating new hypotheses. However, without further study, case reports can only be considered suggestive.

A.03.b. Analyses

The results of epidemiologic studies and clinical trials are frequently presented as a relative risk (see Table 2).

Relative risk is the rate of disease in a group exposed to a potential risk factor, divided by the rate of disease in the unexposed group. For example, if the annual rate of myocardial infarction in women who smoke is 220 per 100,000 and the annual rate in women who do not smoke is 110 per 100,000, the relative risk associated with smoking would be determined as follows:

Relative risk (RR) equals the rate in exposed people divided by the rate in those not exposed.

$$ RR = \frac{220}{100,000/year} \div \frac{110}{100,000/year} = 2.00 $$

This means that compared with unexposed women, the rate of myocardial infarction for smoking women is twice that of nonsmoking women.

Table 2. Relative risk nomenclature

The *relative risk* (RR) tells the estimated magnitude of the change in risk related to the presence versus the absence of a factor of interest.

A relative risk *less than* 1.0 (<1) means that the factor lowers risk. For example, a RR of 0.50 means that there is a 50% reduction in risk among those with versus without the factor. An RR of 0.3 means a 70% reduction in risk.

A relative risk *greater than* 1.0 (>1) means that the factor increases risk. For example, an RR of 1.2 means that there is a 20% increase in risk in the group with versus those without the factor. An RR of 2.0 means a doubling of risk.

The *P value* is the probability of obtaining the observed relative risk (or a more extreme value) by chance.

The *confidence interval,* usually cited with the relative risk, indicates the range within which the true magnitude of the measured effect lies with a certain degree of assurance. A 95% confidence interval (CI) gives the range of values that have a 95% probability of containing the true relative risk. When a 95% CI does not contain the number 1.0 (eg, 0.40-0.80 or 1.12-1.37), the measured relative risk is significant by at least $P < 0.05$. The wider the CI, the more variability in the data.

The *odds ratio* is an estimate used in case-control studies that approximates the relative risk.

The impact of relative risk depends on incidence. This can be quantified by *attributable risk* (or risk difference). This is the difference in the incidence rates in the exposed and unexposed groups (the groups with and without the risk factor being studied). The attributable risk serves to quantify the effect of exposure and, thus, gives a measure of its public health impact. For example, in the calculation presented earlier, the attributable risk (AR) would be as follows:

$$ AR = \frac{220}{100,000/year} - \frac{110}{100,000/year} = \frac{110}{100,000/year} $$

This means that for every 100,000 women who smoke, there would be 110 additional cases of myocardial infarctions per year. Depending on the baseline rates of disease, the attributable risk can vary greatly, given the same relative risk. For example, if the baseline rate of a disease is 6 per 100,000 per year and smoking doubled the risk to 12 per 100,000 per year, the relative risk would be 2.0; however, the attributable risk would be only 6 per 100,000 per year.

A *meta-analysis* is an analytic technique used to pool the results from many smaller studies. Pooling studies has the effect of increasing the sample size, thereby gaining statistical power. Thus, a meta-analysis may pool the results of clinical trials that are too small to have statistical significance but that may show significance when pooled. Specific criteria (eg, completeness of data) are established to determine which studies will be included in the analysis. Observational studies may also be pooled in a meta-analysis. It must be remembered that any biases present in the contributing studies will be present in the meta-analysis.

Bibliography

Hennekins CH, Buring JE, Mayrent SL. *Epidemiology in Medicine.* Boston, MA: Little Brown and Co; 1987.

Last JM. *A Dictionary of Epidemiology.* 2nd ed. New York, NY: Oxford University Press; 1988.

LeLorier J, Gregoire G, Benhaddad A, Lapierre J, Derderian F. Discrepancies between meta-analyses and subsequent large randomized, controlled trials. *N Engl J Med* 1997;337:536-542.

McKinlay SM. Issues in design, measurement, and analysis for menopause research. *Exp Gerontol* 1994;29:479-493.

Moher D, Cook DJ, Eastwood S. Olkin I, Rennie D, Stroup DF. Improving the quality of reports of meta-analyses of randomised controlled trials: the QUOROM statement. Quality of reporting of meta-analyses. *Lancet* 1999;354:1896-1900.

As a woman moves from the reproductive phase of life through the menopause transition into the postmenopausal phase, many changes can be observed. Some are related to menopause, others to aging. It may be difficult to differentiate between the two. Several hormonal systems manifest age-related changes that may or may not have their onset during the menopause transition. Additionally, medical conditions such as obesity, diabetes, thyroid disorders, and hypertension often develop during midlife.

B.01. Stages of reproductive aging

Chronological age is an inaccurate predictor of reproductive age. Since women vary widely in timing of the menopause transition, a more specific way to determine their reproductive age would be useful. A standardized definition of the stages of reproductive aging has recently been proposed to facilitate care of women as well as clinical research (see Fig 1 on page 9). The stages are based on menstrual cycle pattern, hormone levels, and symptoms. The major categories are reproductive, menopause transition, and postmenopause.

B.01.a. Reproductive interval

The normal menstrual cycle involves three successive phases: follicular (or proliferative), periovulatory, and luteal (or secretory)(Fig 2).

Menses coincides with the beginning of the follicular phase. At the onset of the menstrual cycle, circulating levels of estrogen and progesterone are low, signaling the hypothalamus and pituitary to release follicle-stimulating hormone (FSH). FSH initiates the process of follicular maturation, and the follicle (fluid-filled sac containing an ovum or egg) increases estrogen production, stimulating new endometrial growth. At the end of the follicular phase, the endometrium has thickened 3-fold, and a primordial follicle has matured in preparation for the release of an ovum.

During the periovulatory phase, increased estrogen from the mature follicle triggers a sharp increase in luteinizing hormone (LH), causing release of the ovum. After this release, LH continues to stimulate the residual ovarian follicle, transforming it into the corpus luteum.

The luteal phase is marked by increased secretion of progesterone from the corpus luteum to support and enrich the thickened endothelium in preparation for implantation and pregnancy. If fertilization of the ovum does not occur, the corpus luteum regresses, estrogen and progesterone levels decline, and menses (ie, shedding of the endometrial lining and uterine bleeding) occurs.

The cyclical release of FSH and LH from the pituitary gland is tightly regulated and easily disturbed. When the pituitary gland does not release appropriate quantities of FSH or LH, ovulation may not occur, potentially disrupting the cycle.

In the normal ovarian cycle, circulating serum estradiol levels fluctuate from less than 10 to 100 pg/mL (37-370 pmol/L) in the early follicular phase, 200 to 800 pg/mL (730-2,930 pmol/L) at midcycle, and 200 to 340 pg/mL (730-1,250 pmol/L) during the luteal phase.

During the menstrual cycle, ovarian production of estradiol, the primary estrogen produced, ranges from 36 µg/day in the follicular phase to 250 µg/day in the luteal phase. More than 95% of the circulatory estradiol comes from the dominant follicle and corpus luteum; most of the remaining amount is derived from peripheral conversion of estrone.

Estrone is the second most abundant estrogen in females. Estrone is derived primarily from the metabolism of estradiol and from peripheral aromatization of androstenedione in adipose tissue and muscle, although ovarian and adrenal secretions supply a small amount. During the menstrual cycle, serum estrone levels vary from 30 to 180 pg/mL (110-670 pmol/L). In premenopausal women, the ratio of circulating estradiol to estrone is greater than 1.0.

The major gonadal peptides involved in the feedback loop are inhibin A and inhibin B. During the menstrual cycle, inhibin A levels are low for most of the follicular phase then rise in midcycle, subsequently falling and again rising to reach the highest levels during the luteal phase, in parallel with the secretion of estradiol and progesterone. Inhibin B levels rise and fall in the first half of the follicular phase, also show a midcycle peak, then subsequently fall to their lowest concentrations during the luteal phase. It is hypothesized that inhibin B and FSH form a closed-loop feedback system during the first half of the cycle, with the levels of inhibin B providing a fine-tuning regulation of FSH levels. Thus, the ovary employs two negative feedback signals: estradiol and the inhibins.

In reproductive-age women, circulating androgens are produced in the ovaries, the adrenal glands, and through peripheral conversion of circulating androstenedione and DHEA to testosterone. Five androgens are clinically important: testosterone, dihydrotestosterone (DHT), androstenedione, dehydroepiandrosterone (DHEA), and dehydroepiandrosterone sulfate (DHEA-S).

Androgens circulate in blood bound to proteins and in the unbound state. DHEA-S is bound strongly to albumin, resulting in a very low metabolic clearance rate. DHEA and

Figure 2. The menstrual cycle

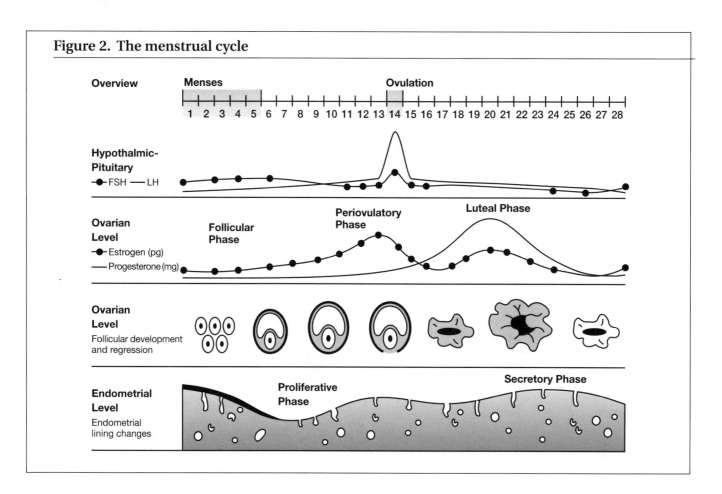

androgen are bound weakly to albumin and their metabolic clearance rates are higher.

One-quarter of circulating testosterone originates in the ovaries, one-quarter in the adrenals, and one-half from peripheral conversion of androstenedione. Testosterone levels range from 0.7 to 2.8 nmol/L (0.2-0.81 ng/mL). During the menstrual cycle, there is a slight but significant preovulatory rise in testosterone concentration.

DHEA, the predominant adrenal androgen, has a very short half-life, whereas DHEA-S, the sulfated metabolite of DHEA, circulates longer and is more readily measured. Circulating levels of DHEA-S peak in early adulthood and then fall steadily after age 40. DHEA-S levels are about 40% lower in women than in men.

B.01.b. Menopause transition

The menopause transition is characterized by erratic hormone secretion presenting as menstrual cycle irregularity and, finally, complete cessation of menses. Both central nervous system control mechanisms and decline of follicles within the ovary may contribute to the initiation and progression of the menopause transition.

During the late reproductive stage, elevation of FSH (>10 IU/L) in the early follicular phase (between days 2 and 5) of the menstrual cycle is the first measurable sign of reproductive aging. Eventually, the accelerated loss of follicles and resultant decline of inhibin B lead to elevation of FSH levels.

The ovary contains the maximum number of germ cells during fetal development, and follicular loss begins in utero. Women are born with 1 to 2 million follicles. By menopause, they have only a few hundred to a few thousand remaining. Most follicular loss results from atresia (cell death and degeneration), not ovulation (<500 follicles over a lifetime). The rate of fall in the number of follicles is linear until approximately age 37, following which there is a steeper decline until menopause. However, the rate of atresia varies from woman to woman.

As numbers of ovarian follicles decline, levels of inhibin B fall, allowing FSH to rise and, for a time, sustain follicular development and ovulatory function. The higher levels of FSH recruit relatively more follicles per cycle, which might contribute to accelerated follicular atresia after age 37. Over-production of estradiol by this enlarged cohort of recruited follicles may be responsible for common midlife symptoms such as bloating, irritability, mastalgia, menorrhagia, and growth of uterine fibroids. Other symptoms in the late reproductive phase may include vasomotor symptoms, insomnia, migraines, and premenstrual dysphoria. These symptoms may occur in the face of regular menstrual cycles.

The formal onset of the menopause transition is marked by a change in menstrual cycle length of at least 7 days. Later in the menopause transition, as the number of ovarian follicles decreases, those remaining often respond poorly to FSH and LH. As a result, ovulation is erratic and cycle irregularity develops. Some cycles may be anovulatory (ie, no follicle released) whereas several follicles may be released during some cycles (perhaps accounting for in the increased incidence of twins born to midlife women). In the late menopause transition, as ovulation becomes more irregular, the rhythmic cyclical fluctuations in estrogen and progesterone are disrupted, and women experience irregular uterine bleeding and episodes of amenorrhea. Symptoms of genital atrophy and problems in sexual function may arise at this time. By the late menopause transition, estrogen levels are often very low.

Despite the resulting decline in fertility, women should be aware that pregnancy is possible until menopause occurs and is confirmed either by 12 consecutive months of amenorrhea or having consistently elevated levels of FSH (≥30 mIU/mL).

In reproductive-age women, the ovary is the major source of estrogen. During the menopause transition, a marked decline in ovarian secretion of estrogen occurs. The greatest decline in estrogen concentrations takes place during the first year postmenopause, which is followed by a more gradual decline during the next few years.

Progesterone production depends on the integrity of the menstrual cycle. Early in the menopause transition, progesterone levels are usually normal. In anovulatory cycles, progesterone levels are low. During the menopause transition, progesterone is sometimes lower than normal even during ovulatory cycles.

Testosterone concentrations during the menopause transition have been reported to be unchanged or to decrease slightly. In one small study, the midcycle rise in bioavailable testosterone and androstenedione, characteristic of younger regularly cycling women (19-37 years old), was consistently and significantly absent in older regularly cycling women (43-47 years old), while total testosterone did not differ significantly in any cycle stage between older and younger women. A prospective longitudinal study from Australia did not show a difference

in total testosterone levels in the same women in the years before and after their final menstrual period. A longitudinal study from Norway reported a 15% decrease in testosterone after menopause. Data from the Rancho Bernardo Study suggest that a decline in testosterone at menopause may be transient and followed by normalization of testosterone levels in older women.

DHEA and DHEA-S are not influenced by menopause, since these androgens are secreted mainly by the adrenals. The concentration of DHT does not appear to be affected by aging or menopause. There are no significant changes in metabolic clearance rates at menopause or with age. The pathways of metabolism are not altered at menopause, but aromatization of DHEA, androgen, and testosterone to estrone and estradiol all increase with age. Thus, androgen metabolism in general is affected more by age than by declining ovarian function.

B.01.c. Postmenopause stages

The hallmark for postmenopause is the final menstrual period (FMP). Early postmenopause is defined as 5 years since the FMP. This period encompasses a further dampening of ovarian hormones to a permanent level. Late postmenopause begins 5 years after the FMP and continues until death.

The classic endocrine findings during postmenopause include elevated FSH levels (10- to 15-fold), increased LH levels, FSH levels greater than LH levels, and marked reductions in serum concentrations of estradiol and estrone. Characteristic high gonadotropin levels after menopause progressively decline with age. Postmenopausal estradiol levels are 10% or less of concentrations attained during reproductive life and range from less than 10 to 37 pg/ml (37-140 pmol/L). Estrone levels range from 6 to 63 pg/mL (22-233 pmol/L). The ratio of estradiol to estrone reverses, and estrone becomes the predominant circulating estrogen. Estrone is derived primarily from peripheral conversion (ie, aromatization) of androstenedione. Estrogen levels, therefore, may be higher in obese women because aromatization increases as a function of the mass of adipose tissue.

Transient elevations of estradiol in postmenopause may reflect activity in a residual follicle, but such activity does not result in ovulation. Progesterone levels remain low after menopause. Because of the reduction in estradiol concentration after menopause, the ratio of estrogen to androgen is decreased.

Recent studies have highlighted the possible clinical significance of very low estradiol levels, previously not reported because they were so low (ie, <37 pmol/L or <10 pg/mL). In one large clinical trial, postmenopausal women assigned to placebo with endogenous estradiol levels greater than 10 pmol/L (2.7 pg/mL) had a 6.8-fold higher rate of breast cancer than that of women with undetectable estradiol levels. In a large observational study, a 3.6-fold increased risk of breast cancer was reported for women with bioavailable estradiol at least 6.83 pmol/L (1.9 pg/mL). Similar correlates have been reported for risk of osteoporotic fractures and performance on tests of cognitive function.

The postmenopausal ovary continues to produce androstenedione and testosterone. In the Rancho Bernardo study, women aged 50 to 89 with intact ovaries had total but not bioavailable (free) testosterone levels that increased with age, reaching premenopausal levels by age 70, with relatively stable levels thereafter. Total testosterone levels were reported to average about 0.6 nmol/L (0.17 ng/mL).

Surgical menopause results in lower testosterone levels. In the same Rancho Bernardo study, women experiencing bilateral oophorectomy and hysterectomy had total and bioavailable testosterone levels that did not vary with age and were 40% to 50% lower (total testosterone: 0.3 nmol/L or 0.09 ng/mL) than levels in women with intact ovaries. Levels of bioavailable estradiol, estrone, and sex hormone-binding globulin were essentially the same regardless of oophorectomy status.

Adrenal androgens continue to fall with progressive age, with lower levels in women than in men. Conversely, cortisol levels rise with increasing age, and serum concentrations at all ages are higher in women than in men.

Bibliography

Burger HG. The endocrinology of the menopause. *J Steroid Biochem Mol Biol* 1999;69:31-35.

Burger HG. Inhibin and reproductive aging. *Exp Gerontol* 2000;35:33-39.

Burger GH, Dudley EC, Cui J, Dennerstein L, Hopper JL. A prospective longitudinal study of serum testosterone, dehydroepiandrosterone sulfate, and sex hormone-binding globulin levels through the menopause transition. *J Clin Endocrinol Metab* 2000;85:2832-2838.

Cauley JA, Lucas FL, Kuller LH, Stone K, Browner W, Cummings SR. Elevated serum estradiol and testosterone concentrations are associated with a high risk for breast cancer. Study of Osteoporotic Fractures Research Group. *Ann Intern Med* 1999;130:270-277.

Cummings SR, Duong T, Kenyon E, Cauley JA, Whitehead M, Krueger KA. Serum estradiol level and the risk of breast cancer during treatment with raloxifene. *JAMA* 2002;287:216-220.

Executive summary: Stages of Reproductive Aging Workshop (STRAW) Park City, Utah, July 2001. *Menopause* 2001;8:402-407.

Laughlin GA, Barrett-Connor E. Sexual dimorphism in the influence of advanced aging on adrenal hormone levels: the Rancho Bernardo Study. *J Clin Endocrinol Metab* 2000;85:3561-3568.

Laughlin GA, Barrett-Connor E, Kritz-Silverstein D, von Muhlen D. Hysterectomy, oophorectomy, and endogenous sex hormone levels in older women: the Rancho Bernardo Study. *J Clin Endocrinol Metab* 2000;85:645-651.

Longcope C. Endocrine function of the postmenopausal ovary. *J Soc Gynecol Investig* 2001;8(1 suppl):S67-68.

Mitchell ES, Woods NF, Marielle A. Three stages of the menopausal transition from the Seattle Midlife Women's Health Study: toward a more precise definition. *Menopause* 2000;7:334-349.

Mushayandebvu T, Castracane VD, Gimpel T, Adel T, Santoro N. Evidence for diminished midcycle ovarian androgen production in older reproductive aged women. *Fertil Steril* 1996;65:721-723.

Overlie I, Moen MH, Morkrid L, Skjaeraasen JS, Holte A. The endocrine transition around menopause — a five-year prospective study with profiles of gonadotropins, estrogens, androgens and SHBG among healthy women. *Acta Obstet Gynecol Scand* 1999; 78:642-647.

Santoro N, Brown JR, Adel T, Skurnick JH. Characterization of reproductive hormonal dynamics in the perimenopause. *J Clin Endocrinol Metab* 1996;81:1495-1501.

Wise PM. Neuroendocrine modulation of the "menopause": insights into the aging brain. *Am J Physiol* 1999;277(6 part 1):E965-E970.

B.02. Hypothalamic-pituitary-ovarian axis

The normal menstrual cycle is controlled by a complex interplay of the hypothalamic-pituitary-ovarian axis. The hypothalamus releases gonadotropin-releasing hormone (GnRH) in a pulsatile fashion, stimulating the pituitary gland to produce FSH and LH. Those hormones stimulate the ovary to secrete estrogen and progesterone. During the monthly cycle, the pattern of pulsatile release of GnRH, pituitary hormones, and subsequent ovarian hormone levels vary at different times (see Fig 2).

As reproductive aging ensues, the hypothalamic-pituitary-ovarian axis changes. The first sign is an increase in FSH. Whether this is due to central aberrations or ovarian alterations is subject to conjecture. There is speculation that perturbations of central nervous system "clocks" may precede signs of ovarian aging. Specifically, a slowing of the GnRH pulse generator might contribute to FSH elevation. Alternatively (or maybe concurrently), ovarian function declines and the negative feedback of ovarian steroids and inhibin is progressively diminished, resulting in increases in FSH secretion.

A rise in FSH can be detected as early as the late stage of the reproductive interval (prior to any menstrual irregularity), although FSH is highly variable. Postmenopause, FSH levels continue to increase and plateau within 1 year. Although FSH levels decline somewhat after several years, they remain elevated above premenopausal concentrations, even in elderly women.

During the menopause transition, LH levels usually remain in the normal range, but estradiol induction of the midcycle LH surge may be compromised. After menopause, LH levels rise and also plateau in about 1 year. The loss of gonadal feedback following menopause also alters the forms of LH and FSH secreted, slowing clearance and prolonging half-life.

Following menopause, the steady age-related decline in serum levels of LH and FSH provides clear evidence for neuroendocrine changes independent of those due to loss of ovarian feedback. A decrease in the frequency of the GnRH pulse generator activity is one finding that might explain the continuous decline in postmenopausal LH and FSH. While the capacity of the hypothalamus to secrete GnRH is not diminished with age, the dynamics of GnRH control and the pattern of secretion are altered.

Preliminary studies do not indicate an age-related change in the degree to which GnRH contributes to gonadotropin secretion. Also, there is no evidence that an increase in gonadotropin clearance contributes to the decline in serum gonadotropin levels with aging. Preliminary evidence does suggest that the capacity of the pituitary to secrete gonadotropins may diminish with age, but this remains to be confirmed.

Bibliography

Birken S, O'Connor J, Kovalevskaya G, Lobel L. Gonadotropins and menopause: new markers. In Lobo RA, Kelsey J, Marcus R, eds. *Menopause: Biology and Pathobiology.* San Diego, CA: Academic Press; 2000:61-76.

Hall JE, Gill S. Neuroendocrine aspects of aging in women. *Endocrinol Metab Clin North Am* 2001;30:631-646.

Longcope C. The endocrinology of the menopause. In Lobo RA, ed. *Treatment of the Postmenopausal Woman: Basic and Clinical Aspects.* 2nd ed. Philadelphia, PA: Lippincott Williams & Wilkins; 1999:35-40.

Wise PM. Neuroendocrine modulation of the "menopause": insights into the aging brain. *Am J Physiol* 1999;277(6 part 1):E965-E970.

B.03. Receptor activity

Hormones, such as estrogen, are released from the cells in which they are produced and are carried in the bloodstream throughout the body to target cells in many tissues, where they trigger a response. Ovarian hormones diffuse freely into cells, but activity within a cell is dependent on the presence of a specific hormone receptor — molecules that bind to the hormones.

Two distinct estrogen receptors (ER) have been identified: ER-alpha (ER-α) and ER-beta (ER-β). The two receptors have different tissue distributions in the body. In general, ER-α are more common in the reproductive system (eg, uterus, breast) and liver; ER-β are more common in other tissues (eg, bone, blood vessels, lungs, and urogenital tract). Both ER-α and ER-β are present in the ovary and the central nervous system.

New insights into the structure and function of the estrogen receptor reveal that it is capable of binding to a variety of substances, or ligands. Different ligands have different affinities for ER-α and ER-β. For example, 17β-estradiol binds actively and extensively to both ER-α and ER-β, whereas ER-β seems to have a higher affinity for phytoestrogens. In addition to binding to natural and synthetic estrogens (estrogen agonists), the estrogen receptor also binds to antiestrogens (estrogen antagonists) and to selective estrogen-receptor modulators, or SERMs (eg, tamoxifen and raloxifene), which act as either estrogen agonists or antagonists depending on the SERM and the target tissue.

Ligand binding to the estrogen receptor initiates receptor activation. Depending on the ligand, the shape or conformation of the estrogen receptor changes in a unique way specific to that ligand. Depending on the tissue in which the ligand-receptor complex resides, tissue-specific cofactors interact with both the receptor and specific locations on the target gene, known as estrogen response elements. The DNA receptor-ligand complex will either turn on (activate) or turn off (repress) gene transcription depending on the ligand, the tissue, and the cofactors (coactivators or corepressors). Alternatively, rapidly acting estrogen receptors on cell membranes might be responsible for rapid, nongenomic effects (no DNA binding required for action). Finally, certain growth factors are capable of activating the estrogen receptor in the absence of estrogen (or other ligands), a process known as ligand-independent activation. Thus, the estrogen receptors modulate a potentially enormous number of different actions by different mechanisms in different tissues throughout the body.

Estrogen-receptor ligands, whether native estrogen, phytoestrogens, or synthetic SERMs, influence target tissues throughout the body. However, more study is needed to understand the extent of agonist/antagonist effects.

Bibliography

Gruber CJ, Tschugguel W, Schneeberger C, Huber JC. Production and actions of estrogen. *N Engl J Med* 2002;346:340-352.

Kuiper GG, Carlsson B, Grandien K, et al. Comparison of the ligand binding specificity and transcript tissue distribution of estrogen receptors alpha and beta. *Endocrinology* 1997;138:863-870.

Longcope C. The endocrinology of the menopause. In Lobo RA, ed. *Treatment of the Postmenopausal Woman: Basic and Clinical Aspects.* 2nd ed. Philadelphia, PA: Lippincott Williams & Wilkins; 1999:35-40.

McDonell, DP. Molecular pharmacology of estrogen and progesterone receptors. In Lobo RA, Kelsey J, Marcus R, eds. *Menopause: Biology and Pathobiology.* San Diego, CA: Academic Press; 2000:3-11.

Nilsson S, Makela S, Treuter E, et al. Mechanisms of estrogen action. *Physiol Rev* 2001;81:1535-1565.

The menopause transition (perimenopause) usually begins in a woman's 40s. During this time, women report increasing symptoms, with the most prevalent being vasomotor symptoms (hot flashes), sleep disturbances, and vaginal dryness. Many factors contribute to perimenopausal health complaints, including the impact of life changes (eg, stress, shifts in home environment) and physiologic changes related to menopause and those related to aging. The clinical significance of subtle hormonal changes that may occur in a woman's 30s is not known.

Most symptoms that occur at perimenopause as disturbances of varying severity are termed *acute* since they will not typically continue long into the postmenopause. These changes are, for the most part, perfectly normal and natural; thus, some prefer not to call perimenopausal disturbances "symptoms."

Other changes resulting from lowered hormone levels may have long-term consequences, including increased risk for diseases such as osteoporosis and, possibly, cardiovascular disease.

Knowledge about perimenopausal changes is limited, as it is largely derived from studies among Caucasian woman over the age of 45. The Study of Women's Health Across the Nation (SWAN) will provide information about the multiethnic and multiracial population of US women aged 40 to 55.

A wide range of health changes are attributed to menopause. A discussion of the primary ones follows.

C.01. Decline in fertility

Many women in industrialized countries worldwide are delaying childbearing. In terms of fertility and maternity, those aged 35 years or older are considered to be of advanced maternal age. A significant decline in fertility occurs in women around age 35 to 38, or 10 to 15 years before menopause. In addition, advanced maternal age is associated with increased risk for spontaneous miscarriage (50% by age 45), increased risk for chromosomal abnormalities in the fetus (1 in 40), and increased risk for pregnancy complications (premature labor, still birth, need for cesarean section).

The functional activity of the ovary changes more with age than almost any other organ in the human body. There is a subtle but real increase in follicle-stimulating hormone (FSH) and a decrease in inhibin A and B, which is responsible for the feedback regulation of FSH throughout the menstrual cycle. Declining secretion of inhibin B appears to contribute significantly to the rising FSH levels observed during the menopause transition and after menopause. The increase in FSH reflects the quality and quantity of aging follicles. Once the oocyte pool decreases to approximately 1,000 follicles, menopause ensues.

In addition to oocyte quality, which is the primary determinant of reproductive potential, age-related uterine changes may contribute to decreased fertility without creating any major change in the characteristics of the menstrual cycle. Decreased fertility may occur without any obvious changes in a women's menstrual experience.

Research for assisted reproductive technologies has provided significant information regarding aging and fertility. It is now thought that the functional ovarian reserve as directly measured by a basal day 3 serum FSH is the most important indicator of age-related infertility. Ovarian reserve describes a woman's reproductive potential as it relates to the processes of follicular depletion and oocyte quality. Although there is some intercycle variability, women with elevations of FSH in one cycle usually have elevations in subsequent cycles.

If a planned treatment or surgery has the potential to induce menopause, the healthcare practitioner needs to discuss childbearing options with the woman before the procedure. More options are becoming available for women who are unable to conceive "naturally." Whether a woman will be able to use the fertility technologies will depend on her unique circumstances, including her age, general health, health conditions requiring treatment or surgery, the type of treatment or surgery, and her ability to afford the fertility method.

Despite a decline in fertility during perimenopause, women should be aware that pregnancy is still possible. The perimenopausal woman is not totally protected from an unplanned pregnancy until she has reached menopause (ie, no menstrual periods for 12 consecutive months) or until levels of FSH are consistently elevated (>30 mIU/mL).

It is important for women to know that fertility becomes significantly compromised long before overt clinical signs occur. The relationships among the monotropic FSH rise, accelerated follicular atresia, shortened follicular phase, and oocyte quality remain to be determined. Current research in assisted reproductive technologies will continue to define these issues and offer options to women with decreased fertility.

Bibliography

Bopp BL, Seifer DB. Oocyte loss and the perimenopause. *Clin Obstet Gynecol* 1998;41:898-911.

Klein J, Sauer MV. Assessing fertility in women of advanced reproductive age. *Am J Obstet Gynecol* 2001;185:758-770.

Klein NA, Soules MR. Endocrine changes of the perimenopause. *Clin Obstet Gynecol* 1998;41:912-920.

Nugent D. The effects of female age on fecundity and pregnancy outcome. *Hum Fertil* 2001;4:43-48.

Speroff L, Glass RH, Kase NG, eds. *Clinical Gynecologic Endocrinology and Infertility.* 6th ed. Philadelphia, PA: Lippincott, Williams & Wilkins; 1999.

Yen SC, Jaffe RB, eds. *Reproductive Endocrinology: Physiology, Pathophysiology, and Clinical Management.* 3rd ed. St. Louis, MO: WB Saunders, Co; 1999.

C.02. Irregular uterine bleeding

Changes in both menstrual flow and frequency are the hallmarks of the menopause transition. Approximately 90% of women experience 4 to 8 years of menstrual cycle changes before menopause. Most report irregular menses that are attributed to decreased frequency of ovulation and erratic levels of ovarian secreted hormones. Initial menstrual cycle changes as women approach menopause can be subtle, and a variety of menstrual patterns are possible (see Table 1).

Some terms used to describe menstrual periods and menstrual patterns include:

- *dysmenorrhea* — painful menses;
- *menorrhagia* — prolonged or excessive uterine bleeding occurring at the regular intervals of menstruation, a loss of 80 mL or more of blood each menstrual cycle, or bleeding that lasts longer than 7 days;
- *oligomenorrhea* — decreased frequency of menstrual periods;
- *hypomenorrhea* — decreased menstrual flow;
- *polymenorrhea* — bleeding that occurs every 21 days or less;
- *metrorrhagia* — bleeding that occurs between periods;
- *menometrorrhagia* — frequent bleeding that is excessive and irregular in amount and duration;
- *amenorrhea* — the absence of menses.

Bleeding irregularities reported in one population-based study included changes in menstrual flow only (23%), in both frequency and flow (28%), in frequency only (9%), and absence of menses for at least 3 months (13%). A chart review of 500 perimenopausal patients found that alterations in menstrual flow fit one of three patterns: oligomenorrhea and/or hypomenorrhea (70%); menorrhagia, metrorrhagia, and/or hypermenorrhea (18%); and sudden amenorrhea (12%).

Each woman will report a pattern that is irregular for her. There is no universal definition of irregular. Changes in menstrual patterns and flow are considered normal, natural phenomena of the menopause transition and must be differentiated from *abnormal* uterine bleeding. Heavier-than-usual bleeding (blood loss >80 mL, especially with blood clots or anemia), prolonged bleeding (>7 days), frequent menstrual periods (cycle length <21 days), and bleeding or spotting between menses and/or after sexual intercourse are abnormal and require investigation (see Section M).

Bibliography

Burger HG, Dudley EC, Hopper JL, et al. The endocrinology of the menopausal transition: a cross-sectional study of a population-based sample. *J Clin Endocrinol Metab* 1995;80:3537-3545.

Frazer IS. Changes in the menstrual pattern during the perimenopause. In: Lobo RA, ed. *Treatment of the Postmenopausal Woman: Basic and Clinical Aspects.* 2nd ed. Philadelphia, PA: Lippincott Williams & Wilkins; 1999:69-74.

The North American Menopause Society. Clinical challenges of perimenopause: consensus opinion of The North American Menopause Society. *Menopause* 2000;7:5-13.

Seltzer VL, Benjamin F, Deutsch S. Perimenopausal bleeding patterns and pathologic findings. *J Am Med Womens Assoc* 1990;45:132-134.

Speroff L. Management of the perimenopausal transition. *Contemp OB/GYN* 2000;45:16-37.

Treolar AE, Boynton RE, Behn BG, et al. Variation of the human menstrual cycle through reproductive life. *Int J Fertil* 1967;12 (1 part 2):77-126.

Table 1. Possible menstrual changes during perimenopause

Lighter/heavier bleeding (avg blood loss, 40 mL; <20 mL)

Bleeding for fewer/more than 4 days (<2 days)

Cycle shorter/longer than 28 days (<7 days)

Skipped menstrual periods

No changes

C.03. Vasomotor symptoms

The symptoms of vasomotor instability are commonly termed *hot flashes.* A hot flash is a sudden, transient sensation that ranges from warmth to intense heat. During a hot flash, skin temperature rises as blood flows to the skin; this change is particularly marked in the fingers and toes, where skin temperature can increase 1 to 7°C. A sudden wave of heat sensation spreads over the body, particularly on the upper body and face (creating flushing). Although a woman in this stage of a hot flash feels hot, core body temperature drops because of the heat lost via evaporative cooling (perspiration) and increased blood flow to the skin, resulting in the woman feeling chilled. A few women have the chill without the flash.

Some experts distinguish the hot *flash* from the hot *flush;* however, the terms can be used interchangeably. NAMS prefers hot flash.

The hot flash is the second most frequent perimenopausal symptom (after irregular menses), reported by as many as 85% of perimenopausal women. It is considered the hallmark of perimenopause, even though there are other causes for a hot flash.

Hot flashes that occur with drenching diaphoresis (ie, perspiration) during sleep are termed *night sweats.*

Hot flashes can occur infrequently (monthly, weekly) or frequently (hourly). Approximately 10% to 15% of women have very frequent hot flashes. Women who have hot flashes usually do so for 3 to 5 years, but some women have hot flashes only for a few months. Some women report hot flashes years and even decades before menopause. Typically, these hot flashes occur in concert with menses. Postpartum women may also report severe hot flashes. Hot flashes tend to last longer and be more severe with surgically induced menopause.

Hot flashes usually have a consistent within-woman pattern. Some hot flashes are easy to ignore, others are annoying or embarrassing, while some can be debilitating. It has been estimated that about 15% of women experience severe hot flashes. About 25% of US women experience sufficient discomfort to seek help from their healthcare provider. The available treatments do not "cure" hot flashes, but they can offer symptomatic relief.

Hot flashes typically stop without treatment, but there is no reliable method for determining when this will occur. As previously mentioned, for some women, hot flashes continue to occur for many years past menopause.

Table 2. Potential hot flash triggers	
A warm environment	Alcohol
Stress	Caffeine
Hot or spicy foods	Certain medications
Hot drinks	

Few studies have evaluated the effect of hot flashes on quality of life, although the potential for hot flashes to disrupt daily activity and sleep quality is widely recognized.

Hot flashes often increase with stress and may be associated with palpitations and feelings of anxiety. The unsettling feeling that precedes a hot flash can trigger an anxiety (or panic) attack in women with a history of panic attacks.

The reporting of hot flashes varies among women of different cultures. Between 75% and 85% of women in North American and northern Europe report experiencing hot flashes, in contrast to 25% of women in Japan. In the United States, the prevalence of vasomotor complaints is similar between African American and Caucasian women. Data from the Study of Women's Health Across the Nation (SWAN) suggested that African American women have more hot flashes than Caucasian women, although some researchers have criticized the selection of women for this study as not being representative of the entire US population.

The precise cause of hormone-related hot flashes is not known. It is not strictly accurate to say that hot flashes are caused by low or fluctuating estrogen levels, although exogenous estrogen administration has been shown to diminish the frequency of hot flashes in a dose-dependent manner. Another hypothesis for the cause of hot flashes points to a decreasing ability of estrogen to bind to estrogen receptors.

A number of factors, called "triggers," affect the frequency and/or severity of hot flashes (see Table 2).

In addition, cigarette smoking and a maternal history of hot flashes have been associated with higher incidences of hot flashes.

Clinicians should not presume that approaching menopause is the only cause of hot flashes. Other potential (although rare) causes include thyroid disease, epilepsy, infection, insulinoma, pheochromocytoma, carcinoid syndromes, leukemia, pancreatic tumors, autoimmune disorders, and mast-cell disorders. When hot flashes are not relieved by estrogen therapy, further investigation is warranted.

Bibliography

Avis NE, Stellato R, Crawford, et al. Is there a menopausal syndrome? Menopausal status and symptoms across racial/ethnic groups. *Soc Sci Med* 2001;52:345-256.

Bachmann GA. Vasomotor flushes in postmenopausal women. *Am J Obstet Gynecol* 1999;180(3 part 2):S312-S316.

Kronenberg F. Hot flashes. In: Lobo RA, ed. *Treatment of the Postmenopausal Woman: Basic and Clinical Aspects.* 2nd ed. Philadelphia, PA: Lippincott Williams & Wilkins; 1999:157-177.

Kronenberg F. Hot flashes: phenomenology, quality of life, and search for treatment options. *Exp Gerontol* 1994;29:319-336.

The North American Menopause Society. Clinical challenges of perimenopause: consensus opinion of The North American Menopause Society. *Menopause* 2000;7:5-13.

Schwingl PJ, Hulka BS, Harlow SD. Risk factors for menopausal hot flashes. *Obstet Gynecol* 1994;84:29-34.

Staropoli CA, Flaws JA, Bush TL, Moulton AW. Predictors of menopausal hot flashes. *J Womens Health* 1998;9:1149-1155.

C.04. Sleep disturbances

Adequate sleep is the amount and quality of sleep needed to maintain alertness during desired waking hours. One-third to one-half of women 40 to 54 years old report sleep problems. A National Sleep Foundation survey (1998) revealed that, when compared with premenopausal women, peri- and postmenopausal women sleep less, have more frequent insomnia symptoms, and are more than twice as likely to use prescription sleeping aids. It also indicated that most people do not volunteer information about sleep disturbances to their healthcare clinician, and most clinicians do not ask about sleep disturbances.

Poor sleep (ie, inadequate quantity or poor quality) contributes to somatic and mood/cognition symptoms and is associated with fatigue, lethargy, inability to concentrate, lack of motivation, difficulty performing tasks, increased tension and irritability, and dysphoria. It has also been linked to chronic illness, especially cardiac problems, and mood state disorders, such as depression.

Insomnia (reported poor sleep) in midlife women can include difficulty falling asleep or staying asleep through the night or awaking prematurely without being able to resume sleep. Insomnia can be transient (lasting only a few days) or short-term (lasting not more than 3 to 4 weeks), usually accompanying acute emotional life situations or environmental changes. Chronic or persistent sleep difficulties (defined as occurring at least 3 nights per week for a month or longer) require medical intervention. Chronic insomnia manifests as mental and physical stress arousal at bedtime with or without poor sleep efficiency, as assessed by polysomnography (PSG). In the context of poor PSG sleep efficiency, insomnia is referred to as *psychophysiologic.* With normal PSG sleep efficiency, insomnia is referred to as *subjective insomnia* or *sleep state misperception.*

Reports of insomnia increase as women transition through midlife. Perceived declines in sleep quality may be attributed to general aging effects, the onset of sleep-related disorders (eg, apnea), high stress and social strain, as well as ovarian hormone changes.

Most studies of menopausal status and sleep reveal that physiologic sleep disturbances emerging at menopause occur mainly in women most bothered by nighttime hot flash and/or night sweat activity. However, women reporting sleep problems to clinicians may not have abnormal physiological sleep changes. Besides ovarian hormonal changes, many midlife women also experience significant life challenges (eg, job-related stress, loss of life partners through divorce or death, caregiving for young and/or old family members, or development of chronic illness). Since stress and sleep are highly linked, subjective insomnia for many women may be attributed to high life-stress activation (mental and physiological).

Sleep-related disordered breathing (SDB) is classified on a continuum from increased airway resistance, manifested as snoring or airflow reductions (hypopneas), to periodic airflow cessations (apneas), which characterize the sleep apnea/hypopnea syndrome. All manifestations are potentially dangerous, having been linked to cardiovascular disease. Episodes of SDB are associated with sleep arousals and varying desaturated oxygen blood levels. A high frequency of sleep disruptions and arousals leads to fragmented sleep with reports of excessive daytime sleepiness and unrefreshing sleep.

Classical indicators of SDB include reports of loud snoring, excessive daytime sleepiness, disrupted or restless sleep, witnessed apneas, and an increased tendency for automobile and work-related injuries. Physical features of obesity (most important predictor), a large neck circumference (often for men), and crowded oropharynx (with or without obesity) are common. Women appear similar to men in reporting snoring and daytime sleepiness, but they report less restless sleep or witnessed apneas. Women are more likely than men to report morning headaches and fatigue. Women appear more likely to exhibit an upper respiratory resistance and less of a complete breathing pause component to their SDB pattern.

Postmenopausal women have been observed to display more SDB episodes than premenopausal women, but comparisons of pre-, peri-, and postmenopausal women have shown no clear differences in apnea/hypopnea, arousal, or arterial desaturation episodes. Body weight and facial morphology have more importance than ovarian hormone factors in the SDB patterns of midlife women, but a functional breathing difference over and above an anatomical factor has also been associated with menopausal status.

Insomnia can also be secondary to painful chronic illnesses, such as arthritis, fibromyalgia, gastrointestinal disturbances, cardiovascular disease, respiratory disease, and neurological and psychiatric conditions, as well as thyroid abnormalities and allergies. Drugs that can disturb sleep include thyroid medication, theophylline, phenytoin, and levadopa.

Healthcare providers are encouraged to assess sleep quality in all women in perimenopause and beyond.

Bibliography

Baker A, Simpson S, Dawson D. Sleep disruption and mood changes associated with menopause. *J Psychosom Res* 1997;43:359-369.

Carskadon MA, Bearpark HM, Sharkey KM, et al. Effects of menopause and nasal occlusion on breathing during sleep. *Am J Respir Crit Care Med* 1997;155:205-210.

Cela V, Naftolin F. Clinical effects of sex steroids on the brain. In: Lobo RA, ed. *Treatment of the Postmenopausal Woman: Basic and Clinical Aspects.* 2nd ed. Philadelphia, PA: Lippincott Williams & Wilkins; 1999:247-262.

Dancey DR, Hanly PJ, Soong C, Lee B, Hoffstein V. Impact of menopause on the prevalence and severity of sleep apnea. *Chest* 2001;120:151-5.

Erlik Y, Tataryn IV, Meldrum DR, Lomax P, Bajorek JG, Judd HL. Association of waking episodes with menopausal hot flushes. *JAMA* 1981;245:1741-1744.

Gislason T, Benediktsdottir B, Bjornsson JK, Kjartansson G, Kjeld M, Kristbjarnarson H. Snoring, hypertension, and the sleep apnea syndrome: an epidemiologic survey of middle-aged women. *Chest* 1993;103:1147-1151.

Katz D, McHorney CA. Clinical correlates of insomnia in patients with chronic illness. *Arch Intern Med* 1998;158:1099-1107.

Kuh DL, Wadsworth M, Hardy R. Women's health in midlife: the influence of the menopause, social factors and health in earlier life. *Br J Obstet Gynaecol* 1997;104:923-933.

Owens JF, Matthews KA. Sleep disturbance in healthy middle-aged women. *Maturitas* 1998;30:41-50.

Shaver J, Giblin E, Lentz M, Lee K. Sleep patterns and stability in perimenopausal women. *Sleep* 1988;11:556-561.

van Diest R. Subjective sleep characteristics as coronary risk factors: their association with type A behavior and vital exhaustion. *J Psychosom Res* 1990;34:415-426.

2002 Sleep in America Poll. Washington, DC: National Sleep Foundation; 1998. Accessible at http://www.sleepfoundation.org/2002poll.html.

C.05. Urogenital changes

Urogenital problems frequently affect women after midlife (see Table 3).

Table 3. Potential urogenital changes at midlife and beyond
Dryness and/or irritation of the vagina
Itching and/or irritation of the vulva
Discomfort during sexual activity
Urinary urgency or the need to urinate more frequently
Urine leakage when coughing or sneezing
Pelvic relaxation and accompanying symptoms

C.05.a. Vulvovaginal changes

During their lifetimes, approximately one-third of women experience some vulvovaginal problems, such as an unusual vaginal discharge (often with an unpleasant odor) that may cause redness, irritation, and itching of the vulva (outer genital area). Discharge and itching can be caused by vaginitis (inflammation of the vagina). While not a serious condition, vaginitis can be bothersome, uncomfortable, and sometimes recurrent. Vaginitis typically does not resolve on its own, and requires some type of treatment.

There are many other possible causes of vulvovaginal complaints (see Table 4).

Table 4. Possible causes of vulvovaginal complaints

- Hormonal changes, especially low estrogen levels

- Vaginal infection, including candidiasis (ie, yeast) and trichomoniasis

- Bacterial vaginosis, an overgrowth of normal vaginal bacteria

- Medications, such as antibiotics, that contribute to candidiasis

- Sexually transmitted diseases

- Allergic reactions to chemicals in soaps, bubble baths, spermicides, condoms, feminine hygiene sprays, deodorant tampons/pads

- Douching

- Irritation from tampons or birth control devices (eg, diaphragm or cervical cap) left inside the vagina too long

- Skin conditions, such as eczema or Lichen sclerosus

- Certain diseases, such as inflammatory bowel disease (Crohn's disease)

- Injury to pelvic nerve fibers (leading to persistent vulvar pain)

As women reach menopause, decreased estrogen levels may result in vulvovaginal changes, although not all women develop troublesome symptoms.

Estrogen loss causes vaginal epithelial thinning, which leads to increasingly fragile vaginal mucosa characterized by decreased elasticity, disappearance of rugae (ie, small folds of the mucous membrane), and pallor. Vaginal blood flow and cervical and vaginal secretions diminish, resulting in decreased lubrication. Vaginal shortening and narrowing occur. Pruritus and irritation subsequently ensue. Cytologic examination reveals a loss of superficial cells and an increase of basal and parabasal cells.

The problem may progressively worsen in susceptible women. The vaginal walls can exhibit inflammation and small petechiae (ie, pinpoint, nonraised, round, purple-red spots caused from intradermal or submucous hemorrhage). All of these changes increase the likelihood of trauma, infection, and pain. This can result in dyspareunia and/or pain during a pelvic examination, as well as tears and bleeding from vaginal penetration. These effects are less likely to occur in women who experience regular sexual stimulation, which promotes blood flow to the genital area.

The condition described above is *vaginal atrophy* (or *atrophic vaginitis* when there is an inflammatory episode).

Loss of estrogen results in a decrease in vaginal fluid and an increase in the vaginal pH from a healthy acidic environment to an unhealthy alkaline one, creating a more susceptible habitat for vaginal infection. In reproductive-age women, the vaginal flora is dominated by lactobacilli. In postmenopausal women, diverse flora enter the vagina, including pathogenic organisms commonly found in urinary tract infections.

Other vulvovaginal conditions that are seen in midlife and beyond include contact dermatitis (chemical irritation), dermatoses (skin diseases) of the vulva (eg, eczema), vestibulitis (inflammation of the vestibular gland), vulval dystrophy, and vulvodynia (pain in the vulva), all of which need to be diagnosed and treated. These conditions are not directly related to menopause.

C.05.b. Urinary complaints

Urinary complaints, including urinary incontinence and recurrent urinary tract infection, become more common in postmenopause. Urinary and fecal incontinence are not an inevitability of aging and should not be considered normal. Urinary tract infection is primarily caused by a bacterial pathogen. However, all these complaints may be partially caused by the effects of menopause.

Incontinence. Urinary incontinence (ie, persistent, involuntary leakage of urine) of all forms affects 10% to 30% of US women between the ages of 50 and 64, compared with only 1.5% to 5% of men the same age.

A national Canadian poll suggested that 1.5 million Canadians (7% of the population) had experienced an episode of incontinence in the previous year. More women than men were affected, with an increasing prevalence associated with increasing age (from 2% in those aged 35 years and under, to 12% in those older than 55).

The prevalence of urge incontinence appears to increase with the number of years postmenopause, whereas stress incontinence is most common during perimenopause, with no significant increase during the years beyond.

Studies designed to determine the relationship between menopause and incontinence have found conflicting results. The female urethra and trigone of the bladder (ie, triangular portion of the mucous membrane at the base of the bladder), because of their shared embryologic origin with the vagina, contain estrogen receptors and are affected by decreased levels of circulating estrogen. (Studies have not consistently documented the presence of progesterone receptors in the urethra or bladder.) Some forms of urinary incontinence may occur as a result of decreased bladder and urethral tissue tone due to aging and trauma. Although many women relate the onset of their incontinence with menopause, at least one study has demonstrated that the prevalence of incontinence increased with age but not with the time of menopause.

Regardless of the cause, women reaching midlife and beyond may need to urinate more frequently (called frequency), have sudden urges to urinate even though the bladder may not be full (urgency), may urinate several times during the night (nocturia), or notice urine leakage upon coughing, laughing, sneezing, or lifting (stress incontinence). Another type of incontinence occurs with a sudden strong desire to void (urge incontinence). Others experience urine leakage during sexual intercourse or orgasm. Some women may experience painful urination.

While urinary incontinence can occur at any time, a woman's likelihood of becoming incontinent increases with age due to a number of factors, including:

- Decreased endogenous estrogen levels;

- Infections of the bladder (cystitis) and of the urethra (urethritis);

- Defects of the pelvic muscles, nerves, and ligaments due to natural aging;

- Previous damage from childbirth injury, particularly deliveries requiring use of forceps;

- Irritation of the bladder with smoking, drinking alcohol, and/or caffeine;

- Certain prescription medications (eg, diuretics and some tranquilizers);

- Obesity;

- Other medical conditions (such as multiple sclerosis, stroke, Parkinson's disease).

Fecal incontinence has been observed in 15% to 26% of women with urinary incontinence. Both conditions arise from neuromuscular dysfunction of the pelvic floor. Fecal incontinence, like urinary incontinence, may be partly due to lowered estrogen levels. An abundance of estrogen receptors is found in the anorectum.

Urinary tract infection. Lack of estrogen results in shortening and shrinking of the distal portion of the urethra, minimizing its defense against offending pathogens and increasing the risk of urinary tract infections (UTIs).

As endogenous estrogen levels decline, epithelial cell glycogen production also decreases, causing increased alkalinity of the vaginal, urethral, and bladder environment. This places women at even greater risk for developing vaginitis, leukorrhea, and UTIs. In the case of UTIs, vaginal estrogen therapy can restore the vaginal environment and reduce the incidence of recurrent UTIs.

A recent case-controlled study of postmenopausal women found that urinary incontinence, presence of a cystocele, and elevated postvoid residual were strongly associated with recurrent bladder infections. This study supports observations made in clinical practice. Urinary incontinence leads to two behavioral changes that can contribute to bladder infections — chronic use of incontinence pads and decreased fluid intake. Pads provide an opportunistic environment for bacterial growth, and fluid restriction not only alters voiding behavior, but may promote constipation as well. It is important to consider the interrelationship of these conditions when evaluating postmenopausal women.

Bibliography

Bachmann GA, Ebert G, Burd ID. Vulvovaginal complaints. In: Lobo RA, ed. *Treatment of the Postmenopausal Woman: Basic and Clinical Aspects.* 2nd ed. Philadelphia, PA: Lippincott Williams & Wilkins; 1999:195-201.

Bachmann G. Urogenital ageing: an old problem newly recognized. *Maturitas* 1995;22(suppl):S1-S5.

Brown JS, Grady D, Ouslander JG, Herzog AR, Varner RE, Posner SF. Prevalence of urinary incontinence and associated risk factors in postmenopausal women. Heart & Estrogen/Progestin Replacement Study (HERS) Research Group. *Obstet Gynecol* 1999;94:66-70.

DeMarco EF. Urinary tract disorders in perimenopausal and postmenopausal women. In: Lobo RA, ed. *Treatment of the Postmenopausal Woman: Basic and Clinical Aspects.* 2nd ed. Philadelphia, PA: Lippincott Williams & Wilkins; 1999:213-227.

Drutz H, Bachmann G, Bouchard C, Morris B. Towards a better recognition of urogenital aging. *J SOGC* 1996;18:1017-1031.

Grady D, Brown JS, Vittinghoff E, Applegate W, Varner E, Snyder T. Postmenopausal hormones and incontinence: the Heart and Estrogen/Progestin Replacement Study. *Obstet Gynecol* 2001; 97:116-120.

Griebling TL, Nygaard IE. The role of estrogen replacement therapy in the management of urinary incontinence and urinary tract infection in postmenopausal women. *Endocrinol Metab Clin North Am* 1997;26:347-360.

Hillier SL, Lau RJ. Vaginal microflora in postmenopausal women who have not received estrogen replacement therapy. *Clin Infect Dis* 1997;25(suppl 2):S123-S126.

Iosif CS, Batra SC, Ek A, Astedt BI. Estrogen receptors in the human female urinary tract. *Am J Obstet Gynecol* 1981;141:817-820.

Jackson S, Shepherd A, Brookes S, Abrams P. The effect of oestrogen supplementation on post-menopausal urinary stress incontinence: a double-blind placebo-controlled trial. *Br J Obstet Gynaecol* 1999;106:711-718.

Johnson S. Canadian consensus on menopause and osteoporosis: urogenital health. *J SOGC* 2001;23: 973-977.

Khullar V, Damiano R, Toozs-Hobson P, Cardozo L. Prevalence of faecal incontinence among women with urinary incontinence. *Br J Obstet Gynaecol* 1998;105:1211-1213.

Milsom I, Ekelund P, Molander U, Arvidsson L, Areskoug B. The influence of age, parity, oral contraception, hysterectomy and menopause on the prevalence of urinary incontinence in women. *J Urol* 1993;149:1459-1462.

Raz R, Gennesin Y, Wasser J, et al. Recurrent urinary tract infections in postmenopausal women. *Clin Infect Dis* 2000;30:152-156.

Raz R, Stamm WE. A controlled trial of intravaginal estriol in postmenopausal women with recurrent urinary tract infections. *N Engl J Med* 1993;329:753-756.

C.06. Central nervous system changes

During the menopause transition, various central nervous system changes may be observed that may or may not be related to menopause: headache, increased premenstrual dysphoria and mood swings, depression, anxiety, and changes in cognition.

C.06.a. Headache

Most headaches are minor and not reported to healthcare providers. However, an estimated 23 million Americans suffer from severe headaches. The following are the three most common types of headaches:

- *Tension-type headache.* This type of headache is described as a steady squeezing or pressing pain on both sides of the head — a feeling as if a band is being tightened around the head. Tension-type headaches can be acute or chronic, last from 30 minutes to 1 week, and are not aggravated by exertion. Women reportedly experience them more frequently than men.

- *Cluster headache.* Cluster headaches, which are less common than tension-type or migraine headaches, affect men four to six times more often than women. They are described as being very severe, with non-throbbing pain felt behind one eye, which may be accompanied by inflammation, watering of the eye, and/or severe pain on that side of the face. Cluster headaches usually last up to 3 hours, and occur periodically over several weeks or months, sometimes disappearing for months to years.

- *Migraine headache.* In the United States, migraines affect about 18% of women and 6% of men, occurring most often between the ages of 25 and 55. Typically, migraines cause a moderate to severe, throbbing pain that is worse on one side of the head and is usually aggravated by physical activity. Other symptoms, such as nausea, vomiting, and sensitivity to light and noise, are often present. Migraines last 4 to 72 hours and may occur rarely or up to several times a week.

There are two types of migraine headaches: those with aura and those without aura. An aura is typically visual, with flashing lights, wavy lines, or other visual changes, and begins less than an hour before the headache. A person may temporarily lose vision, have speech problems, or experience numbness, tingling, or weakness in an extremity, although this is rare. Migraines without aura are much more common than migraines with aura. Both types of migraines may have other symptoms, such as mood changes, fatigue, nausea, vomiting, facial congestion, and diarrhea. These symptoms may occur up to a day or two before a headache.

Causes of headaches include sinus infections, dental problems, allergies, or colds. Although most headaches are not serious, the following characteristics may be an indication of a more serious problem, such as hypertension or a brain tumor:

- Occurrence of a new, "worst-ever" headache;

- Progressively worsening headache;

- More severe headache pain than usual;

- Headache that causes nocturnal awakening;

- Stiff neck accompanied by a high fever;

- Confusion, dizziness, weakness;

- Presence of a focal neurological symptom.

Common factors that may trigger a migraine headache include the following:

- Consumption of alcoholic beverages, caffeine, tyramine-containing foods (eg, chocolate, yogurt, sour cream, aged cheese, red wine), foods containing nitrite preservatives (eg, hot dogs, sausage, bacon, bologna, smoked fish), and foods containing monosodium glutamate (MSG, a flavor-enhancer sometimes added to Chinese food as well as processed or frozen foods);

- Change in eating pattern (eg, fasting or skipping meals, not drinking enough water);

- Change in sleeping pattern (eg, getting too much or too little sleep);

- Emotional changes (eg, stress, anxiety, anger, or excitement);

- Environmental changes (eg, noise, bright lights, changes in barometric pressure, or inhaling fumes;

- Use of hormone replacement therapy, especially with a progestin.

Some data suggest that hormonal fluctuations may play a role in headaches. Reproductive-aged women may notice headaches associated with their menstrual periods (sometimes called menstrual migraines), a time of fluctuating estrogen levels. Migraines often improve during pregnancy when estrogen levels are more stable. Use of oral contraceptives (which alter hormonal levels monthly) may also trigger headaches, particularly during the placebo week.

During the menopause transition, hormonal changes may increase the prevalence or intensity of headaches. Women with a history of menstrual headaches may find that their headaches become worse at perimenopause. Following menopause, about two-thirds of women experience remission of their migraines.

Tracking headaches in a "headache diary" for a few weeks may help pinpoint the cause(s). Data to record include the time a headache was experienced, the symptoms, and the potential triggers (eg, particular foods, noise, or stress). Identifying patterns may help determine strategies to prevent headaches.

C.06.b. Mood swings

Epidemiologic studies suggest a greater incidence of mood disturbances in perimenopausal women than in postmenopausal women. Many perimenopausal women report distressing symptoms of irritability, tearfulness, insomnia, fatigue, and decreased memory and concentration. Mood changes have been observed in up to 10% of perimenopausal women participating in some longitudinal, community-based studies.

Most women become accustomed to their own hormonal rhythm during their reproductive years. During perimenopause, the rhythm changes. Hormone fluctuations, although a normal consequence of ovarian activity declines, can still be stress-provoking. Many women find that the unexpected timing and extent of these changes create upset and a sense of loss of control.

The psychological disturbances reported most often by perimenopausal women — irritability, "blue moods," and fatigue — have not been directly linked to diminished ovarian hormone levels. However, sleep deprivation related to menopausal night sweats often results in fatigue, irritability, and moodiness.

Transient depressed mood during perimenopause is often associated with depressed mood during the premenopausal years, a longer menopause transition, or more severe menopause-related symptoms. Perimenopausal women seeking help for mood changes are usually less healthy, have more hot flashes and psychosomatic complaints, and are more likely to have a history of premenstrual symptoms.

Some midlife women who report the beginning or worsening of premenstrual syndrome (PMS) may be experiencing the onset of perimenopause. Monitoring symptoms with daily charting will help determine if symptoms are confined to the luteal phase, meeting the criteria for premenstrual dysphoric disorder (PMDD).

Other common causes of mood disturbances during the menopause transition include the following:

- Untreated vasomotor symptoms;

- Recurrence of major depression or new episode of depression;

- Nutritional deficiencies;

- Hypothyroidism;

- Medications for acute or chronic disease treatment;

- Stressful life events;

- Adjustment to age-related social changes;

- Socioeconomic status.

In a 1998 NAMS/Gallup poll of recently postmenopausal US women, respondents indicated that they felt happier and more fulfilled at this time of their life than at any other. Nevertheless, growing older may be difficult for some women. Women in midlife may experience changes in self-concept, self-esteem, and body image. Often, hormone related changes coincide with other stressors and losses in their lives (see Table 5). Many women begin to think about their own mortality and become introspective about the meaning and purpose of their lives. Although these changes may provide an opportunity for positive transformation and growth, some women may need supportive assistance to adapt.

Table 5. Potential stressors at midlife

- Undesired childlessness

- Floundering relationship with a partner

- Development of personal or partner medical problems

- Changes in physical appearance

- Divorce or widowhood

- Care of young children, struggles with adolescents, or return of grown children to the home

- Concerns about aging parents or other family members

- "Sandwich generation" phenomena (ie, responsibility for both children and elders)

- Career and education issues

When evaluating mood disturbances during the menopause transition, it is important to consider all possible causes. If emotional symptoms persist after hormonal treatment has alleviated the vasomotor symptoms, consideration should be given to a trial with an antidepressant or more intensive mental health evaluation and treatment.

C.06.c. Depression and anxiety

Clinical depression affects more than 15 million people in North America. Clinical depression causes pain and suffering, and it is a leading cause of death worldwide. Data indicate that women experience depression and anxiety disorders at a higher rate than do men. These disorders frequently occur in connection with reproductive events such as puberty, menses, postpartum, and menopause, although they may be unrelated to these events. The incidence of clinical depression in women peaks in their 30s, not their 40s.

Women with a history of psychiatric illness may experience an exacerbation of this illness at menopause. However, mental health problems such as depression and anxiety are not inevitable as hormone production decreases. In fact, only a small percentage of menopause-aged women develop symptoms of dysphoria and feeling "blue," and an even smaller percentage develop full depression. Studies have shown that women with mood swings or dysphoria are affected by other aspects of the menopause, such as hot flashes and sleep loss, or the influence of perimenopausal hormone fluctuations on the brain. Most women pass through the menopause transition without significant emotional or psychiatric problems.

Depression. Some of the somatic and psychological symptoms of perimenopause may be difficult to distinguish from depression. The use of standardized mood-rating scales, along with a careful history, will help clarify the diagnosis. Women who experience depression at menopause are more likely to have had depressive episodes during premenopause, PMDD, or postpartum affective disorders.

The word *depression* can sometimes be misleading because it may refer to a symptom or a number of syndromes, each of which is managed differently. Depression is a term used to describe the following three conditions of varying severity:

- *Depressed mood.* A normal, brief period of feeling blue or sad that is commonly experienced and rarely requires treatment. This is sometimes called *dysphoria.*

- *Depression as a symptom.* Sometimes called an adjustment reaction, this type of depression may be due to a wide variety of medical or psychological problems, or to intense reactions to life events (eg, divorce, losing a job, death of a loved one). It is usually short-term and most often does not require treatment, although it can progress to clinical depression. Depression that occurs most of the day, more days than not, for at least two years is called *dysthymia.*

- *Clinical depression.* This is a pathological disorder believed to result from a chemical imbalance in the brain. A clinical (major) depression requires treatment. Women with a history of clinical depression seem to be particularly susceptible to another depression at menopause.

The Diagnostic and Statistical Manual (4th ed) of the American Psychiatric Association (DSM-IV) provides valid and reliable criteria for determining diagnoses.

Anxiety. Anxiety — an agitated sense of anticipation, dread, or fear — is a universally experienced emotion. During the menopause transition, the various physical and psychological changes, including new stressors, may cause anxiety.

As with the term depression, the term *anxiety* can have many meanings. It can refer to a symptom or indicate a more precisely defined disorder, such as phobias, generalized anxiety disorder, panic disorder, agoraphobia (eg, fear of open spaces), or posttraumatic stress. Many of these conditions may have preceded the onset of the menopause transition. Careful observation will clarify if anxiety worsens or improves during this time.

Although anxiety usually resolves on its own without treatment, it may accompany and be a warning sign of a pathological condition such as panic attacks (characterized by shortness of breath, chest pain, dizziness, heart palpitations, and/or feelings of "going crazy" or being out of control). Sometimes the unsettling feelings preceding a hot flash can trigger a panic attack in susceptible women. Symptoms of anxiety can be related to depression or adjustment reaction.

Relaxation and stress-reduction techniques, counseling, psychotherapy, and/or prescription drug treatment usually provide relief for both anxiety and depression.

C.06.d. Cognition

Cognition is a general term for the group of mental processes by which knowledge is acquired or used. It includes learning and concentration as well as memory and planning.

From a neuropsychological perspective, *concentration* is closely related to, and overlaps with, concepts of awareness, attention, and vigilance. Concentration refers to the ability to focus on the task at hand while at the same time suppressing awareness of potential distractions. Impaired concentration is a common symptom of brain damage. Even among healthy people, the ability to concentrate is influenced by fatigue, mood, and a variety of physical symptoms. Difficulty concentrating is a common complaint in peri- and postmenopausal women.

Concentration affects *memory.* There are different kinds of memory. Memory usually refers to the ability to learn new information and to recall this information after time. Another kind of memory involves the memory for words, names, and general facts. Poor concentration means that new information is learned less efficiently and that recall strategies are used less efficiently.

Estrogen, progesterone, and androgen modulate brain function, even in regions that do not serve a reproductive role. Subsets of neurons within the brain have receptors for these sex steroids, as do other cell types. Estrogen effects on neurotransmitter systems, including acetylcholine, serotonin, noradrenalin, and dopamine, have the potential to influence processes involved in concentration. Effects on acetylcholine, as well as other actions within the hippocampus (a brain region essential to the formation of conscience new memories), have the potential to affect learning and memory.

The menopause transition is associated with concentration and memory impairment that may be caused, in part, by sleep disturbances, hot flashes, and various midlife stressors. However, most studies fail to show a clear association between hot flashes and difficulty with concentration and memory.

The rapidity of the transition from the reproductive state to menopause may be a factor. The adaptation of neuronal systems, dependent on estrogen, may be compromised by an abrupt decline in estrogen, as following surgical menopause. Menopause-related symptoms are more frequent and intense following surgical menopause than natural menopause and, therefore, may represent the clinical manifestation of dysfunctional estrogen-dependent neural systems.

Bibliography

American Psychiatric Association. *Diagnostic and Statistical Manual of Mental Disorders. Primary Care Version.* 4th ed. Washington, DC: American Psychiatric Association; 1995.

Avis NE, Brambilla D, McKinlay SM, Vass K. A longitudinal analysis of the association between menopause and depression: results from the Massachusetts Women's Health Study. *Ann Epidemiol* 1994;4:214-220.

Bromberger JT, Matthews KA. A longitudinal study of the effects of pessimism, trait anxiety, and life stress on depressive symptoms in middle-aged women. *Psychol Aging* 1996;11:207-213.

Cela V, Naftolin F. Clinical effects of sex steroids on the brain. In: Lobo RA, ed. *Treatment of the Postmenopausal Woman: Basic and Clinical Aspects.* 2nd ed. Philadelphia, PA: Lippincott Williams & Wilkins; 1999:247-262.

Classification and diagnostic criteria for headache disorders, cranial neuralgias and facial pain. Headache Classification Committee of the International Headache Society. *Cephalalgia* 1998;8(suppl 7):1-96.

Dahlof CG, Dimenas E. Migraine patients experience poorer subjective well-being/quality of life even between attacks. *Cephalalgia* 1995;15:31-36.

Dennerstein L, Dudley EC, Hopper JL, Guthrie JR, Burger HG. A prospective population-based study of menopausal symptoms. *Obstet Gynecol* 2000;96:351-358.

Drake EB, Henderson VW, Stanczyk FZ, et al. Associations between circulating sex steroid hormones and cognition in normal elderly women. *Neurology* 2000;54:599-603.

Fettes I. Migraine in the menopause. *Neurology* 1999;53(4 suppl 1): S29-S33.

Groeneveld FP, Bareman FP, Barentsen R, et al. Vasomotor symptoms and well being in the climacteric years. *Maturitas* 1996;23:293-299.

Halbreich U. Role of estrogen in postmenopausal depression. *Neurology* 1997;48(suppl 7):S16-S19.

Hallstrom T, Samuelsson S. Mental health in the climacteric: the longitudinal study of women in Gothenburg. *Acta Obstet Gynecol Scand Suppl* 1985;130:13-18.

Henderson VW. *Hormone Therapy and the Brain: A Clinical Perspective on the Role of Estrogen.* New York, NY: Parthenon Publishing; 2000.

Hunter M. The south-east England longitudinal study of the climacteric and postmenopause. *Maturitas* 1992;14:117-126.

Kaufert PA, Gilbert P, Tate R. The Manitoba project: a re-examination of the link between menopause and depression. *Maturitas* 1992;14:143-155.

Kessler RC. Gender differences in major depression. In: Frank E, ed. *Gender and Its Effects on Psychopathology.* Washington, DC: American Psychiatric Press; 2000.

Klein P, Versi E, Herzog A. Mood and menopause. *Br J Obstet Gynaecol* 1999;106:1-4.

Kuh DL, Wadsworth M, Hardy R. Women's health in midlife: the influence of the menopause, social factors and health in earlier life. *Br J Obstet Gynaecol* 1997;104:923-933.

Landau C, Milan FB. Assessment and treatment of depression during the menopause: a preliminary report. *Menopause* 1996;3:201-207.

Lipton RB, Stewart WF, Diamond S, Diamond ML, Reed M. Prevalence and burden of migraine in the United States: data from the American Migraine Study II. *Headache* 2001;41:646-657.

MacGregor EA. Menstruation, sex hormones, and migraine. *Neurol Clin* 1997;15:125-141.

Matthews KA, Kuller LH, Wing RR, Meilahn EN. Biobehavioral aspects of menopause: lessons from the healthy women study. *Exp Gerontol* 1994;29:337-342.

McKinlay JB, McKinlay SM, Brambilla D. The relative contribution of endocrine changes and social circumstances to depression in mid-aged women. *J Health Soc Behav* 1987;28:345-363.

Neri I, Granella F, Nappi R, et al. Characteristics of headache at menopause: a clinico-epidemiologic study. *Maturitas* 1993;7:31-37.

Panay N, Studd JW. The psychotherapeutic effects of estrogens. *Gynecol Endocrinol* 1998;12:353-365.

Pearlstein TB. Hormones and depression: what are the facts about premenstrual syndrome, menopause, and hormone replacement therapy? *Am J Obstet Gynecol* 1995;173:646-653.

Rasmussen BK, Jensen R, Schroll M, Olesen J. Epidemiology of headache in a general population — a prevalence study. *J Clin Epidemiol* 1991;44:1147-1157.

Rubinow DR, Roca CA, Schmidt PJ. Estrogens and depression in women. In: Lobo RA, ed. *Treatment of the Postmenopausal Woman: Basic and Clinical Aspects.* 2nd ed. Philadelphia, PA: Lippincott Williams & Wilkins; 1999:189-194.

Rubinow DR, Schmidt PJ, Roca CA. Estrogen-serotonin interactions: implications for affective regulation. *Biol Psychiatry* 1998;44:839-850.

Rubinow DR, Schmidt PJ. Androgens, brain, and behavior. *Am J Psychiatry* 1996;153:974-984.

Schmidt PJ, Rubinow DR. Menopause-related affective disorders: a justification for further study. *Am J Psychiatry* 1991;148:844-852.

Schmidt PJ, Rubinow, DR. Neuroregulatory role of gonadal steroids in humans. *Psychopharmacol Bull* 1997;33:219-220.

Sherwin BB. Estrogen effects on cognition in menopausal women. *Neurology* 1997;48(suppl 7):S21-S26.

Sherwin BB. Hormones, mood, and cognitive functioning in postmenopausal women. *Obstet Gynecol* 1996;87(suppl 2):20S-26S.

Stewart DE, Boydell K, Derzko C, Marshall V. Psychologic distress during the menopausal years in women attending a menopause clinic. *Int J Psychiatry Med* 1992;22:213-220.

Stewart W, Schechter I, Rasmussen BK. Migraine prevalence: a review of population-based studies. *Neurology* 1994;44(6 suppl 4):S17-S23.

Utian WH, Boggs PP. The North American Menopause Society 1998 Menopause Survey. Part I. Postmenopausal women's perceptions about menopause and midlife. *Menopause* 1999;6:122-128.

Woods NF, Mitchell ES, Adams C. Memory functioning among midlife women: observations from the Seattle Midlife Women's Health Study. *Menopause* 2000;7:257-265.

Woods NF, Mitchell ES. Patterns of depressed mood in midlife women: observations from the Seattle Midlife Women's Health Study. *Res Nurs Health* 1996;19:111-123.

Yaffe K, Grady D, Pressman A, Cummings S. Serum estrogen levels, cognitive performance, and risk of cognitive decline in older community women. *J Am Geriatr Soc* 1998;46:816-821.

C.07. Sexual function effects

Sexual desire decreases with age in both sexes, and low desire is particularly common in women in their late 40s and 50s. Sexual concerns are often an issue for women at midlife and beyond, although they frequently are not reported to their healthcare providers.

Menopause contributes to changes in sexual function through the change in gonadal hormone production and consequent changes in function as a result of that decline. The degree of impact of the declining hormones varies from woman to woman, including women with the same level of hormonal decline, indicating that sexual function is more likely multifactorial in cause (see Table 6).

With sexual arousal, lubrication occurs as a result of secretions from the vaginal glands and transudate from the subepithelial vasculature. Changes in the epithelial lining of the vagina occur relatively rapidly as estrogen levels decline. Subsequent vascular, muscular, and connective tissue changes occur over time. Decreased vascularization of surrounding tissue makes it more difficult for engorgement and lubrication. The vagina also loses its elasticity, which can result in discomfort during sexual activity.

Decreased estrogen is responsible for most of these changes, but testosterone, too, is an important factor in midlife sexual changes affecting women. Testosterone is necessary for a normal sex drive in both men and women, playing a role in motivation, desire, and sexual sensation. By the time most women reach their 60s, their testosterone levels are half of what they were before age 40. However, during perimenopause, as estrogen levels are declining, women also experience a decrease in sex hormone-binding globulin (SHBG), which binds both estrogen and testosterone. Some perimenopausal women may notice an increase in sexual desire and activity, perhaps because the declining levels of SHBG free up more testosterone. Oral estrogen increases SHBG levels, which lowers the free testosterone levels and may decrease sexual desire.

One of the most significant and universal changes that occurs with age is a decline in the drive component of sexual desire. Desire refers to one's interest in being sexual and is determined by the interaction of three related but separate components: drive, beliefs/values/expectations, and motivation.

Table 6. Potential factors influencing women's sexual function

- Previous attitudes. In general, women who enjoyed sex in their younger years will continue to do so during and beyond midlife, while those who have not enjoyed sex previously may view any midlife reduction in sexual activity as a relief rather than a loss. Some women, however, have increased interest in sex.

- No available partner.

- Partners may lose interest in sex or have decreased capacity for sexual activity (especially those with erectile dysfunction).

- Age-related changes. With age, sexual drive generally decreases gradually in both men and women. However, a decline does not mean an abrupt halt, and the rate and extent of any decline is individual.

- A woman's perception of her body. Menopause usually occurs at a time when women are experiencing changes in their physical appearance. Women who accept these changes and maintain a positive outlook about their bodies usually have a strong sense of self-esteem that contributes to sexual health.

- Health concerns. Following surgical procedures such as removal of a breast or uterus, a woman may feel unattractive and may avoid initiating sexual encounters. Also, her partner may be fearful that sexual activity will cause her pain.

- Incontinence. This syndrome can lead to sexual avoidance.

- Sleep disturbances. These often result in fatigue and irritability, thereby affecting sexual desire.

- Stressors, such as family and relationship issues.

- Medications. Some drugs such as antihypertensives or antidepressants can decrease sexual desire and orgasmic capacity.

- A male partner's ability to achieve erections through erectile dysfunction therapy (eg, with sildenafil), after no intercourse for months or years, may result in extreme vaginal discomfort for the woman due to lack of lubrication and elasticity.

- Diminished androgen levels.

Drive is the biologic component of desire, resulting from neuroendocrine mechanisms. Drive is typically manifested by sexual thoughts, feelings, fantasies or dreams, increased erotic attraction to others in proximity, seeking out sexual activity (alone or with a partner), and genital tingling or increased genital sensitivity. Drive declines in both men and women as a function of aging, although the exact neuroendocrine mechanisms that are responsible for drive are not fully understood.

For some women, declining levels of free testosterone, related to declining ovarian function or surgical menopause, may result in a noticeable decrease in sexual drive.

The second component of desire reflects an individual's *expectations, beliefs, and values* about sexual activity. The more positive the person's beliefs and values are about sexuality, the greater the person's desire to behave sexually.

The third component of desire is *psychological and interpersonal motivation.* Motivation is driven by emotional or interpersonal factors and is characterized by a willingness of a person to behave sexually with a given partner. This component tends to have the greatest impact overall on desire and is the most complex and elusive.

For many women, particularly postmenopausal women, drive declines and may no longer be the initial step in the response cycle. The classic Masters and Johnson model first developed in 1966 suggested a linear model of the sexual response cycle: desire leading to arousal and plateau then to orgasm and resolution. More recently, an alternative model to understanding the sexual response cycle has suggested that for many women, desire comes after arousal and that many women begin from a point of sexual neutrality. Arousal may come from a conscious decision or as a result of seduction or suggestion from a partner.

According to the DSM IV, there are six female sexual dysfunctions. Hypoactive sexual desire disorder is the most prevalent female sexual dysfunction. Hypoactive sexual desire disorder is defined as persistently or recurrently deficient (or absent) sexual fantasies, and/or desire for sexual activity that causes personal distress. It is the sexual dysfunction that is often assumed to correspond with menopause due to loss of testosterone that occurs with ovarian hormone decline.

In June 2001, a panel of experts reviewed the existing literature on androgen deficiency in women and proposed a new syndrome called female androgen insufficiency (FAI). FAI is defined as a pattern of clinical symptoms in the presence of decreased bioavailable testosterone and normal estrogen status. The clinical symptoms include impaired sexual function, mood alterations, and diminished energy and well-being.

The reason the term *insufficiency* (and not *deficiency*) is used is that not enough is known about normal levels of androgens in women to be able to state what is considered a deficiency. There are no consistent laboratory assessments. Most commercially available methods are inaccurate or unreliable. Equilibrium dialysis is the current gold standard, but it is not readily available in most laboratories.

Another problem with androgen insufficiency is that not all women experience symptoms even when they may have declining levels of free testosterone. Also, it is much too comfortable a diagnosis. Healthcare providers appreciate having a simple biologic factor that is responsible for a specific problem. Unfortunately, this is often not the case with regard to female sexual dysfunction, particularly with aging women and decreased sexual desire. Female sexuality and hypoactive desire disorder are very complicated and cannot be summed up by a simple biologic theory. Even when androgen insufficiency may be involved, there are a number of other psychosocial factors that are at least as important, if not more important, in understanding the problem.

The Massachusetts Women's Health Study, a large, population-based trial, showed that a woman's menopause status has a smaller impact on sexual functioning than other factors, such as health, sociodemographic variables, psychological aspects, a partner's health and sexual dysfunction, and lifestyle. Although menopause (but not serum estrogen levels) was significantly associated with decreases in several sexual function measurements, including lower sexual desire and declines in arousal, the impact was not as great as that of the other factors. The Melbourne Women's Midlife Health Project found similar results.

Declining estrogen levels have been associated with a decline in sexual function, while declining testosterone levels have been associated with a decline in libido. The menopause-associated estrogen loss leads to vaginal dryness, urogenital atrophy, and dyspareunia. These changes may appear during perimenopause, but they are more common during the first few years after menopause. In perimenopause, hot flashes can result in chronic sleep disturbance, which may affect psychologic function. Negative changes in mood and well-being as well as poor self-esteem may also be relevant to sexual dysfunction associated with menopause.

Some experts believe that changes in sexual desire, decreased sexual frequency, and diminished responsiveness may be a result of either diminished estrogen effects on the cardiovascular system, which impair arterial blood flow, or decreased estrogenic effects on the central and peripheral nervous system, which impair touch and vibration perception.

Diminished endogenous progesterone appears to have no adverse effects on sexual function, although some types of progestogen therapy can indirectly affect sexual function and/or sexual activity by its negative influence on mood or by causing frequent uterine bleeding.

Most experts agree that a woman's libido is more associated with androgen (testosterone). Conditions that accelerate declining androgen production are found in Table 7.

Table 7. Conditions that accelerate declining androgen production in women

Bilateral oophorectomy. Surgical removal of both ovaries in women prior to spontaneous menopause decreases circulating levels of testosterone by as much as 40% to 50%.

Hysterectomy without oophorectomy. Up to 40% of women may experience ovarian atrophy within 3 years of the hysterectomy.

Pituitary/adrenal insufficiency. Androgen depletion is seen with Sheehan's syndrome and Addison's disease. In addition to decreased libido, symptoms include muscle wasting, loss of pubic and axillary hair, osteoporosis, and immune disorders.

Corticosteroid therapy. Androgen depletion is seen with Cushing's syndrome. In addition to decreased libido, symptoms include muscle wasting, loss of pubic and axillary hair, osteoporosis, and immune disorders.

Chronic illness. Low androgen concentration is also seen in those with anorexia nervosa, advanced cancer, and burn trauma.

Bibliography

Avis NE, Stellato R, Crawford S, Johannes C, Longcope C. Is there an association between menopause status and sexual functioning? *Menopause* 2000;7:297-309.

Bachmann GA. Influence of menopause on sexuality. *Int J Fertil Menopausal Stud* 1995;40(suppl 1):16-22.

Basson R, Berman J, Burnett A, et al. Report of the international consensus development conference on female sexual dysfunction: definitions and classifications. *J Urol* 2000;163:888-893.

Buckler HM. The perimenopausal state and incipient ovarian failure. In: Lobo RA, ed. *Treatment of the Postmenopausal Woman: Basic and Clinical Aspects.* 2nd ed. Philadelphia, PA: Lippincott Williams & Wilkins; 1999:47-60.

Buster JE, Casson PR. Where androgens come from, what controls them, and whether to replace them. In: Lobo RA, ed. *Treatment of the Postmenopausal Woman: Basic and Clinical Aspects.* 2nd ed. Philadelphia, PA: Lippincott Williams & Wilkins; 1999:141-154.

Dennerstein L, Lehert P, Burger H, Dudley E. Factors affecting sexual functioning of women in the mid-life years. *Climacteric* 1999;2:254-262.

Executive summary: Stages of Reproductive Aging Workshop (STRAW): Park City, Utah, July 2001. *Menopause* 2001;8:402-407.

Horton K, Gath D, Dave A. Sexual function in a community sample of middle aged women with partners: effects of age, marital, socioeconomic, psychiatric, gynecological and menopause factors. *Arch Sex Behav* 1994;3:375-395.

Hunter MS. Emotional well-being, sexual behaviour and hormone replacement therapy. *Maturitas* 1990;12:299-314.

Judd HL, Lucas WE, Yen SS. Effect of oophorectomy on circulating testosterone and androstenedione levels in patients with endometrial cancer. *Am J Obstet Gynecol* 1974;118:793-798.

Kaunitz AM. The role of androgens in menopausal hormonal replacement. *Endocrinol Metab Clin North Am* 1997;26:391-397.

Levine SB. *Sexual Life.* New York, NY: Plennum Press; 1992.

Lobitz WC, Lobitz GK. Resolving the sexual intimacy paradox: a developmental model for the treatment of sexual desire disorders. *J Sex Marital Ther* 1996;22:71-84.

Sarrel PM. Sexuality and menopause. *Obstet Gynecol* 1990; 75(4 suppl):26S-30S.

Sherwin BB. Impact of the changing hormonal milieu on psychologic functioning. In: Lobo RA, ed. *Treatment of the Postmenopausal Woman: Basic and Clinical Aspects.* 2nd ed. Philadelphia, PA: Lippincott Williams & Wilkins; 1999:179-187.

C.08. Skeletal system effects

Osteoporosis is the most common bone disease affecting humans. It is characterized by reduced bone mass accompanied by architectural deterioration of the skeleton, which leads to an increased risk for fracture. The disease has no warning signs. Often, the first indication of osteoporosis is a fracture. Falls or other injuries can often break osteoporotic bones, but sometimes osteoporotic bones, such as vertebrae, become so fragile that they collapse without any obvious precipitating trauma.

Bone strength reflects the integration of bone density (determined in each individual by peak bone mass and amount of bone loss, expressed as grams of mineral per area or volume) and bone quality (architecture, turnover, damage accumulation such as microfractures, and mineralization).

Bone loss commonly occurs as women age, but osteoporosis is not always the result of bone loss. If a high peak bone mass is not reached during the early years, osteoporosis may develop. Therefore, to prevent osteoporosis, achieving optimal peak bone mass is just as important as preventing bone loss.

Osteoporosis can be defined as either primary or secondary:

- *Primary osteoporosis* can occur in both women and men at all ages, but often follows menopause in women.

- *Secondary osteoporosis* is a result of medications (eg, glucocorticoids), certain medical conditions (eg, hypogonadism), or diseases (eg, celiac disease).

Most cases of osteoporosis occur in postmenopausal women, and the incidence increases with age. In the United States, approximately 8 million women have osteoporosis, defined as femoral bone mineral density (BMD) greater than 2.5 standard deviations below the mean of young, healthy white women. Another 22 million women have low bone mass, defined as BMD between 1 and 2.5 standard deviations below the mean.

Osteoporosis rates vary with ethnicity. In the United States, the highest rates are in whites and those of Asian descent and the lowest in blacks. In those aged 50 and older, an estimated 20% of non-Hispanic white and Asian women have osteoporosis, with 52% having low bone mass. For Hispanic women, 10% have osteoporosis and 49% have low bone mass. For African American women, 5% have osteoporosis another 35% have low bone mass.

Age also increases osteoporosis rates, which rise from 4% in women 50 to 59 years old to 52% for women 80 and older.

In the United States, white women older than age 50 have nearly a 40% risk for osteoporotic fracture in their remaining lifetime, with two-thirds of the fractures occurring after age 75.

Up to 90% of all hip and spine fractures in elderly white women (aged 65 to 84 years) can be attributed to osteoporosis. The estimated lifetime risks of hip, vertebral, and forearm fracture for a 50-year-old white woman are 17.5%, 15.6%, and 16.0%, respectively. Black women have about one-third the fracture rate of white women, a difference usually attributed to their higher bone mass.

Osteoporotic hip fractures have a particularly devastating toll, resulting in greater disability, cost, and mortality than all other osteoporotic fracture types combined. Hip fractures cause up to a 20% increase in mortality within a year of the incident. Approximately 25% of women require long-term care after a hip fracture, and 50% will have some long-term loss of mobility.

Fractures at other sites, however, can also result in serious morbidity. Vertebral fractures may cause substantial pain as well as loss of height and exaggerated thoracic kyphosis. The pain and deformity can greatly restrict normal movement, including simple movements such as bending and reaching. An important consequence of vertebral fractures is that they greatly increase (5- to 7-fold) the risk of subsequent vertebral fracture. Thoracic fractures can restrict lung function, and fractures of the lower back can cause nonvertebral disorders, especially digestive problems. Tooth loss is another potential complication of osteoporosis and low bone mass.

Osteoporosis takes a psychological toll as well. Depression is common in women with osteoporosis. Hip and vertebral fractures and their consequences of pain, loss of mobility, and loss of independence can lead to depression and anxiety. The fear, anger, frustration, and loss of self-esteem that these women may experience can have significant effects on their personal relationships.

Prevention and treatment of osteoporosis are important factors in maintaining postmenopausal dental health. Tooth loss has been associated with osteoporosis through a sequence that begins with atrophy of bony tooth sockets leading to gum retraction and exposure of nonenamel tooth surfaces, periodontal pocket development, bacterial invasion, and clinical periodontitis. Women with postmenopausal osteoporosis lose a substantial amount of cancellous bone early, followed by a slower loss of cortical bone. Cortical bone makes up the dense outer shell of bone that encases the cancellous bone (also called trabecular bone), which forms the internal honeycomb-like structure. The sequence is similar to that of bone disease associated with hyperparathyroidism, which has been associated with loss of dental lamina dura.

C.08.a. Relationship with menopause

Studies have demonstrated that lack of estrogen plays a key role in primary osteoporosis. The decline in circulating levels of 17β-estradiol is the predominant factor influencing the increased bone loss associated with menopause. Bone loss at the spine begins about 1.5 years before the last menstrual period and totals approximately 10.5% over 8 years. Bone mass at the hip has an age-related rate of decline of about 0.5% per year before and after menopause, and it sustains an additional estrogen-related loss of approximately 5% to 7% across the menopause transition (defined in this study as the 2 to 3 years before menopause and the first 3 to 4 years after menopause). Bone mass continues to decline in women older than age 70. This effect may be accelerated by secondary hyperparathyroidism caused by an age-related drop in calcium absorption. Overall, women lose about one-third of their BMD between menopause and age 80.

Surgical menopause is associated with an increased risk of osteoporosis when compared with women who experience menopause spontaneously.

C.08.b. Pathophysiology

Bone remodeling is the process of bone resorption (ie, breakdown) and bone formation. At the cellular level, osteoclasts promote bone resorption by stimulating the production of enzymes that dissolve bone mineral and proteins. Osteoblasts promote bone formation by creating a protein matrix consisting primarily of collagen, which is soon calcified, resulting in remineralization of bone.

Bone remodeling is the process of bone resorption and bone formation. At the cellular level, osteoclasts promote bone resorption by stimulating the production of enzymes that dissolve bone mineral and proteins. Osteoblasts promote bone formation by creating a protein matrix consisting primarily of collagen, which is soon calcified, resulting in mineralized bone.

In normal bone remodeling, bone resorption is balanced by bone formation. Bone loss occurs when there is an imbalance between bone removal and bone replacement, resulting in a decrease in bone mass and an increase in the risk for bone fracture.

Bone mass increases rapidly throughout childhood. After a slowing of bone mineral accumulation in the late teens, bone mass continues to increase during the 20s, the time of peak bone mass. Adequate nutrition and exercise in childhood are essential to reach one's optimal bone mass.

Sometime in midlife, bone loss begins. In women over age 70, bone loss may be accelerated by various factors, including secondary hyperparathyroidism caused by a decline in calcium absorption. It is the increase in bone loss during the menopausal years, combined with a woman's lower bone mass compared with that of men and the longer female life expectancy, that make osteoporotic fractures predominantly a woman's condition.

Dramatic changes in bone architecture accompany this loss in bone, greatly increasing the risk of fracture. Every standard deviation of reduction in bone mineral density results in a 2-fold or greater risk of fracture.

The point at which a woman has increased fracture risk depends on many factors, including age, genetics, nutrition, activity levels, peak bone mass, smoking, frailty, ability to prevent falls, and hormonal status.

Reduction in estrogen affects bone primarily through reduced skeletal turnover and a reduced rate of bone loss.

Bibliography

Assessment of Fracture Risk and Its Application to Screening for Postmenopausal Osteoporosis: Report of a WHO Study Group. (Technical report series 843.) Geneva, Switzerland: World Health Organization; 1994.

Boyce BF, Hughes DE, Wright KR, et al. Recent advances in bone biology provide insight into the pathogenesis of bone diseases. *Lab Invest* 1999;79:83-94.

Chrischilles EA, Butler CD, Davis CS, Wallace RB. A model of lifetime osteoporosis impact. *Arch Intern Med* 1991;151:2026-2032.

Coelho R, Silva C, Maia A, et al. Bone mineral density and depression: a community study in women. *J Psychosom Res* 1999;46:29-35.

Daniell HW. Postmenopausal tooth loss: contributions to edentulism by osteoporosis and cigarette smoking. *Arch Intern Med* 1983; 143:1678-1682.

Eastell R. Treatment of postmenopausal osteoporosis. *N Engl J Med* 1998;338:736-746.

Hui SL, Perkins AJ, Zhou L, et al. Bone loss at the femoral neck in premenopausal white women: effects of weight change and sex-hormone levels. *J Clin Endocrinol Metab* 2002;87:1539-1543.

Klotzbuecher CM, Ros PD, Landsman PB, Abbott TA, Berger M. Patients with prior fractures have an increased risk of future fractures: a summary of the literature and statistical synthesis. *J Bone Miner Res* 2000;15:721-739.

Krall EA, Garcia RI, Dawson-Hughes B. Increased risk of tooth loss is related to bone loss at the whole body, hip, and spine. *Calcif Tissue Int* 1996;59:433-437.

Lindsay R, Cosman F. Pathophysiology of bone loss. In: Lobo RA, ed. *Treatment of the Postmenopausal Woman: Basic and Clinical Aspects.* 2nd ed. Philadelphia, PA: Lippincott Williams & Wilkins; 1999:305-314.

Lindsay R, Silverman SL, Cooper C, et al. Risk of new vertebral fracture in the year following a fracture. *JAMA* 2001;285:320-323.

Looker AC, Orwoll ES, Johnston CC Jr, et al. Prevalence of low femoral bone density in older US adults from NHANES III. *J Bone Miner Res* 1995;12:1761-1768.

Looker AC, Wahner HW, Dunn WL, et al. Updated data on proximal femur bone mineral levels of US adults. *Osteoporos Int* 1998;8:468-489.

Melton LJ 3rd, Thamer M, Ray NF, et al. Fractures attributable to osteoporosis: report from the National Osteoporosis Foundation. *J Bone Miner Res* 1997;12:16-23.

National Institutes of Health Consensus Development Panel on Osteoporosis Prevention, Diagnosis, and Therapy. *JAMA* 2001;285:785-795.

National Institutes of Health Consensus Development Panel on Optimal Calcium Intake. Optimal calcium intake. *JAMA* 1994;272:1942-1948.

National Osteoporosis Foundation. *America's Bone Health: The State of Osteoporosis and Low Bone Mass.* Washington, DC: National Osteoporosis Foundation; 2002.

National Osteoporosis Foundation. Osteoporosis: *Physician's Guide to Prevention and Treatment of Osteoporosis.* Belle Mead, NJ: Excerpta Medica; 1998.

The North American Menopause Society. The role of calcium in peri- and postmenopausal women: consensus opinion of The North American Menopause Society. *Menopause* 2001;2:84-95.

The North American Menopause Society. Management of postmenopausal osteoporosis: position statement of The North American Menopause Society. *Menopause* 2002;2:84-101.

Recker RR, Lappe J, Davies K, Heaney R. Characterization of perimenopausal bone loss: a prospective study. *J Bone Miner Res* 2000;15:1965-1973.

The Society of Obstetricians and Gynaecologists of Canada. The Canadian consensus conference on menopause and osteoporosis. *J SOGC* 1998;20:2-64.

Wactawski-Wende J, Grossi SG, Trevisan M, et al. The role of osteopenia in oral bone loss and periodontal disease. *J Periodontol* 1996;67(suppl 10):S1076-S1084.

US Congress Office of Technology Assessment. *Hip Fracture Outcomes in People Age 50 and Over — Background Paper.* Washington, DC: US Government Printing Office; 1994. Publication OTA-BP-H-120.

C.09. Cardiovascular system effects

In the United States, cardiovascular disease (CVD) is the number one cause of mortality in both men and women. Among US women, the mortality rate from CVD is greater than the next 14 causes of death combined. Since 1984, CVD has caused more deaths in women than in men.

The median age of mortality from CVD in women is 74 years. The age-adjusted mortality rate for CVD is 140 per 100,000 in white women and 160 per 100,000 in black women.

After age 50, more than half of all deaths in women are caused by some form of CVD. Many more women die from heart disease than from breast cancer, although before age 65, more lives are lost to breast cancer.

In part because women suffer myocardial infarctions (MI; ie, heart attack) at older ages than men do, they are more likely to die from an MI within a few weeks. About 38% of women will die within 1 year after having a recognized MI. Within 6 years of an MI, 35% of women will have another MI, 6% of women will experience sudden death, and 46% of women will be disabled with heart failure.

Cardiovascular disease is a term used to describe many conditions:

- Hypertension (ie, high blood pressure);

- Atherosclerosis (ie, plaque deposits in blood vessels, resulting in reduced blood flow);

- Coronary artery disease (sometimes called coronary heart disease). This can result in MI and angina pectoris. This type of CVD was responsible for the greatest percentage (49%) of all deaths from CVD among US men and women in 1997.

- Stroke. These arterial occlusions in the brain were responsible for the second greatest percentage (17%) of all deaths from CVD among US men and women in 1997;

- Arrythmias (ie, abnormal heart beats);

- Valvular heart disease including rheumatic fever and rheumatic heart disease;

- Congenital cardiovascular defects;

- Congestive heart failure.

Proper function of the myocardium (ie, muscle of the heart) depends on a positive balance of oxygen and nutrient supply and demand. Angina is most often associated with the narrowing of coronary arteries, resulting from the formation of atherosclerotic plaques in the proximal coronary arteries. Chronic narrowing of the lumen of the coronary artery is the result of a continuous process of plaque formation, disruption, reorganization, and reformation that begins early in life, and it may lead to stable angina. Genetic, metabolic, behavioral, and environmental factors can all contribute to the process of narrowing of the coronary arteries. An MI usually occurs when a previously narrowed artery suddenly becomes completely occluded with a blood clot.

Diseased blood vessels outside the heart can lead to conditions such as stroke and hypertension. In addition, poor circulation can lead to peripheral vascular disease with difficulty walking, and even to amputation.

C.09.a. Relationship with menopause

Cardiovascular disease is uncommon in premenopausal women. After menopause, a woman's risk increases (especially after age 65), leading some to suggest that estrogen provides cardioprotective benefits. The extent to which diminished estrogen levels increase CVD risk in women has not been definitively established.

There does seem to be a relationship between premature menopause and increased incidence of CVD morbidity and mortality. Menopause before age 35 has been associated with a 2- to 3-fold increased risk of MI. The Nurses' Health Study found an overall significant association between younger age of menopause and higher risk of CVD among women who experienced natural menopause and never used estrogen or hormone replacement therapy (ERT/HRT); this increased risk was observed only among current smokers, not among participants who never smoked.

When examining the possible reasons for the increase in CVD in postmenopausal women, the most prevalent finding is that cholesterol levels change after menopause. Low-density lipoprotein cholesterol (LDL) and very low-density lipoprotein increase, and there is enhanced oxidation of LDL. In a cross-sectional analysis of 9,309 women who had never used ERT, the increases in total cholesterol, LDL, and triglycerides from premenopause to postmenopause were 4.4%, 4.0%, and 3.2%, respectively (after adjusting for covariates such as smoking and age), although results from prospective studies underway may tell a different story. Levels of high-density lipoprotein cholesterol (HDL) may decrease over time, but these changes are relatively insignificant compared with LDL increases.

The direct vascular effects that occur after menopause are considered important. Estrogen and progesterone receptors have been found in vascular tissues, including coronary arteries. Coagulation balance may also play a role in the hormone/vascular interaction and menopause changes. Certain fibrinolytic factors (eg, antithrombin III and plasminogen) increase along with some procoagulation factors (eg, factor VII and fibrinogen). After menopause, blood flow in all vascular beds decreases, prostacyclin decreases, endothelin levels increase, and vasoconstriction occurs in response to acetylcholine challenges or arteries constrict in response to acetylcholine challenges. Circulating plasma levels of nitric oxide increase and levels of angiotensin-converting enzyme decrease.

Postmenopausal women who are healthy and not obese experience a decrease in carbohydrate tolerance as insulin resistance increases. Stress reactivity is exaggerated in postmenopausal women compared with younger women. However, the role of diminished estrogen in these results has not been definitively determined.

Bibliography

American Heart Association. *2001 Heart and Stroke Statistical Update.* Dallas, TX: American Heart Association; 2000.

de Aloysio D, Gambacciani M, Meschia M, et al. The effect of menopause on blood lipid and lipoprotein levels. The ICARUS Study Group. *Atherosclerosis* 1999;147:147-153.

Gorodeski GI, Utian WH. Epidemiology and risk factors of cardiovascular disease in postmenopausal women. In: Lobo RA, ed. *Treatment of the Postmenopausal Woman: Basic and Clinical Aspects.* 2nd ed. Philadelphia, PA: Lippincott Williams & Wilkins; 1999:331-359.

Herrington DM. Sex hormones and normal cardiovascular physiology in women. In: Julian DG, Wenger NK, eds. *Women and Heart Disease.* London, Eng: Martin Dunitz Publishers; 1997:243-264.

Hu FB, Grodstein F, Hennekens CH, et al. Age at natural menopause and risk of cardiovascular disease. *Arch Intern Med* 1999;159: 1061-1066.

Jensen J, Nilas L, Christiansen C. Influence of menopause on serum lipids and lipoproteins. *Maturitas* 1990;12:321-331.

Poehlman ET, Toth MJ, Ades PA, Rosenn CJ. Menopause-associated changes in plasma lipids, insulin-like growth factor I and blood pressure: a longitudinal study. *Eur J Clin Invest* 1997;27:322-326.

Saba S, Link MS, Homoud MK, Wang PJ, Estes NA. Effect of low estrogen states in healthy women on dispersion of ventricular repolarization. *Am J Cardiol* 2001;87:354-356.

Stampfer MJ, Colditz GA, Willett WC. Menopause and heart disease. *Ann N Y Acad Sci* 1990;592:193-203.

C.10. Other changes/complaints

Perimenopausal women often report other health changes that they may or may not attribute to approaching menopause. Among these changes are weight gain, heart palpitations, and joint pain, as well as changes of the skin, eyes, hair, and teeth/oral cavity. With some, the decline in ovarian hormones does play a role, but so does the aging process.

C.10.a. Weight gain

During the menopause transition, many women gain weight. The average amount of weight gained during this period averages approximately 5 lbs (2.25 kg). This increase is sometimes attributed to menopause or to treatment for menopause-related conditions, including use of ERT/HRT. However, the notion that menopause or hormone therapy is responsible for weight gain is not supported by scientific evidence.

Menopause-related weight gain appears to be most related to aging and lifestyle. Several pieces of evidence support this conclusion. Body fat accumulates throughout adult life, and most women in the Western world will continue to accumulate body fat during peri- and postmenopause, adding to the fat already there. Lean body mass decreases with age, and this loss seems to accelerate after menopause, especially given the more sedentary lifestyle of older women. Women who decrease their physical activity during and after the menopausal transition seem to suffer from accelerated loss of lean body mass. Burning fewer calories through less physical activity also increases fat mass and weight gain.

Although research suggests that age, rather than menopause, is associated with weight gain, there is some evidence that menopause may be related to changes in body composition and/or fat distribution. Several studies have shown that menopause is associated with increased fat in the abdominal region. Current research is focusing more on changes in body composition and placement of body fat than on actual weight gain.

In the Postmenopausal Estrogen/Progestin Interventions (PEPI) trial, women receiving estrogen with or without progestogen weighed, on average, 1 kg less than placebo recipients at the end of the 3-year trial. No weight difference was noted between the HRT and ERT regimens. When self-assessing weight gain and appetite increases, women using HRT were more likely to note weight loss and decreased appetite than placebo recipients, while women who used unopposed ERT did not perceive more weight gain than placebo recipients.

C.10.b Palpitations

Recent literature has suggested that decreased estrogen levels slow the rate of ventricular repolarization, possibly rendering postmenopausal women more susceptible to cardiac arrhythmias. These findings may, in part, explain the higher rate of arrhythmias seen in these women, although the clinical relevance of these findings has not been confirmed. Measures of atrioventricular conduction time and cardiac repolarization time after hysterosalpingo-oophorectomy (ie, excision of the uterus, uterine tubes, and ovaries) are not modified by ERT/HRT.

During vasomotor episodes, heart rate increases of 4 to 35 beats per minute can occur, and some women may interpret the perceived increase as palpitation. Palpitations also are a common symptom in anxiety disorders including generalized anxiety, phobias, panic disorder, and agitated depression.

Although it is unlikely that palpitations in this age group are related to serious coronary abnormalities, caution should be exercised. An electrocardiographic examination should be conducted if symptoms are accompanied by exercise intolerance, shortness of breath, or chest pain. Individuals with a high personal risk of coronary disease or with a strong family history of early cardiac death — men who have died under the age of 50 or women who have died under the age of 60 — should also be assessed.

C.10.c. Joint pain

Another change noticed at midlife is painful joints. There are no studies linking menopause and joint pain. Osteoarthritis, the most common form of joint disease, increases in frequency with aging and particularly affects women in the postmenopausal age group. Considerable research is ongoing to clarify the relationship between hormones and immune function, including arthritis. There are numerous data to support the role of sex hormones (estrogen, in particular) as modulators of immune cell actions.

C.10.d. Skin changes

The dermis forms the main bulk of the skin. The fibers present in the dermis consist of two main types of fibrous protein: collagen (97.5%) and elastin (2.5%). Collagen fibers are responsible for the main mass and the resilience of the dermis.

The skin actually ages relatively well. It is only with exposure to extrinsic factors, primarily sunlight and, to some extent, tobacco smoke, that a more marked aging of the skin occurs. Sun exposure is also largely responsible for variations in pigmentation. These variations manifest as a variety of darker spots on the skin, and as light spots often seen on the backs of the forearms and on the face. In sun-damaged locations in the dermis, elastin becomes fragmented as a direct consequence of ultraviolet light absorption. Dark clumps can be seen in stained specimens of elastin, giving it an appearance that clearly differs from that of fine elastin fibers seen in young skin.

Hormones play an important role in skin physiology. The androgen hormones modulate sebum production. Acne can result from androgen-induced excessive sebum production. The effects of androgens on acne are more evident in adult women than in adolescents. Clinically, the adult variety of acne is mostly on the lower face, particularly along the chin, jawline, and neck. Lesions are predominantly papulonodular and are often tender. Circulating androgens are typically in the normal range, but levels have been shown to be significantly higher in women with acne than in women without acne.

Estrogen has a number of functions in the skin, where estrogen receptors are present in significant numbers. Cross-sectional data have shown a highly significant correlation between the declines in skin collagen and skin thickness and the years since menopause. The decline in skin collagen content after menopause occurs at a much more rapid rate in the initial postmenopausal years than in the later ones. Some 30% of skin collagen is lost during the first 5 years after menopause, with an average decline of 2% per postmenopausal year over a period of 20 years. These statistics are similar to that of bone loss after menopause. Increases in skin laxity and wrinkling as well as decreases in skin elasticity also are seen after menopause. No significant correlation has been found between skin thickness and skin collagen content and the actual chronological age of a woman, adding to the evidence suggesting that years since menopause is a more important factor than age affecting skin parameters.

C.10.e. Ocular changes

Various ocular changes may occur during the menstrual cycle, pregnancy, and at menopause. Visual performance may be altered by increased corneal, lid, and conjunctival edema during certain phases of the menstrual cycle and during perimenopause. These effects may reduce contact lens tolerance. Hormonal and menopausal status may adversely affect clinical outcomes following refractive surgery, which is now recognized to cause dry eyes (keratoconjunctivitis sicca) in a segment of people, both male and female.

Ocular complaints reported by postmenopausal women include dryness, burning, pressure, sensitivity to light, blurred vision, increased lacrimation, tired eyes, swollen or reddened eyelids, foreign-body sensation, and scratchiness. Presbyopia often starts just prior to menopause and requires many women to wear reading glasses.

Dry eye syndrome is one of the most common ocular manifestations of menopause and is characterized by symptoms of ocular irritation such as dryness, pressure, foreign-body sensation, scratchiness, and burning as well as light and cold intolerance. The signs of ocular surface damage include redness, aberrant mucus production, and even corneal scarring. Any event that contributes to abnormalities of tear stability or flow can induce or exacerbate dry eye. These include environmental triggers, such as low humidity or wind; autoimmune diseases, such as Sjögren's syndrome or rheumatoid arthritis; and the use of certain drugs, such as diuretics, antihistamines, or psychotropics.

Studies in animal models have revealed that lacrimal gland function is significantly influenced by sex hormones. Androgens specifically have been shown to exert essential and specific effects on maintaining normal glandular functions and suppressing inflammation. It has been proposed that the pathology of dry eye may be initiated when systemic androgen levels fall below the threshold necessary to support secretory function and maintain an anti-inflammatory environment. The decrease in systemic androgen levels that comes with aging may have a direct effect on dry eye syndrome.

Cataract formation becomes more common with age in men and women, although there is conflicting information regarding any sex predilection. Animal studies have shown that estrogen provides protection against cataract formation. Furthermore, retrospective analyses of large population-based studies suggest a protective effect in postmenopausal women using ERT.

C.10.f. Hair changes

Some women in midlife begin to have thinning of hair on the scalp (*androgenic alopecia*) and/or unwanted growth of hair on the face (*hirsutism*). Since menopause occurs in midlife, some women associate these changes with perimenopause/menopause. The actual causes of both scalp hair thinning and growth of unwanted hair in women are unknown, but both appear to be genetic and hormone related. It has been postulated that the increase in the ratio of androgen to estrogen during the midlife transition may influence hair changes in some women. Additionally, hair loss may be associated with excessive dieting, iron deficiency, hypothyroid dysfunction, lupus, sudden hormonal shift (ie, post total abdominal hysterectomy TAH), scalp wounds, burns or infections, intense prolonged stress, and, possibly, vitamin B_{12} deficiency.

Thinning of the hair usually begins between the ages of 12 and 40 years in both sexes, and approximately half the population expresses this trait to some degree before the age of 50. Alopecia occurs as often in women as in men and affects 50% of women under 50 years of age.

Androgenic alopecia. Most women with androgenic alopecia have normal menses, pregnancies, and endocrine function, including normal serum androgen levels. Hormonal evaluation is indicated if hair loss is sudden or other symptoms of androgen excess such as irregular menses, in reproductive years, a history of infertility, hirsutism, severe cystic acne, virilization, or galactorrhea are present.

Some medications, such as cancer chemotherapy agents, cause hair thinning or loss. Thinning can occasionally be associated with antihyperlipidemic agents or systemic retinoids. While rare, use of testosterone preparations, DHEA, and possibly oral contraception with high androgenicity can be a factor in androgenic alopecia in women.

Hirsutism. Excessive hair growth in androgen-sensitive skin areas is called hirsutism. Except for rare cases of virilizing tumors or adrenal hyperplasia due to enzymatic defects, hirsutism is mainly caused by ovarian androgen overproduction (the polycystic ovary syndrome) or by peripheral hypersensitivity to normal androgen circulating levels (idiopathic hirsutism). The role of androgens in women with hirsutism is further evidenced by the reduction in hair density that can be attained with antiandrogen treatments, including oral contraceptives with low androgenicity.

Another hair-related phenomenon of concern to many women is the appearance of fine hairs ("peach fuzz") on the face — most commonly on the upper lip and chin but sometimes generalized in appearance. Large "rogue hairs" can sometimes be found on the chin, growing very quickly. The growth of unwanted hair is a common phenomenon, and sometimes occurs long before menopause.

A number of methods are available for removal of unwanted hair. Hair removal can be accomplished with yellow-light lasers, which can be effective for large areas and may be repeated every year, if needed. Standard epilating needles are effective for removal of larger hairs, such as those on the upper lip, and bleaching is an effective alternative to actual removal of the hair. Women may also choose to remove hair with waxing treatments or by shaving.

C.10.g. Dental/oral cavity changes

After menopause, tooth loss and the need for dentures increase, as do gingival inflammation and bleeding.

Tooth loss has been associated with systemic osteoporosis in both dentate and edentulous individuals. The rate of systemic bone loss in postmenopausal women has been shown to be a predictor of tooth loss. For each 1% per year decrease in whole body BMD, the risk for tooth loss more than quadrupled. A study of women with severe osteoporosis found them to be three times more likely to have no teeth than healthy, age-matched controls. In ERT/HRT users, longitudinal studies have found higher tooth counts and reduced risk of tooth loss, thereby implying a relationship to menopause.

In contrast to the apparent association of tooth loss and osteoporosis, there is controversy regarding whether a relationship exists between low BMD and periodontal disease. Long-term, age- and risk factor-matched studies are needed to further delineate a link. Nevertheless, prevention and treatment of osteoporosis are important factors in maintaining postmenopausal dental health.

Fluctuations of sex hormones during menopause have been implicated as factors in inflammatory changes in gingiva. Estrogen affects cellular proliferation, differentiation, and keratinization of the gingival epithelium. Thinning of the oral epithelium is reflected in increased gingival recession, enhanced susceptibility to tissue injury, and sensitivity (eg, burning mouth and tongue, root sensitivity, generalized increased tissue sensitivity). Hormone receptors have been identified in basal and spinous layers of the epithelium and connective tissue implicating gingival and other oral tissues as targets that manifest hormone deficiencies.

The complaint of a burning sensation in the mouth can be a symptom of another disease (such as anemia or diabetes) or a syndrome in its own right of unknown etiology. It has been suggested that, when no underlying dental or medical causes are identified and no oral signs are found, the term *burning mouth syndrome* (BMS) should be used. The prominent feature is burning pain which can be localized to the tongue and/or lips but can be more widespread and involve the entire oral cavity. A Cochrane Review reports that prevalence rates in general populations vary from 0.7% to 15%. Many of these patients show evidence of anxiety, depression, and personality disorders, which has lead to treating BMS as an emotional problem. However, new research shows that BMS may be the result of nerve damage. When nerves that carry taste signals are damaged, especially in people with sensitive taste buds, the brain seems to magnify mouth pain. A small percentage of women reaching menopause report BMS. It has not been associated with menopause.

Bibliography

Bjorkelund C, Lissner L, Andersson S, Lapidus L, Bengtssen C. Reproductive history in relation to relative weight and fat distribution. *Int J Obes Relat Metab Disord* 1996;20:213-219.

Brincat M, Kabalan S, Studd JW, Moniz CF, de Trafford J, Montgomery J. A study of the decrease of skin collagen content, skin thickness, and bone mass in the postmenopausal woman. *Obstet Gynecol* 1987;70:840-845.

Brincat MP, Galea R. Collagen: the significance in skin, bone, and carotid arteries. In: Lobo RA, ed. *Treatment of the Postmenopausal Woman: Basic and Clinical Aspects.* 2nd ed. Philadelphia, PA: Lippincott Williams & Wilkins; 1999:179-187.

Brincat M, Moniz CJ, Kabalan S, et al. Decline in skin collagen content and metacarpal index after the menopause and its prevention with sex hormone replacement. *Br J Obstet Gynaecol* 1987;94:126-129.

Castelo-Branco C, Duran M, Gonzalez-Merlo J. Skin collagen changes related to age and hormone replacement therapy. *Maturitas* 1992;15:113-119.

Crawford SL, Casey VA, Avis NE, McKinlay SM. A longitudinal study of weight and the menopause transition. *Menopause* 2000;7:96-104.

Cumming RG, Mitchell P. Hormone replacement therapy, reproductive factors, and cataract. The Blue Mountains Eye Study. *Am J Epidemiol* 1997;145:242-249.

Freeman EE, Munoz B, Schein O, West SK. Hormone replacement therapy and lens opacities: the Salisbury Eye Evaluation Project. *Arch Ophthalmol* 2001;119:1687-1692.

Grossi SG, Jeffcoat MK, Genco RJ. Osteopenia, osteoporosis, and oral disease. In: Rose LF, Genco RJ, Cohen DW, Mealey BL, eds. *Periodontal Medicine.* St Louis, MO: BC Decker, Inc; 2000:167-182.

Guttridge NM. Changes in ocular and visual variables during the menstrual cycle. *Ophthalmic Physiol Opt* 1994;14:38-48.

Hales AM, Chamberlain CG, Murphy CR, McAvoy JW. Estrogen protects lenses against cataract induced by transforming growth factor-beta (TGFbeta). *J Exp Med* 1997;185:273-280.

Henry F, Pierard-Franchimont C, Cauwenbergh G, Pierard GE. Age-related changes in facial skin contours and rheology. *J Am Geriatr Soc* 1997;45:220-222

Johnson SL, Graves GR, Kendler DL, Fluker MR. Medical and special conditions: the Canadian consensus on menopause and osteoporosis. *J SOGC* 2001;23:1096-1101.

Krall EA, Dawson-Hughes B, Hannan MT, Wilson PW, Kiel DP. Postmenopausal estrogen replacement and tooth retention. *Am J Med* 1997;102:536-542.

Krall EA, Dawson-Hughes B, Papas A, Garcia RI. Tooth loss and skeletal bone density in healthy postmenopausal women. *Osteoporos Int* 1994;4:104-109.

Krall EA, Garcia RI, Dawson-Hughes B. Increased risk of tooth loss at the whole body, hip, and spine. *Calcif Tissue Int* 1996;59:433-437.

Kritz-Silverstein D, Barrett-Connor E. Long-term postmenopausal hormone use, obesity, and fat distribution in older women. *JAMA* 1996;275:987-988.

McCarthy CA, Ng I, Waldron B, et al. Relation of hormone and menopausal status to outcomes following excimer laser photorefractive keratectomy in women. Melbourne Excimer Laser Group. *Aust NZ J Ophthalmol* 1996;24:215-222.

Milewicz A, Tworowska U, Demissie A. Menopausal obesity — myth or fact? *Climacteric* 2001;4:273-283.

Norman RJ, Flight IH, Rees MC. Estrogen and progestin hormone replacement therapy for peri-menopausal and post-menopausal women: weight and body fat distribution. *Cochrane Database Syst Rev* 2000;(2):CD001018.

Paganini-Hill A. Benefits of estrogen replacement therapy on oral health. The Leisure World Cohort. *Arch Intern Med* 1995; 155:2325-2329.

Pierard-Franchimont C, Cornil F, Dehavay J, et al. Climacteric skin ageing of the face: a prospective longitudinal comparative trial on the effect of oral hormone replacement therapy. *Maturitas* 1999; 32:87-93.

Poehlman EAT, Tchernof A. Traversing the menopause: changes in energy expenditure and body composition. *Coron Artery Dis* 1998; 9:799-803.

Reinhardt RA, Payne JB, Maze CA, Patil KD, Gallagher SJ, Mattson JS. Influence of estrogen and osteopenia/osteoporosis on clinical periodontitis in postmenopausal women. *J Periodontol* 1999; 70:823-828.

Sowers ME, Crutchfield M, Jannausch ML, Russel-Aulet M. Longitudinal changes in body composition in women approaching midlife. *Ann Hum Biol* 1996;23:253-265.

Sullivan DA, Dartt DA, Meneray MA, eds. *Lacrimal Gland, Tear Film, and Dry Eye Syndrome*. New York, NY: Plenum Press, 1998.

Venning VA, Dawber MA. Patterned androgenic alopecia in women. *J Am Acad Dermatol* 1988;18:1073-1077.

von Wowern N, Klausen B, Kollerup G. Osteoporosis: a risk factor in periodontal disease. *J Periodontol* 1994;65:1134-1138

Wactawski-Wende J. Periodontal diseases and osteoporosis: association and mechanisms. *Ann Periodontol* 2001;6:197-208.

Wing RR, Matthews KA, Kuller LH, Meilahn EN, Plantinga PL. Weight gain at the time of menopause. *Arch Intern Med* 1991; 151:97-102.

Worzola K, Hiller R, Sperduto RD, et al. Postmenopausal estrogen use, type of menopause, and lens opacities: the Framingham Studies. *Arch Intern Med* 2001;161:1448-1454.

Zadrzewska JM, Glenny AM, Forssell H. Interventions for the treatment of burning mouth syndrome. *Cochrane Database Syst Rev* 2001;3:CD002779.

Women who experience abnormal physiologic symptoms related to menopause present a clinical challenge to healthcare professionals. This section addresses some of the short- and long-term effects associated with premature menopause, induced menopause, and temporary menopause. It also addresses dementia.

D.01. Premature menopause

Premature menopause is irreversible cessation of menses in women younger than age 40. Premature menopause and premature ovarian failure (POF) can be synonymous. (In 1990, it was estimated that 1% of women under the age of 40 had POF.) However, menopause is, by definition, the very last menses. Premature ovarian failure (ie, hypergonadotropic amenorrhea), while having all the characteristics of menopause, may be transient. About 5% to 25% of women with idiopathic or presumed autoimmune POF will undergo at least one spontaneous remission. Among women with POF who have a normal karyotype, half may still have remaining ovarian follicles that function intermittently. Women with POF have an estimated 5% to 10% chance for spontaneous pregnancy.

Because the diagnosis of premature menopause means the end of "natural" childbearing, the psychological impact may be devastating. For some women, fertility is linked with womanhood, femininity, and/or sexual desirability. Addressing the psychological impact is as important as assessing the physical impact. Donor oocyte programs are an option for women who still desire pregnancy, although this option may not be available to some women, adding to the psychological distress.

D.01.a. Signs and symptoms

There is no characteristic menstrual history preceding premature menopause or premature ovarian failure. Cessation of menses may be abrupt, or present as oligomenorrhea or irregular uterine bleeding. Onset may come postpartum or after cessation of an oral contraceptive. Flushing may occur with regular menses. A positive family history is usually present in less than 10% of cases. When primary amenorrhea is associated with pubertal delay, a chromosomal defect is highly likely.

D.01.b. Etiology

The differential diagnosis is rather extensive and includes a variety of causes (Table 1).

Table 1. Potential causes of premature ovarian failure

Prodromal premature menopause
Karyotypic abnormality
Pure gonadal dysgenesis
Iatrogenic
Autoimmune
    Polyglandular
    IgG, IgA
Miscellaneous
    Enzyme deficiency
    Metabolic syndromes
    Pseudohypoparathyroidism
    Thymic disorders
Idiopathic
Pseudo
    Gonadotropin-producing pituitary adenoma
    Antibodies to the gonadotroph
    Hypothyroidism
    Isolated gonadotropin deficiency

Follicle depletion. Recent advances in the genome project are associated with numerous new findings of gene locus on the X chromosome related to ovarian failure. Fetuses with a single X chromosome, as in Turner's syndrome, develop normal ovaries with a normal complement of primordial follicles, but accelerated atresia often leads to ovarian failure. Most women with galactosemia (an autosomal recessive condition) eventually develop ovarian failure, along with hepatocellular damage, renal cellular damage, cataracts, and mental retardation.

Irradiation and many forms of chemotherapy may induce ovarian failure. The greatest of these reactions are on rapidly proliferating cells. Because prepubertal ovaries may be more resistant to insult, gonadotropin suppression has been suggested as a means for protection, although further study is necessary to determine its efficacy. The increasing use of uterine artery embolization for myomata is another possible modality for iatrogenic ovarian failure. Patients undergoing this procedure should be informed about this possible risk.

Table 2. Possible emotions linked to premature menopause

- A sense of feeling old, regardless of actual age, in a society that values youth and fertility

- A sense of embarrassment about going through menopause at a young age

- A feeling that she has lost control over bodily functions

- A lasting feeling of grief and loss for the children she hoped to conceive, similar to that experienced after the death of a loved one

- A feeling that she has somehow failed or is no longer a "complete woman" — that her inability to have children is her fault

- Concerns about her partner's reaction to her inability to conceive and, sometimes, a feeling of uncertainly about whether her partner will continue to love her

- Concerns about relationships and sexuality, such as fear of losing the ability to elicit or feel sexual desire, fear of rejection by her sexual partner, and a fear of discomfort during intercourse

- Concerns about finding someone who will love her even though she is unable to have children

- Feelings of isolation and loneliness, as if no one understands what she is going through

- Concerns about the long-term effects of estrogen loss (eg, increased risk of osteoporosis)

- Feelings of jealousy, anger, and resentment when friends or family members become pregnant — and guilt over having those feelings

- Irritability and fatigue caused by menopause-related hot flashes that interfere with sleep, making coping more difficult

Inflammatory causes of ovarian failure include viral (classically mumps) and bacterial diseases. In a patient with mumps parotitis, this diagnosis is suspected when associated with ovarian pain and lower abdominal tenderness. Cause-and-effect relationships between febrile illness and ovarian failure have not been established.

D.01.c. Diagnosis

After 4 months of amenorrhea, FSH levels that fall in the postmenopausal range at least 1 month apart are strong indicators of ovarian failure. However, 1 year of amenorrhea is still required to meet the standard definition of menopause. The prodromal form should be considered in any young woman complaining of vasomotor symptoms to avoid needless delay in the diagnosis. The progestogen challenge test can be misleading. Other laboratory screening will not detect endocrine or autoimmune disorders. Ultrasound is not clinically useful.

Obtaining a careful medical history is helpful, including prior ovarian surgery, chemotherapy, or irradiation, as well as a history in themselves or their family of autoimmune disorders, such as hypothyroidism, Addison's disease, diabetes, Graves' disease, vitiligo, systemic lupus, rheumatoid arthritis, Sjögren's syndrome, or inflammatory bowel disease.

The physical examination should include atrophic vaginal changes, an indicator of estrogen status. However, because intermittent estrogen stimulation is possible, this symptom is not definitive. A search should include other genetic or autoimmune stigmata.

Women who reach menopause earlier than anticipated may experience a range of emotions related to a diagnosis of premature menopause (see Table 2). Counseling about menopause, its acute and long-term consequences, and emotional issues is essential. Referral to a therapist may be indicated.

Bibliography

Coulam C. Immunology of ovarian failure. *Am J Reprod Immunol* 1991;25:169-174.

Eaker ED, Castelli WP. Coronary heart disease and its risk factors among women in the Framingham Study. In: Eaker E, Packard B, Wagner NK, Clarkson TB, Tyoler HA, eds. *Coronary Heart Disease in Women.* New York, NY: Haymarket Doyma; 1987:122-132.

Gorodeski GI, Utian WH. Epidemiology and risk factors of cardiovascular disease in postmenopausal women. In: Lobo RA, ed. *Treatment of the Postmenopausal Woman: Basic and Clinical Aspects.* 2nd ed. Philadelphia, PA: Lippincott Williams & Wilkins; 1999:331-359.

Hadjidakis D, Kokkinakis E, Sfakianakis M, Raptis SA. The type and time of menopause as decisive factors for bone mass changes. *Eur J Clin Invest* 1999;29:877-885.

Kalantaridou SN, Davis SR, Nelson LM. Premature ovarian failure. *Endocrinol Metab Clin North Am* 1998;27:989-1006.

Kim SS, Battaglia DE, Soules MR. The future of human ovarian cryopreservation and transplantation: fertility and beyond. *Fertil Steril* 2001;75:1049-1056.

The North American Menopause Society. Clinical challenges of perimenopause: consensus opinion of The North American Menopause Society. *Menopause* 2000;7:5-13.

Pouilles JM, Tremollieres F, Bonneu M, Ribot C. Influence of early age at menopause on vertebral bone mass. *J Bone Miner Res* 1994;9:311-315.

Rebar RW, Cedars MI, Liu JH. Premature ovarian failure: a model for the menopause? In: Lobo RA, ed. *Perimenopause.* New York, NY: Springer-Verlag; 1997:7-11.

Rebar RW, Connelly HV. Clinical features of young women with hypergonadotropic amenorrhea. *Fertil Steril* 1990;53:804-808.

Ryu RK, Chrisman HB, Omary RA, et al. The vascular impact of uterine artery embolization: prospective sonographic assessment of ovarian arterial circulation. *J Vasc Interv Radiol* 2001;12:1071-1074.

Vega EM, Egea MA, Mautalen CA. Influence of the menopausal age on the severity of osteoporosis in women with vertebral fractures. *Maturitas* 1994;19:117-124.

Zinn AR. The X chromosome and the ovary. *J Soc Gynecol Invest* 2001;8(suppl 1):S34-S36.

D.02. Induced menopause

Induced menopause occurs as a result of surgical intervention (bilateral oophorectomy) or ovarian damage from other medical means, such as chemotherapy or radiation therapy. With induced menopause of any type, levels of all ovarian hormones, including estrogen, progesterone, testosterone, and androstenedione, drop rapidly. Women experiencing induced menopause do not go through the transition to menopause. They are subjected to an abrupt withdrawal of ovarian hormones which may result in an exacerbation of symptoms.

The different causes of induced menopause — surgery, chemotherapy, and pelvic radiation — produce different effects. One effect is infertility.

D.02.a. Effect on fertility

Surgery. Bilateral oophorectomy ("surgical menopause") results in a rapid decline in ovarian hormone levels, usually occurring within days after surgery. Fertility ends immediately.

Hysterectomy is the surgical removal of the uterus for benign conditions (eg, endometriosis, uterine fibroids) or for various forms of cancer (eg, endometrial, ovarian, cervical). Depending on the woman's age and diagnosis, unilateral or bilateral salpingo-oophorectomy may be performed simultaneously. Hysterectomy ends menses and the woman's ability to carry a fetus, but it does not cause menopause.

Rarely, hysterectomy results in menopause (or earlier menopause), even with conservation of ovaries. This may be due to interference with the blood supply to the ovaries related to the surgical procedure.

All women who undergo treatments or surgery that may result in infertility should discuss childbearing issues with their healthcare practitioners prior to treatment. Medical options for women who are unable to conceive naturally can be discussed. Surrogacy is a potential option for some women. Freezing of ova or ovarian tissue sections is being studied for its potential in facilitating future procreation.

Chemotherapy. Chemotherapy is a systemic treatment that affects normal cells in addition to cancer cells. Among the cells most likely to be affected are those of the reproductive system, including the ovaries. These effects usually occur over time, not immediately. The more gradual the reduction in ovarian hormones, the more likely the menopause-related symptoms will be moderate as opposed to severe.

The ovaries of younger women (age <30 years) are more likely to recover from chemotherapy. These women may experience temporary ovarian failure, with subsequent resumption of menstruation and fertility. In women aged 30 and older, ovarian damage is more likely to be permanent. Certain chemotherapeutic agents, such as alkylating agents, appear to be more toxic. Pretreatments with gonadotropin-releasing hormone (GnRH) analogues to suppress the ovaries may provide some protection from toxic chemotherapeutics.

Pelvic radiation therapy. Radiation therapy affects the reproductive system only when it is used to treat the pelvic area. Unlike chemotherapy, which exposes the entire body to anticarcinogenic agents, radiation therapy affects only the tumor and the surrounding area. Pelvic radiation therapy is more likely to cause menopause if the ovaries receive high doses of radiation (such as for the treatment of cervical cancer). If smaller doses of pelvic radiation are used (such as for Hodgkin's disease), the ovaries may recover.

Following pelvic radiation therapy, estrogen levels often decline quickly and dramatically. Menopause-related symptoms may be more intense than those experienced after chemotherapy. These symptoms may occur within 3 to 6 months of treatment or concurrently.

Women who experience induced menopause from chemotherapy or pelvic radiation for hormone-sensitive cancers (eg, breast, uterine) may be unable to use estrogen therapy because of potential effects on their tumors, and must rely on progestogens or alternate therapies for symptom relief and well-being. Since they are also at risk for osteoporosis, bone mineral density testing is recommended. Heart disease risk may also be increased.

D.02.b. Effect on menopause symptoms

The sudden loss of ovarian hormones associated with induced menopause may result in more intense menopause-related symptoms. Almost all women experience hot flashes, which tend to be more severe and may last longer than the hot flashes associated with spontaneous menopause. Some women also experience mood changes, lack of energy, depression, and insomnia, although it may be unclear whether all of these symptoms are due to the original disease process, treatment stress, or loss of estrogen production.

Younger women undergoing induced menopause must be appropriately counseled and medically supported to cope with the earlier onset of menopausal symptoms and to prevent the potential consequences of hormone depletion.

D.02.c. Effect on sexual function

The different causes of induced menopause produce different effects on sexual function, with most effects due to the sudden drop in ovarian hormones.

The extent of the ovarian damage caused by chemotherapy and radiation will determine the amount of testosterone the ovaries continue to produce. If testosterone levels decline significantly, a loss of sexual drive may occur. Sexual interest also may decline as a result of acute symptoms, such as hot flashes and lack of sleep. Emotional responses to the situation and/or depression may also adversely affect sexual interest.

A significant drop in estrogen levels may cause severe vaginal symptoms, such as vaginal dryness, irritation, and atrophy. This may result in dyspareunia and increased risk for vaginal infections. The changes in the epithelial lining of the vagina occur relatively rapidly as estrogen levels decline. Subsequent vascular, muscular, and connective tissue changes also occur. Decreased vascularization of the surrounding tissues denies the vagina of necessary nutrients and inhibits engorgement and lubrication. The vagina also loses elasticity and narrows, particularly in women who are sexually abstinent.

Induced menopause and aging may also affect the clitoris. Possible changes include a decrease in clitoral perfusion, diminished engorgement during the desire and arousal phases, and a decline in the neurophysiologic response, including slowing of nerve impulses and decreased touch perception, vibratory sensation and reaction time. In some women, the clitoris may noticeably diminish in size.

Concurrent declines in muscle tension may increase the time it takes from arousal to orgasm, diminish the peak of orgasm, and cause a more rapid resolution to a nonstimulated state. While decreased estrogen levels are responsible for most of these changes, androgen levels also decline, especially as a result of induced menopause, and have an important impact on sexual health.

The possible changes in sexual function associated with induced menopause should be discussed with women prior to any procedure or treatment. Subsequent attention should be paid to local estrogenization of vulvar/vaginal tissues as well as to psychological factors, such as the impact of the illness or treatment on the couple and any possible concomitant depression.

Surgery. Surgical procedures vary greatly in the effects on the vagina. Some have no direct effect on the vaginal tissues, whereas others could adversely affect coital function (due to shortened vaginal length, painful neuroma or fibroma at the vaginal vault incision).

Hysterectomy is one of the most common surgical procedures performed. By age 64, an estimated 40% of US women will have undergone hysterectomy. A literature review conducted in 2000 evaluating the effect of hysterectomy on sexual function found that, for most women, removal of the uterus did not adversely affect sexuality. However, the reviewers noted that most studies were poorly designed. In the 2-year Maryland Women's Health Study, sexual function was not impaired by hysterectomy. In fact, most women reported that their sexual activity and overall libido improved.

In many cases, hysterectomy leads to enjoyable sexual activity for the first time in many years, as women enjoy freedom from pelvic pain, dyspareunia, heavy bleeding, and worries about contraception. During intercourse and orgasm, some women may notice a change in sensation but, in general, these changes do not interfere with sexual functioning or achieving orgasm.

Some women, however, report decreased orgasmic ability, possibly because of a loss of uterine contractions that had led to pleasure and/or because of a loss of "cervical tapping" that was a trigger for orgasm. There is some evidence that a subtotal hysterectomy (removal of body of uterus while leaving the cervix in place) decreases risk for diminished sexual pleasure.

Women with pre-existing sexual problems and/or depression may continue to experience problems postoperatively. It is important to diagnose and treat preoperative depression as well as establish baseline sexual function. These may improve with the surgery or remain problematic.

Following unilateral oophorectomy, many women experience no adverse change in sexual function. However, after bilateral oophorectomy, some women may report decreased sexual drive or a decreased sense of well-being. This has been attributed to the drop in serum testosterone as well as estrogen levels. Even with conservation of both ovaries, up to 30% of hysterectomized women may experience a loss or decrease in ovarian function within 3 years.

Chemotherapy. Agents used for chemotherapy may irritate the vaginal and uterine lining, which often become dry and inflamed. Vaginal yeast infections are common during chemotherapy, especially in women taking steroids or broad-spectrum antibiotics. Fatigue and nausea may interfere with sexual interest as can poor body image related to hair loss and other potential cancer and/or chemotherapy-related physical changes.

Pelvic radiation therapy. Pelvic radiation may cause vaginal itching, burning, and dryness. Vaginal tenderness may occur during treatment or persist for a few weeks afterwards. The walls of the vagina may become tough and fibrous, and lose elasticity. Pelvic radiation may make the vaginal lining thin and fragile, more prone to vaginal sores or ulcers. Vaginal scarring from radiation therapy may shorten the vagina, making intercourse impossible. Some women experience pain related to the vagina's decreased caliber or lack of fluid, which may result in vaginismus (the muscles around the opening of the vagina become tense and spasmodic, preventing penetration).

During pelvic radiation treatment, some women are advised not to have intercourse. Most women are able to resume intercourse within a few weeks after treatment ends. In this population, the appropriate use of topical estrogen may enhance the healing process and sexual function. Alternative treatments to support vaginal health and sexual function should be discussed if estrogen is contraindicated.

D.02.d. Effect on mental health

Women who experience induced menopause may have additional emotional concerns related to the illness, perhaps life-threatening, that has been (or is being) treated. Coupled with menopause-related effects, the side effects of the treatments can be overwhelming (see Table 3). For example, cancer therapies often produce an array of side effects, including fatigue, alopecia, and flu-like symptoms. For women who experience induced menopause at a young age, especially as a result of treatment for a serious illness, these feelings may be intensified.

Table 3. Possible concerns of women following induced menopause	
Impact of illness	Decline in sexual function
Side effects of treatments	Disease risk in later years
Infertility	Emotional health
Induced menopause symptoms	Inability (for some) to use ERT

Emotional and physical health are closely linked. Physical illness or discomfort may cause emotional distress, which may negatively affect the body's ability to heal and remain healthy.

Induced menopause that results from treatment or surgery for a benign condition will be associated with different concerns than menopause that results from treatment for a life-threatening disease, such as cancer.

In younger women, procedures that cause permanent infertility may precipitate a range of emotions. In addition, women who undergo surgical menopause may have lingering feelings of doubt about the necessity of the surgery.

Women who have been treated for cancer are likely to have significant fears about disease recurrence or death (see Table 4).

Women who undergo cancer treatment often have a variety of emotional concerns that may affect sexual desire. Weight changes, hair loss, and physical changes that may be perceived as disfigurement may have a negative impact on body image. Women may fear rejection by their partners. Both women and their partners might fear that vaginal penetration will cause pain.

Both the woman who undergoes a hysterectomy and her partner must be reassured that removal of the uterus will not result in loss of sexual desire or sexual function.

Table 4. Concerns related to cancer and cancer therapy

- Fears about cancer returning or developing a new cancer

- Fear of death

- Fear of pain or discomfort related to the illness and/or treatment

- Fear of being disfigured, disabled, and/or becoming dependent on others

- Feelings related to lack of information or "information overload"

- Concerns about body image due to changes caused by the illness/treatment; in some cases, women may grieve for a lost body part/organ

- Apprehension about sexual function, intimacy, and relationships (fear of rejection)

- Feelings of guilt about family members having to deal with the illness

- A feeling of hopelessness and uncertainty about the future after cancer treatment

- Anger for getting cancer

- Fears about using ERT because of a possible link between ERT and some cancers

D.02.e Effect on long-term health

Loss of endogenous estrogen often causes symptoms that adversely affect quality of life and may increase the risk for osteoporosis and coronary heart disease. It also has an impact on urogenital function, which includes bladder, urethral, and vaginal health. Women who experience induced menopause during their premenopausal years will spend more years without the protection of estrogen, increasing their lifetime risk for these diseases. The younger a woman is when she goes through induced menopause, the longer she is without estrogen.

Healthcare providers must make a commitment to support women following induced menopause in their efforts to maintain their health and well-being. Available pharmacologic treatments should be discussed according to the cause of the woman's induced menopause. It is imperative that the woman's healthcare team collaborate in developing the recommended treatment plan and providing ongoing care.

Bibliography

Cawood EH, Bancroft J. Steroid hormones, the menopause, sexuality and well-being of women. *Psychol Med* 1996;26:925-936.

Davis SR. Androgens and female sexuality. *J Gend Specif Med* 2000;3:36-40.

Farrell SA, Kieser K. Sexuality after hysterectomy. *Obstet Gynecol* 2000;95:1045-1051.

Gath D, Cooper P, Bond A, Edmonds G. Hysterectomy and psychiatric disorder: II. Demographic psychiatric and physical factors in relation to psychiatric outcome. *Br J Psychiatry* 1982;140:343-350.

Heim C, Newport DJ, Heit S, et al. Pituitary-adrenal and autonomic responses to stress in women after sexual and physical abuse in childhood. *JAMA* 2000;284:592-597.

Khastgir G, Studd J. Hysterectomy, ovarian failure, and depression. *Menopause* 1998;5:113-122.

Kjerulff KH, Rhodes JC, Langenberg PW, Harvey LA. Patient satisfaction with results of hysterectomy. *Am J Obstet Gynecol* 2000;183:1440-1447.

Laumann EO, Paik A, Rosen RC. Sexual dysfunction in the United States: prevalence and predictors. *JAMA* 1999;281:537-544.

Meirow D. Reproduction post-chemotherapy in young cancer patients. *Mol Cell Endocrinol* 2000;169:123-131.

Myers LS. Methodological review and meta-analysis of sexuality and menopause research. *Neurosci Biobehavioral Rev* 1995; 19:331-341.

Rhodes JC, Kjerulff KH, Langenberg PW, Guzinski GM. Hysterectomy and sexual functioning. *JAMA* 1999;282:1934-1941.

Ryan MM. Hysterectomy: social and psychosexual aspects. *Bailliere's Clin Obstet Gynaecol* 1997;11:23-36.

Ryan MM, Dennerstein L, Pepperell R. Psychological aspects of hysterectomy: a prospective study. *Br J Psychiatry* 1989;154:516-522.

Sherwin BB. Affective changes with estrogen and androgen replacement therapy in surgically menopausal women. *J Affect Disord* 1988;14:177-187.

Sherwin BB. Impact of the changing hormonal milieu on psychologic functioning. In: Lobo RA, ed. *Treatment of the Postmenopausal Woman: Basic and Clinical Aspects.* 2nd ed. Philadelphia, PA: Lippincott Williams & Wilkins; 1999:179-188.

Sherwin BB, Gelfand MM. The role of androgen in the maintenance of sexual functioning in oophorectomized women. *Psychosom Med* 1987;49:397-409.

Sherwin BB, Gelfand MM, Brender W. Androgen enhances sexual motivation in females: a prospective, crossover study of sex steroid administration in the surgical menopause. *Psychosom Med* 1985;47:339-351.

D.03. Temporary menopause

Temporary menopause describes a span of time when normal ovarian function is interrupted and temporary amenorrhea results. Some women experience temporary menopause after chemotherapy or pelvic radiation therapy. Women who over-exercise or over-diet may experience amenorrhea due to a hypoestrogenic state. Some drug therapies such as GnRH analogues, may also result in temporary menopause.

GnRH analogues. These drugs are indicated for the treatment of fibroids, endometriosis, and severe premenstrual syndrome. They are sometimes used before certain types of surgery, such as myomectomy, and are prominently used for in vitro fertilization cycles along with fertility drugs.

GnRH analogues inhibit secretion of gonadotropins by blocking GnRH receptors at the pituitary. This causes the ovaries to temporarily stop hormone production, inducing a hypoestrogenic state.

Women who take short-acting forms of GnRH analogues (administered daily subcutaneously) usually resume normal ovarian function soon after injections are stopped. After taking the long-acting (depot) forms of the drugs (given as intramuscular injections or as an implant), normal ovarian function may take 2 or more months to resume due to the longer half-life of the depot form of the medication.

Newer agents called GnRH antagonists have quicker onset of action in suppressing the gonadal axis. If used on a continual basis, they will lead to the same clinical situations associated with GnRH analogues.

Bibliography

Couzinet B, Young J, Brailly S, Le Bouc Y, Chanson P, Schaison G. Functional hypothalamic amenorrhea: a partial and reversible gonadotropin deficiency of nutritional origin. *Clin Endocrinol* 1999;50:229-235.

Grinspoon S, Miller K, Coyle C, et al. Severity of osteopenia in estrogen-deficient women with anorexia nervosa and hypothalamic amenorrhea. *J Clin Endocrinol Metab* 1999;84:2049-2055.

Hughes E. Fedorkow D, Collins J, Vandekerckhove P. Ovulation suppression for endometriosis. *Cochrane Database Syst Rev* 2000;(2):CD000155.

Tzafettas JM. Current and potential application of GnRH agonists in gynecologic practice. *Ann NY Acad Sci* 2000;900:435-443.

D.04. Pelvic pathology/abnormal uterine bleeding

Some symptoms attributed to menopause may be the result of pelvic pathology. Perhaps the most common of these is abnormal uterine bleeding.

Terminology describing uterine bleeding is not consistent. In NAMS materials, *abnormal uterine bleeding* (AUB) is defined as excessive and/or erratic bleeding in the presence or absence of intracavity or uterine pathology. It may be associated with structural or systemic abnormalities. *Dysfunctional uterine bleeding* is a term that describes abnormal uterine bleeding of unknown etiology. *Anovulatory uterine bleeding* is defined as menstrual bleeding arising from anovulation or oligo-ovulation. The normal, irregular bleeding of the perimenopause transition is a type of anovulatory uterine bleeding.

AUB has an array of consequences, such as heavy or prolonged menstrual flow, which may lead to social embarrassment, sexual compromise, and diminished quality of life. Pain is not a common presenting symptom unless it is associated with the passage of large blood clots. In some cases, anemia may result, with complaints of fatigue, pica (unusual food cravings), or headaches.

Etiology. Abnormal and anovulatory uterine bleeding may be related to a number of benign and malignant diseases of the reproductive tract and systemic diseases (Table 5). Pregnancy and infection must always be considered. Thyroid abnormalities, hyperprolactinemia, and polycystic ovarian syndrome may cause anovulation and bleeding irregularities. Systemic diseases other than those associated with the endocrine system, such as leukemia, infrequently present with abnormal uterine bleeding as the only sign or symptom.

Below is a discussion of some of the various possible causes of AUB:

- *Hormonal imbalance.* An imbalance in ovarian estrogen and progesterone production, usually related to anovulation, can cause AUB. In some women with amenorrhea, the endometrium is stimulated by continuous exposure to estrogen without sufficient levels of progesterone to allow for complete shedding of the endometrial lining. This may eventually result in irregular or heavy bleeding. If estrogen exposure is continuous, an abnormal overgrowth of cells may develop within the endometrium (endometrial hyperplasia) that could lead to endometrial cancer.

Table 5. Possible causes of abnormal and anovulatory uterine bleeding

Benign reproductive tract conditions
- Anovulation
- Pregnancy
- Leiomyomata uteri
- Endometrial or endocervical polyps
- Adenomyosis
- Endometritis
- Endometriosis
- Pelvic inflammatory disease
- Vaginal/cervical infection

Endometrial neoplasia
- Endometrial hyperplasia without atypia
- Endometrial hyperplasia with atypia
- Endometrial adenocarcinoma

Systemic causes
- Coagulation disorders (thrombocytopenia, von Willebrand's disease, leukemia)
- Hyperprolactemia
- Liver disease
- Thyroid dysfunction
- Obesity
- Anorexia
- Rapid fluctuations in weight
- Chronic illness
- Depression

Other causes
- Steroids
- Progestogen withdrawal
- Contraceptive devices/injections
- Anticoagulants
- Select herbs
- Smoking (through ovarian toxicity)
- Excessive alcohol intake

- *Hormonal contraceptives.* Oral contraceptives (OCs) may result in spotting while using the medication and/or light bleeding at the time of expected menses. Missed OCs may cause breakthrough bleeding. Progestin-only contraceptives often result in irregular bleeding or spotting, which diminishes over time. Progestogen-secreting intrauterine devices (IUDs) reduce bleeding at menses, while unmedicated IUDs may increase menstrual blood loss. Certain medications may interfere with absorption of hormonal contraceptives, resulting in spotting or bleeding, and potentially a decrease in efficacy.

- *Pregnancy.* Until menopause is reached, pregnancy may occur, causing amenorrhea. Spontaneous and therapeutic abortions as well as ectopic pregnancies also cause irregular uterine bleeding in reproductive-age women.

- *Fibroids.* Benign uterine fibroid tumors are commonly associated with abnormal uterine bleeding. While most fibroids are asymptomatic, others produce dramatic changes in menstrual periods (eg, heavier and prolonged periods) as well as a range of other symptoms, such as menstrual cramps, back pain, dyspareunia, and difficulties with bowel movements or urination. Although the cause of fibroids is unknown, estrogen may stimulate their growth. Fibroids often shrink after menopause, when ovarian production of estrogen diminishes; rarely, estrogen replacement therapy may stimulate fibroids to grow again. Fibroids can undergo torsen, degenerate, or become necrotic.

- *Thyroid dysfunction.* Hypothyroidism may result in menorrhagia. Both hypo- and hyperthyroidism are associated with amenorrhea. Although the signs and symptoms of these conditions may be subtle, the functional impairment can be significant.

- *Abnormalities of the endometrium.* Endometrial hyperplasia, noncancerous endometrial polyps, and sometimes endometriosis can result in abnormal bleeding.

- *Cancer.* In a small percentage of cases, certain types of cancer of the uterus or cervix may cause abnormal vaginal bleeding. Regular pelvic exams and Pap smears — plus endometrial biopsy and ultrasound, when appropriate — are effective methods for the diagnosis and successful treatment of these serious diseases. The risk of endometrial cancer increases with each decade of life; endometrial biopsy is compulsory when abnormal uterine bleeding occurs in a postmenopausal woman.

- *Other causes.* Coagulopathies may result in heavy uterine bleeding. Women with renal or liver disease may experience abnormal uterine bleeding. Although bleeding usually originates in the uterus, it is possible for the vagina or the cervix to be the source, particularly when it occurs after intercourse. Vaginal or cervical infections or vaginal atrophy are frequently the cause. (For clarity, the terms uterine bleeding and vaginal bleeding should not be used interchangeably.)

Management strategies for AUB are found in Section M.

References

Burger HG, Dudley EC, Hopper JL, et al. The endocrinology of the menopausal transition: a cross-sectional study of a population-based sample. *J Clin Endocrinol Metab* 1995;80:3537-3545.

Farquhar CM, Lethaby A, Sowter M, et al. An evaluation of risk factors for endometrial hyperplasia in premenopausal women with abnormal menstrual bleeding. *Am J Obstet Gynecol* 1999; 181:525-529.

Frazer IS. Changes in the menstrual pattern during the perimenopause. In: Lobo RA, ed. *Treatment of the Postmenopausal Woman: Basic and Clinical Aspects.* 2nd ed. Philadelphia, PA: Lippincott Williams & Wilkins; 1999:69-74.

Kurman RJ, Kaminski PF, Norris HJ. The behavior of endometrial hyperplasia. A long term study of "untreated" hyperplasia in 170 patients. *Cancer* 1985;56:403-412.

The North American Menopause Society. Clinical challenges of perimenopause: consensus opinion of The North American Menopause Society. *Menopause* 2000;7:5-13.

Seltzer VL, Benjamin F, Deutsch S. Perimenopausal bleeding patterns and pathologic findings. *J Am Med Womens Assoc* 1990;45:132-134.

Speroff L. Management of the perimenopausal transition. *Contemp OB/GYN* 2000;45:16-37.

Treolar AE, Boynton RE, Behn BG, et al. Variation of the human menstrual cycle through reproductive life. *Int J Fertil* 1967; 12(1 part 2):77-126.

Weber AM, Belinson JL, Piedmonte MR. Risk factors for endometrial hyperplasia and cancer among women with abnormal bleeding. *Obstet Gynecol* 1999; 93:594-598.

D.05. Dementia

Dementia represents the loss of memory and other intellectual abilities, severe enough to interfere substantially with usual daily activities. Although dementia may occur at any age, it is typically a disorder of the elderly. Between ages 65 and 90, the prevalence of dementia doubles about every 5 years. The most common cause of dementia is Alzheimer's disease, accounting for over one-half of all cases. The second most common cause is vascular disease affecting the brain, particularly the accumulation of multiple small strokes (multi-infarct dementia), which represents about 15% of the total.

Alzheimer's disease is a neurodegenerative disorder that develops insidiously and progresses gradually over about a decade. This illness is characterized by a profound loss of memory, as well as difficulties with attention, speech and language, judgment, the ability to carry out skilled movements, and perception. Some patients also develop personality changes or troublesome behaviors. About 1.5 to 3 times more women than men have Alzheimer's disease. This is due in part because women live longer than men, but also because women may be at greater risk. The number of cases increases an estimated 5% per year in women older than 65, reaching 50% in women older than 85.

The pathogenesis of Alzheimer's disease is often unknown. Genetic mutations inherited as autosomal dominant traits may cause early-onset disease in which symptoms appear before age 60. Fortunately, this form of the disorder is uncommon. Genes involved in later-onset disease, many of which remain to be identified, act to modify disease susceptibility rather than to cause disease.

It is hypothesized that one consequence of diminished estrogen concentrations after the menopause is an increased risk of Alzheimer's disease. There are a number of potential mechanisms by which estrogen might influence the development or manifestations of this disorder. For example, estrogen modulates acetylcholine and other neurotransmitters, protects against certain kinds of neural damage, and prevents the accumulation of beta-amyloid, an abnormal protein found in Alzheimer's-diseased brain. However, clinical trials have not described a causal relationship between levels of estrogen and Alzheimer's disease.

Observational studies suggest that ERT may have a benefit in delaying brain aging and dementia. Short-term clinical trials of women undergoing surgical menopause suggest that ERT may help preserve memory, although any long-term benefit has not yet been demonstrated in randomized, controlled trials. Limited observational and clinical trial studies suggest that estrogen therapy has little, if any, effect on improving cognitive performance in postmenopausal women. Of note is the possibility that putative benefit may be offset when estrogen is combined with a progestogen.

Research is ongoing to identify a marker, such as apolipoprotein-E, that will predict Alzheimer's disease risk. Also, therapies are being investigated that may slow the progression of this disease — another major area of research.

Bibliography

Aqüero-Torres H, Fratiglioni L, Guo Z, Viitanen M, Winblad B. Mortality for dementia in advanced age: a 5-year follow-up study of incident dementia cases. *J Clin Epidemiol* 1999;52:737-743.

Bachman D, Wole P, Linn R. Prevalence of dementia and probable senile dementia of Alzheimer type in the Framingham study. *Neurology* 1992;42:115-119.

Drake EB, Henderson VW, Stanczyk FZ, et al. Associations between circulating sex steroid hormones and cognition in normal elderly women. *Neurology* 2000;54:599-603.

Ernst RL, Hay JW. The US economic and social costs of Alzheimer's disease revisited. *Am J Public Health* 1994;84:1261-1264.

Fratiglioni L, Wang H-X, Ericsson K, Maytan M, Winblad B. Influence of social network on occurrence of dementia: a community-based longitudinal study. *Lancet* 2000;344:1315-1319.

Henderson VW. *Hormone Therapy and the Brain: A Clinical Perspective on the Role of Estrogen.* New York, NY: Parthenon Publishing; 2000.

Hogervorst E, Williams J, Budge M, Riedel W, Jolles J. The nature of the effect of female gonadal hormone replacement therapy on cognitive function in post-menopausal women: a meta-analysis. *Neuroscience* 2000;101:485-512.

Katzman R. Education and the prevalence of dementia and Alzheimer's disease. *Neurology* 1993;43:13-20

Yaffe K, Grady D, Pressman A, Cummings S. Serum estrogen levels, cognitive performance, and risk of cognitive decline in older community women. *J Am Geriatr Soc* 1998;46:816-821.

Perimenopause provides an ideal opportunity for a comprehensive health evaluation, including a detailed history, complete physical examination, and diagnostic evaluation. As women move through menopause and beyond, regular health examinations are the standard of care.

In general, the clinical evaluation should include the following:

- Detailed medical, psychological, and social history of the woman, including family history.

- Complete physical examination, including breast, pelvic, rectovaginal, and thyroid examinations as well as standard measurements (eg, weight, height, blood pressure).

- Laboratory testing, such as standard blood screens, Papanicolaou (Pap) test, stool guaiac, mammogram, serum cholesterol levels (total, HDL and LDL cholesterol, and triglycerides), thyroid testing, and, when indicated, urine screens and screens for sexually transmitted infections.

- Appropriate testing for differential diagnosis of problems (eg, abnormal uterine bleeding).

- Appropriate testing for specific chronic conditions (eg, diabetes).

This section of the study guide has been prepared with a focus on menopause-related issues. It is not inclusive of all elements of a comprehensive physical examination and laboratory evaluation.

E.01. Primary evaluation

In addition to the many tests and examinations that are important but not covered in this study guide (eg, basic blood screens), the primary evaluation of a woman at midlife or beyond must include information related to menopause issues. The following sections address history-gathering and height/weight measurement.

E.01.a. History

When gathering histories of the woman and her relatives, special attention should be given to the following:

Gynecologic history. Current menstrual status; age at first/last menstrual period; description of periods; presence of uterus/ovaries; date of last examinations, such as Pap smear, mammogram, cholesterol test, bone density test; abnormal results of any of these tests; DES exposure during pregnancy; problems with urination or vaginal discharge; sexual function.

Obstetrical history. Contraceptive method used; number of pregnancies, full-term births, premature births, abortions, and living children; age at time of first birth; complications during pregnancy, delivery, or postpartum.

Medical history. Usual diseases and surgeries, as well as some that may not be obvious, such as stress; fatigue; dizziness; difficulties with sleeping, skin, eyesight, or dental/oral cavity; hair loss/growth; weight loss/gain; frequent falls; loss of height; fractures; domestic violence; psychological therapy. A family medical history should also be obtained.

Symptom history. Ask detailed questions about symptoms that could be related to menopause and rate them according to severity.

Personal habits. Determine self-perceived health status, and information about exercise, diet, stress management, and use of caffeine, alcohol, tobacco, and "recreational" drugs.

Medication history. In addition to asking for current medication use (prescription, nonprescription, and complementary/alternative therapies) and allergies to any medications, ask about current/past use of hormonal contraceptives, current/past use of hormone replacement therapy and any other therapy used to treat menopause (such as herbs, supplements, foods, yoga). Include duration of use, effectiveness, and reason(s) for stopping.

NAMS is developing a comprehensive, multi-page Self-Assessment Form that is geared toward menopause. It is projected to be available on the NAMS Web site (www.menopause.org) by early 2003.

E.01.b. Height

An important component of the clinical evaluation is determining current height and the maximum adult height. Height loss greater than 1.5 inches (3.8 cm) may be associated with vertebral compression fractures and be indicative of osteoporosis. The preferred method for height measurement is a stadiometer. Height should be measured (without shoes) during each visit and, ideally, at approximately the same time of the day.

E.01.c. Weight

Recording a woman's weight is another essential component of clinical evaluation. Clinicians should be aware that weight is a sensitive matter for many women, and weight measurement should be performed discreetly.

Determining the body mass index (BMI) is helpful. The formula for calculating BMI is as follows:

$$BMI = \frac{weight \ in \ kg}{(height \ in \ meters)^2} \times 100$$

BMI gives a measure of adiposity that is relatively independent of height. Table 1 provides an easy conversion from pounds and inches to BMI.

Table 1. Determining body mass index

BMI	20	22	24	26	28	30	32	34
Height (inches)	Body weight (pounds)							
58	96	105	115	124	134	143	153	162
60	102	112	123	133	143	153	163	174
62	109	120	131	142	153	164	175	186
64	116	128	140	151	163	174	186	197
66	124	136	148	161	173	186	198	210
68	131	144	158	171	184	197	210	223
70	139	153	167	181	195	209	222	236
72	147	162	177	191	206	221	235	250
74	155	171	186	202	218	233	249	264
76	164	180	197	213	230	246	263	279

Table 2. Body mass index classification for females

Classification	BMI
Underweight	<18.7
Normal weight	18.7-23.8
Overweight	23.9-28.6
Obese	>28.6

Once the BMI has been calculated, the woman's weight status can be determined (eg, normal, underweight, obese). The World Health Organization has established definitions to classify BMI (see Table 2).

Data from the Third National Health and Nutrition Examination Survey (NHANES III) revealed that obesity is a problem among the US population and is not an age-specific issue. About 28% of women aged 45 to 64 have a BMI equal to or greater than 30, dropping slightly to about 26% at ages 65 to 74, then declining further to about 17% for those over age 75.

Health Canada reports that an estimated 40% of Canadian women are overweight (defined as BMI >25) or obese (defined as BMI >30).

With overweight women, it is helpful to note the fat distribution. The waist-to-hip ratio (WHR) is a means of further classifying body fat distribution as android (waist and stomach) or gynoid (hip) obesity. The ratio estimates the amount of intra-abdominal fat (which is greater with android obesity). A WHR ratio greater than 0.85 is indicative of android obesity and a ratio of less than 0.75 is indicative of gynoid obesity. Some clinicians include a waist and hip measurement as part of the physical examination; most, however, simply determine android or gynoid obesity by observation.

Android obesity is more strongly associated with adverse health conditions than is gynoid obesity. These include insulin resistance, type 2 (noninsulin-dependent) diabetes mellitus, hypertension, stroke, left ventricular hypertrophy, arrhythmias, congestive heart failure, myocardial infarction, angina pectoris, and peripheral vascular disease.

Data from NHANES III indicate that risk for diabetes mellitus increases dramatically as overweight increases, particularly with android obesity. The increase in obesity observed over the past decade in the United States has been accompanied by a 25% increase in the prevalence of type 2 diabetes. In NHANES III, increasing body weight increased the risk for gallstones and cholecystectomy.

The Nurses' Health Study found that women with a WHR of 0.74 or higher had a 2-fold increase in heart disease risk. The investigators concluded that an ideal WHR is less than 0.72. In addition, waist circumference was found to be an independent factor associated with risk of coronary heart disease in women.

Increasing body weight increases the risk for osteoarthritis. Individuals with a body mass index of at least 30 have a markedly increased risk for knee osteoarthritis. However, increased body weight appears to offer protection against the development of osteoporosis.

Obesity, in general, is associated with certain cancers. Compared with normal weight women, obese women have a higher mortality rate from cancers of the endometrium, cervix, gallbladder, colon, ovaries, and breast (in post-menopausal women). An estimated 34% to 56% of cases of endometrial cancer are associated with increased body weight (BMI >29). Almost half of breast cancer cases among postmenopausal women occur in those with a BMI greater than 29. In the Nurses' Health Study, women gaining more than 20 pounds from 18 years of age to midlife doubled their risk for breast cancer compared with women who maintained stable weight. Distinguishing between the effects of diet and obesity is difficult, because high-fat, high-calorie diets may increase risk for some cancers, particularly those of the colon and breast.

Bibliography

Calle EE, Thun MJ, Petrelli JM, Rodriguez C, Heath CW Jr. Body-mass index and mortality in a prospective cohort of U.S. adults. *N Engl J Med* 1999;341:1097-1105.

Eckel RH, Krauss RM. American Heart Association call to action: obesity as a major risk factor for coronary heart disease. AHA Nutrition Committee. *Circulation* 1998;97:2099-2100.

Gallagher D, Visser M, Sepulveda D, Pierson RN, Harris T, Heymsfield SB. How useful is body mass index for comparison of body fatness across age, sex, and ethnic groups? *Am J Epidemiol* 1996;143:228-239.

Harris ML, Flegal KM, Cowie CC, et al. Prevalence of diabetes, impaired fasting glucose, and impaired glucose tolerance in US adults: the Third National Health and Nutrition Examination Survey, 1988-94. *Diabetes Care* 1998;21:518-524.

Manson JE, Willett WC, Stampfer MJ, et al. Body weight and mortality among women. *N Engl J Med* 1995;333:677-685.

National Institutes of Health. Clinical guidelines on the identification, evaluation, and treatment of overweight and obesity in adults: the Evidence Report. *Obes Res* 1998;6(suppl 2):51S-209S.

National Population Health Survey 1994-1995. Ottawa, ON, Canada: Statistics Canada, 1995. Catalogue no. 82-F0001XCB.

National Task Force on the Prevention and Treatment of Obesity. Overweight, obesity, and health risk. *Arch Intern Med* 2000; 160:898-904.

E.02. Ovarian/adrenal function

At present, there is no one test of ovarian function that will predict or confirm menopause. Practitioners must rely on the clinical setting and judicious use of hormone testing to determine if it has been reached.

Tests of ovarian function — follicle-stimulating hormone (FSH), estradiol, luteinizing hormone, progesterone, total and free testosterone, inhibin B — can be important for differentiating various causes of amenorrhea, such as menopause, premature ovarian failure, hypothalamic hypogonadotropic amenorrhea, and anovulatory cycles.

FSH. Since natural menopause is a retrospective diagnosis (ie, 12 months of amenorrhea for which there is no other pathologic or physiologic cause), serum FSH levels have been evaluated as a laboratory marker that would potentially allow earlier diagnosis of menopause as well as impending menopause. In 2001, the FDA approved for marketing a self-test that measures urine FSH levels. In laboratory tests, it was reported to compare favorably to serum FSH tests.

It is generally accepted that a woman has reached menopause if she has consistently elevated levels of FSH greater than 30 mIU/mL (normal FSH levels are noted on Table 3). The difficulty in using FSH as a marker of menopause is that FSH levels in the postmenopausal range can return to premenopausal ranges a few days, weeks, or months later. In the Massachusetts Women's Health Study, 20% of midlife women who experienced 3 months of amenorrhea began menstruating again. A single measurement of FSH greater than 30 mIU/mL in a perimenopausal woman cannot always be considered a definitive diagnosis of menopause. Several FSH measurements consistently greater than 30 mIU/mL may be necessary. Furthermore, FSH levels in women who are in perimenopause are frequently normal.

Table 3. Normal FSH levels in women

	mIU/mL
Postmenopausal	24-170
Menstruating women	
Normal values	2.8-17.2
Midcycle peak	15-35

Source: *A Manual of Laboratory & Diagnostic Tests* 2000.

Hormonal contraceptives may lower FSH levels, making it difficult to diagnose menopause in women who use them. One option is to discontinue the contraceptive, use a nonhormonal method of contraception, and check the FSH level several weeks later. A study of 28 menopausal women placed on oral contraceptives concluded that measuring FSH on the seventh pill-free day was not a sensitive test for confirming menopause. However, a serum FSH:LH ratio greater than 1 or estradiol less than 20 pg/mL (73 pmol/L) on the seventh pill-free day more accurately reflected menopause status.

Much of the recent research on ovarian function tests comes from efforts to assess fertility. FSH has been used as an indicator of "ovarian reserve," a term coined to reflect the remaining reproductive capacity of the ovary. Measuring FSH in the early follicular phase has been used to predict the likelihood of a successful response to infertility treatment and correlates better with treatment outcome than does age.

Changes in FSH levels appear to be preceded by a decline in ovarian production of inhibin B. A lower fertility rate was observed in women who had a normal day 3 FSH but a low inhibin B level compared with women in whom both FSH and inhibin B were normal. As inhibin B levels decline, FSH levels rise. Inhibin B levels are normal in hypothalamic amenorrhea but very low in menopause. The average level of inhibin B in premature ovarian failure is only slightly higher than after menopause. However, the measurement of inhibin B levels is not widely used in clinical practice. Production of inhibin A does not decrease until close to menopause.

While tests of ovarian reserve were designed to predict the success of infertility treatment in the older woman at risk for infertility, there is likely a correlation with the onset of the menopause transition. The Stages of Reproductive Aging Workshop (STRAW) proposed a staging system for menopause and suggested that measuring FSH might be one means of identifying the perimenopausal stages. An elevated early follicular FSH in one cycle would be sufficient to place a woman in the late reproductive stage. Because of the variability during this phase of life, a normal FSH would require a second normal FSH before assuming that the woman was not approaching menopause. Sporadic elevations of estradiol could suppress the FSH and be misleading. Thus, measuring FSH and estradiol together would be more informative. However, neither of these tests will predict menopause.

Estradiol. Estradiol levels are also erratic during perimenopause. It is speculated that the wide variance in estradiol levels may be partly responsible for some of the symptomatology commonly experienced during perimenopause. Normal urinary estradiol values for postmenopausal women are 0 to 4 µg/24 hours. Urinary estradiol values in menstruating women vary between 0 and 14 µg/24 hours depending on the phase of their cycle.

Estrone. In one comparative study, urinary estrone levels were found to be far higher in the perimenopausal group than in either the younger premenopausal group or the older postmenopausal group. However, during perimenopause, estrone levels are erratic. In cases of poor response to hormone therapy, measuring serum estrone can be helpful, as levels below 150 pg/mL (555 pmol/L) 4 hours after oral estrogen suggests abnormal estrogen metabolism.

LH and progesterone. Luteinizing hormone (LH) and progesterone are also markers of ovarian function, although they have limited value in diagnosing perimenopause or menopause when used as isolated tests. The elevation of LH associated with menopause (normal values in postmenopausal women: 35-129 mIU/mL) is a late occurrence, much later than the increase seen with FSH. Progesterone is found at relatively normal yet varying levels during perimenopause, except in the instance of anovulatory cycles. The frequency of anovulatory cycles increases with age.

Androgens. Testosterone levels contribute little to the diagnosis of menopause, as there is only a slight decline in testosterone at midlife. The woman who has undergone bilateral oophorectomy can be presumed to have low levels of testosterone. Measuring testosterone may be of value for the woman with low libido or sexual dysfunction who still has both ovaries and no other identifiable cause of dysfunction.

The recent Princeton consensus statement addresses the need for accurate and reliable measurement of androgens in the diagnosis and treatment of female androgen insufficiency. The expert panel stated that current, commercially available assays are deficient in several respects, particularly in regard to sensitivity and reliability at the lower ranges typical for women. In addition, large databases describing the normal values for women of different ages, races, and reproductive states are unavailable.

The panel recommended that free testosterone (T) concentration, as measured by equilibrium dialysis, be adopted as the "gold standard" for laboratory assessment of bioavailable testosterone in women and that the concentration of circulating sex hormone-binding globulin (SHBG) also be considered. Clinical assessment of both androgen production and androgen availability can be achieved by measuring two of three essential values: either total T and SHBG, free T and SHBG, or free T and total T. Salivary T assays were not recommended for clinical use because they are not sufficiently accurate or reliable.

The consensus statement also concluded that, in women, DHEA-S (the sulfate of dehydroepiandrosterone) is the most useful measure of adrenal androgen production and that these assays are reliable. DHEA-S should be measured if there are concerns regarding an adrenal cause of androgen deficiency. Low DHEA-S has been related to female sexual dysfunction.

The panel cautioned that the diagnosis of female androgen insufficiency is difficult to make. In addition to the problem of suboptimal testosterone assays, symptoms are nonspecific and characteristic of many other medical, psychological, and psychosocial problems, including depression, relationship conflict, and thyroid disease.

Bibliography

Avis NE, McKinlay SM. The Massachusetts Women's Health Study: an epidemiologic investigation of the menopause. *J Am Med Womens Assoc* 1995;50:45-49, 63.

Bachmann G, Bancroft J, Braunstein G, et al. Female androgen insufficiency: the Princeton consensus statement on definition, classification, and assessment. *Fertil Steril* 2002;77:660-665.

Creinin MD. Laboratory criteria for menopause in women using oral contraceptives. *Fertil Steril* 1996;66:101-104.

Executive summary: Stages of Reproductive Aging Workshop (STRAW): Park City, Utah, July 2001. *Menopause* 2001;8:402-407.

Falk RT, Dorgan JF, Kahle L, Potischman N, Longcope C. Assay reproducibility of hormone measurements in postmenopausal women. *Cancer Epidemiol Biomarkers Prev* 1997;6:429-432.

Fischbach F. *A Manual of Laboratory & Diagnostic Tests.* 6th ed. Philadelphia, PA: Lippincott Williams & Wilkins; 2000:235-236, 423-424.

Labrie F, Bélanger A, Cusan L, Gomez JL, Candas B. Marked decline in serum concentrations of adrenal C19 sex steroid precursors and conjugated androgen metabolites during aging. *J Clin Endocrinol Metab* 1997;82:2396-2402.

Lee SJ, Lenton EA, Sexton L, Cooke ID. The Effect of age on the cyclical patterns of plasma LH, FSH, oestradiol and progesterone in women with regular menstrual cycles. *Hum Reprod* 1988;3:851-855.

The North American Menopause Society. Clinical challenges of perimenopause: consensus opinion of The North American Menopause Society. *Menopause* 2000;7:5-13.

Petraglia F, Hartmann B, Luisi S, et al. Low levels of serum inhibin A and inhibin B in women with hypergonadotropic amenorrhea and evidence of high levels of activin A in women with hypothalamic amenorrhea. *Fertil Steril* 1998;70:907-912.

Santoro N, Brown JR, Adel T, Skurnick JH. Characterization of reproductive hormonal dynamics in the perimenopause. *J Clin Endocrinol Metab* 1996;81:1495-1501.

Seifer DB, Scott RT Jr, Bergh PA, et al. Women with declining ovarian reserve may demonstrate a decrease in day 3 serum inhibin B before a rise in day 3 follicle-stimulating hormone. *Fertil Steril* 1999;72:63-65.

E.03. Thyroid function

Hyperthyroidism (high levels of thyroid hormones) and hypothyroidism (low levels of thyroid hormones) affect almost 3% of the US population and are particularly prevalent among women and the elderly.

The primary function of the thyroid gland is to produce hormones that regulate metabolism, primarily increasing the basal metabolism rate. Thyroid hormones also affect protein synthesis, carbohydrate and lipid metabolism, and absorption of vitamins. These hormones are regulated through a complex interaction that includes the hypothalamus, pituitary, and thyroid glands. Much of this regulatory function is controlled by the thyroid-stimulating hormone (TSH) secreted by the anterior pituitary gland.

The thyroid gland takes iodine from the circulating blood, combines it with the amino acid tyrosine, and converts it to the thyroid hormones T_3 (triiodothyronine) and T_4 (thyroxine). The thyroid gland stores T_3 and T_4 until they are released into the bloodstream under the influence of TSH from the pituitary gland. Most thyroid hormones are bound to proteins. The free portion is measured when testing thyroid function.

The clinical expression of both hyper- and hypothyroidism may be similar to many symptoms supposedly related to estrogen insufficiency. Hyperthyroidism may cause hot flashes, heat intolerance, palpitations, tachycardia, and insomnia. Hypothyroidism may cause lethargy, poor memory, cold intolerance, and weight gain.

Thyroid dysfunction can also affect the menstrual cycle. Although an estimated 77% of hypothyroid women have normal periods, about 16% have oligomenorrhea and about 7% have menorrhagia. Hyperthyroidism may be associated with amenorrhea. Although the signs and symptoms of these conditions may be subtle, the functional impairment can be great. Pathophysiologic conditions of the thyroid gland include diffuse enlargement and goiter.

All women at midlife and beyond should be screened for thyroid dysfunction, with testing repeated every 5 years or sooner if symptoms develop. The initial screening test is for thyroid-stimulating hormone (TSH) using a sensitive TSH assay. The range of normal values for TSH in adults is 0.2 to 5.4 mU/L. If the TSH level is abnormal, then thyroid function should be evaluated further.

Bibliography

Fischbach F. *A Manual of Laboratory & Diagnostic Tests.* 6th ed. Philadelphia, PA: Lippincott Williams & Wilkins; 2000:486-497.

E.04. Diabetes risk

A fasting plasma glucose (FPG) test should be run for women who are obese, have elevated cholesterol, have a family history of diabetes, or a personal history of gestational diabetes. The FPG measures the serum glucose levels, which are usually regulated by the hormones glucagon and insulin.

As presented in the consensus opinion from The North American Menopause Society (NAMS), the goal of glucose screening is to identify women who have or who are at risk for diabetes mellitus (DM). Screening should be considered every 3 years for all women aged 45 years and older and for younger women with other risk factors. In addition to age, recognized risk factors for DM include obesity (BMI ≥ 25 kg/m^2) certain ethnic groups (African Americans, Native Americans, Hispanic Americans, Asian Americans, Pacific Islanders, aboriginal people in Canada), family history of diabetes mellitus in a first-degree relative, hypertension, low HDL (≤ 35 mg/dL or ≤ 0.90 mmol/L) and/or high triglycerides (≥ 250 mg/dL or ≥ 2.82 mmol/L), history of gestational DM or macrosomia, previously identified impaired fasting glucose (110-125 mg/dL or 6.1-6.9 mmol/L) or impaired glucose tolerance (2-hour postload glucose 140-199 mg/dL or 7.8-11.0 mmol/L), polycystic ovary syndrome, and habitual physical inactivity. More frequent screening should be considered when risk factors in addition to age are present.

Diabetes mellitus is diagnosed when, on two or more occasions, either the FPG is 126 mg/dL (7.0 mmol/L) or greater or the 2-hour postload glucose is 200 mg/dL (11.1 mmol/L) or greater. Normal levels of FPG are less than 110 mg/dL (6.1 mmol/L). Levels between 110 mg/dL and 126 mg/dL (6.1-7.0 mmol/L) are defined as impaired glucose tolerance.

Bibliography

American Diabetes Association. Clinical practice recommendations 2001: report of the expert committee on diagnosis and classification of diabetes mellitus. *Diabetes Care* 2001;24(suppl 1):S1-S133.

American Diabetes Association. Position statement: screening for diabetes. *Diabetes Care* 2002;25(suppl 1):S21-S24.

The North American Menopause Society. Effects of menopause and estrogen replacement therapy or hormone replacement therapy in women with diabetes mellitus: consensus opinion of The North American Menopause Society. *Menopause* 2000;7:87-95.

Report of the expert committee on the diagnosis and classification of diabetes mellitus. *Diabetes Care* 1997;20:1183-1197.

E.05. Cardiovascular risk

Cardiovascular diseases, especially coronary artery disease, remain the leading cause of death and disability in US and Canadian women. More women than men die of cardiovascular disease (CVD). However, many women are uninformed about the importance of CVD and underestimate their risks.

CVD is a largely preventable disease. Women need to be aware of their personal risk levels and goals for risk factor modification. Recommendations for blood pressure, lipids, and global risk targets are available. Vigilance is needed to ensure optimal achievement of these recommendations, even when evaluating women for conditions other than cardiac disease. In an American Heart Association survey, young women reported being uninformed about heart disease and stroke, and less than 30% indicated that they had had a discussion about these topics with their physician. Developing a standardized procedure for cardiovascular risk factor assessment and management is important to evaluate women at risk for cardiovascular disease.

E.05.a. Blood pressure

High blood pressure is an important condition to identify and manage. Elevated blood pressure is strongly related to the risk of cardiovascular, cerebrovascular, and renal diseases. Treatment and control of elevated blood pressure in the United States has contributed substantially to the reduction in stroke and heart disease mortality during the past 30 years, especially in women.

It is important to obtain blood pressure (BP) measurements under controlled conditions. The recommended technique for measuring BP is summarized below:

- The woman should be seated, back supported, with arm bared and supported at the level of the heart. She should have rested in a quiet room for at least 5 minutes.

- No smoking or caffeine consumption 30 minutes prior to measurement.

- Use the appropriate cuff size with a bladder that encircles at least 80% of the upper arm. With the reduction in availability of mercury sphygmomanometers (which are preferred for measurement accuracy), a validated electronic or calibrated aneroid device may be used.

- Systolic pressure is recorded at the first appearance of sound (first Korotkoff sound), and diastolic pressure is recorded at the disappearance (phase 5) of sound.

- At least one reading should be repeated after 2 minutes. If there is a difference of more than 5 mm Hg between the two readings, additional BP readings should be obtained and averaged.

Using BP readings obtained at two or more sittings, management decisions should be based on the classification of blood pressure for adults from the Sixth Report of the Joint National Committee on Prevention, Detection, Evaluation, and Treatment of High Blood Pressure (see Table 4).

Referral for hypertension management does not require specialty consultation. An evaluation including history, physical examination, and laboratory testing (consisting of urinalysis; complete blood count; blood chemistry, including electrolytes, creatinine, fasting glucose, fasting lipids; and electrocardiogram) should be performed initially to assess associated risks, target organ damage, and identify potential secondary causes. More extensive testing for secondary causes may be conducted depending on suggestive findings on initial screening.

E.05.b. Lipid tests

Elevated serum cholesterol levels, particularly elevated low-density lipoprotein (LDL) cholesterol, are clearly established major risk factors for cardiovascular disease. New guidelines have been established for the evaluation and management of hyperlipidemia, which focus on the primacy of LDL as

the target of evaluation and therapy. The third report of the Expert Panel on Detection, Evaluation and Treatment of High Blood Cholesterol in Adults (ATP III) recommends that a complete *fasting* lipoprotein profile be performed as the initial screening test for all adults. Tests should include a measurement of total cholesterol, LDL cholesterol, high-density lipoprotein (HDL) cholesterol, and triglycerides. The classifications for cholesterol levels recommended by the ATP III are listed in Table 5.

Table 4. Blood pressure screening guidelines for women

Category	Systolic BP (mm Hg)		Diastolic BP (mm Hg)	Recommendations
Optimal	<120	and	<80	
Normal	<130	and	<85	Recheck in 2 yrs
High-normal	130-139	or	89	Recheck in 1 yr
Hypertension				
stage 1	140-159	or	90-99	Confirm within 2 mo
stage 2	160-179	or	100-109	Refer < 1 month
stage 3	≥180	or	≥110	Refer < 1 week

Table 5. Screening recommendations for lipids (fasting)

Serum levels	In mg/dL	In mmol/L	Classification
LDL cholesterol	<100	<2.59	Optimal
	100-129	2.59-3.34	Near optimal/ above optimal
	130-159	3.35-4.11	Borderline high
	160-189	4.12-4.89	High
	≥190	≥4.90	Very high
Total cholesterol	<200	<5.17	Desirable
	200-239	5.17-6.19	Borderline high
	≥240	≥6.20	High
HDL cholesterol	<40	<1.03	Low
	≥60	≥1.55	High

Additional major risk factors should be assessed in determining the specific LDL goal to improve overall cardiovascular risk. The following are considered major risk factors for women: current cigarette smoking, hypertension (BP ≥140/90 mm Hg or on an antihypertensive medication), low HDL cholesterol (<40 mg/dL), family history of premature coronary heart disease (defined as a male parent or sibling with diagnosis or event at age <55 or in a female parent or sibling at age <65), and age of 55 or older (≥45 for men). Additionally, the presence of known cardiovascular disease (including cardiac, peripheral arterial, abdominal aortic aneurysm, and carotid artery), diabetes, or a high risk for developing cardiac disease over 10 years are considered to convey the highest cardiac risk status and require the lowest LDL target (<100 mg), as shown in Table 6.

The ATP III recommends adopting the Framingham Risk Score method to estimate a woman's 10-year risk for developing cardiac events. Points are assigned to various levels of risk, which are then translated into the 10-year estimated risk for cardiovascular events.

Table 6. Risk categories for cardiovascular disease

	LDL goal	
	(mg/dL)	(mmol/L)
Known cardiovascular disease or CHD risk equivalent (diabetes, 10-year risk ≥20%)	<100	<2.59
Multiple major risk factors (2 or more)	<130	<3.36
One or no additional major risk factors	<160	<4.14

E.05.c. Other tests

Newer risk factors such as homocysteine, C-reactive protein, and lipoprotein(a) have been considered by an expert panel for their potential value in screening and modifying cardiovascular risk. However, none has emerged as a convincing means of improving office-based risk assessment. In selected cases, additional risk testing may be beneficial in refining global cardiac risk. Testing for systemic atherosclerosis using the ankle-brachial index (ABI), carotid B-mode ultrasound to measure intima-medial thickness (IMT), electron-beam tomography (EMT) to assess the extent of coronary artery calcification, or treadmill exercise testing in asymptomatic individuals may adjust the risk estimate higher or lower to further guide the intensity of risk factor intervention. Firm guidelines for the application of such additional tests for women are not yet established.

Clinical judgment should be applied when determining whether to proceed with additional testing, primarily when the decision for intervention may not be obvious from the initial clinical and laboratory screening process.

Bibliography

American Heart Association. *2000 Heart and Stroke Statistical Update.* Dallas, TX: American Heart Association; 1999.

Expert Panel on Detection, Evaluation, and Treatment of High Blood Cholesterol in Adults. Executive summary of the third report of the National Cholesterol Education Program (NCEP) Expert Panel on Detection, Evaluation, and Treatment of High Blood Cholesterol in Adults (Adult Treatment Panel III). *JAMA* 2001; 285:2486-2497.

Gorodeski GI, Utian WH. Epidemiology and risk factors of cardiovascular disease in postmenopausal women. In: Lobo RA, ed. *Treatment of the Postmenopausal Woman: Basic and Clinical Aspects.* 2nd ed. Philadelphia, PA: Lippincott Williams & Wilkins; 1999:331-359.

Greenland P, Smith SC, Grundy SM. Improving coronary heart disease risk assessment in asymptomatic people: role of traditional risk factors and noninvasive cardiovascular tests. *Circulation* 2001;104:1863-1867.

Grundy SM, Pasternak R, Greenland P, Smith S, Fuster V. Assessment of cardiovascular risk by use of multiple risk factor assessment equations: a statement for healthcare professionals from the American Heart Association and the American College of Cardiology. *Circulation* 1999;97:1837-1847.

Jacobs DR, Mebane IL, Bangdiwala SI, Cirqin MH, Tyoler HA. High density lipoprotein cholesterol as a predictor of cardiovascular disease mortality in men and women: the follow-up study of the Lipid Research Clinics Prevalence Study. *Am J Epidemiol* 1990;131:32-47.

Manson JE, Colditz, GA, Stampfer MJ, et al. A prospective study of obesity and risk of coronary heart disease in women. *N Engl J Med* 1990;322:882-889.

Mosca L, Grundy SM, Judelson D, et al. Guide to preventive cardiology for women. AHA/ACC scientific statement: consensus panel statement. *Circulation* 1999;99:2480-2484.

Mosca L, Jones WK, King KB, et al. Awareness, perception, and knowledge of heart disease risk and prevention among women in the United States. *Arch Fam Med* 2000;9:506-515.

National Cholesterol Education Program. Second Report of the Expert Panel on Detection, Evaluation, and Treatment of High Blood Cholesterol in Adults (Adult Treatment Panel II). *Circulation* 1994;89:1329-1445.

National Heart, Lung, and Blood Institute. Third report of the expert panel on detection, evaluation, and treatment of high blood cholesterol in adults (adult treatment panel III). Accessible at http://www.nhlbi.nih.gov/guidelines/cholesterol/index.htm.

The North American Menopause Society. A decision tree for the use of estrogen replacement therapy or hormone replacement therapy in postmenopausal women: consensus opinion of The North American Menopause Society *Menopause* 2000;7:76-86.

Pilote L, Hlatky M. Attitudes of women toward hormone therapy and prevention of heart disease. *Am Heart J* 1995;129:1237-1238.

Ridker PM, Hennekens CH, Buring JE, Rifai N. C-reactive protein and other markers of inflammation in the prediction of cardiovascular disease in women. *N Engl J Med* 2000;342:836-843.

Ridker PM, Manson JE, Buring JE, Shih J, Matias M, Hennekens CH. Homocysteine and risk of cardiovascular disease among postmenopausal women. *JAMA* 1999;281:1817-1821.

Robertson RM. women and cardiovascular disease: the risks of misperception and the need for action. *Circulation* 2001; 102:2318-2320.

Schaefer EJ, Lamon-Fava S, Cohn SD, et al. Effects of age, gender, and menopausal status on plasma low density lipoprotein cholesterol and apolipoprotein B levels in the Framingham Offspring Study. *J Lipid Res* 1994;35:779-792.

The Sixth Report of the Joint National Committee on Prevention, Detection, Evaluation, and Treatment of High Blood Pressure. *Arch Intern Med* 1997;157:2413-2446.

Verhoef P, Stampfer MJ, Buring JE, et al. Homocysteine metabolism and risk of myocardial infarction: relation with vitamins B_6, B_{12}, and folate. *Am J Epidemiol* 1996;143:845-859.

Wilson PW, D'Agostino RB, Levy D, et al. Prediction of coronary heart disease using risk factor categories. *Circulation* 1998;97: 1837-1847.

E.06. Osteoporosis risk

All postmenopausal women should be assessed for osteoporosis risk. This assessment requires a history, physical examination, and diagnostic tests. The goals of evaluation are the following:

- Identify risk of fracture;

- Establish the presence of osteoporosis;

- Assess the severity of osteoporosis:

- Rule out secondary causes of osteoporosis;

- Identify modifiable risk factors for falls and injuries.

In addition to age, the major factors that influence bone mass are genetics, lifestyle , and hormonal status.

Genetics. The greatest influence on maximal bone mass is heredity. Studies have suggested that up to 80% of the variability in peak bone mass might be attributable to genetic factors. First-degree relatives of women with osteoporosis also tend to have lower bone mass than those with no family history of osteoporosis. Black women have higher BMD than white women, a difference that further suggests a genetic influence.

Lifestyle. Several lifestyle factors affect the risk of developing osteoporosis, including nutrition, physical activity, cigarette smoking, and heavy alcohol consumption.

- *Nutrition.* A balanced diet plays a crucial role in bone development and maintenance of bone health throughout life. Adequate intakes of calcium are required for a woman to achieve her genetically determined peak bone mass. After peak bone mass is attained, proper nutrition remains important for maintaining optimal bone mass and strength.

  Both calcium and vitamin D have well-known roles in bone metabolism. During and after menopause, several factors increase calcium requirements. By age 65, intestinal calcium absorption declines to less than 50% of that in adolescents. In addition, the renal enzymatic activity that produces vitamin D metabolites (which control calcium absorption) decreases.

- *Physical activity.* Regular exercise has been associated with reduced fracture risk, although few studies have evaluated the effects of exercise on BMD. There is general agreement that weight-bearing exercise confers a positive effect on the skeleton. The effects of exercise on bone mass are attributed to a stimulation of osteoblast activity. Exercise may also reduce the risk for falls, although it is unclear if exercise affects the risk for fracture from falls that do occur.

- *Cigarette smoking.* Smokers tend to lose bone more rapidly, have lower bone mass, and reach menopause up to 2 years earlier than nonsmokers. In addition, some data show postmenopausal smokers have significantly higher fracture rates than nonsmokers. The mechanisms by which smoking might adversely affect bone mass are not known, although evidence suggests that cigarette smoke interferes with calcium absorption and lowers endogenous 17β-estradiol levels.

- *Alcohol consumption.* Heavy alcohol consumption (defined in the Framingham Study as 7 oz or more per week) has been shown to increase risk for falls and hip fracture. Excessive alcohol consumption also has detrimental effects on BMD. However, moderate alcohol consumption in women 65 years of age and older appears to increase BMD and lower the risk for hip fracture.

Hormonal status. The increased rate of bone resorption after menopause clearly indicates a hormonal influence on bone mass in women. Premature menopause, whether spontaneous or induced, increases risk for osteoporosis because more years are spent without the protective effect of endogenous estrogen. However, there is no evidence that this also results in increased risk for osteoporotic fracture.

E.06.a. History/physical examination

The history and physical examination of a postmenopausal woman should focus on the detection of risk factors for osteoporosis and fractures. Risk factors for fracture include low bone mass and osteoporosis, age, previous fracture, family history of fracture, weight less than 127 pounds (<58 kg), frailty, history of falls, and smoking. Risk factors for postmenopausal osteoporosis are listed in Table 7.

After achieving maximum height, most midlife women (and men) will lose 1.0 to 1.5 inches (2.5-3.8 cm) of height as part of their normal aging process, primarily as a result of shrinkage of intervertebral disks. In otherwise asymptomatic women, height loss greater than 1.5 inches (3.8 cm) may be associated with vertebral compression fractures indicative of osteoporosis. Height should be measured using an accurate and precise method, such as a stadiometer.

Acute or chronic back pain should raise suspicion of vertebral fractures. These fractures typically cause fatigue and chronic back pain, especially in the middle back. The mid-back vertebrae T12 and L1 are the most common fracture sites followed by T6 through T9. Multiple vertebral compression fractures result in the most obvious sign of osteoporosis — kyphosis (abnormal curvature of the thoracic spine). Because back pain, height loss, and kyphosis may occur without osteoporosis, vertebral fractures should be confirmed on radiography. Similarly, height loss without back pain requires radiologic evaluation for spine fractures, which may be asymptomatic in two-thirds of the cases. Women with vertebral fracture are at high risk for subsequent fracture, making fracture identification of even greater clinical significance. Wrist fracture, which tends to occur at an earlier age than vertebral or hip fracture, may also be an early clinical expression of osteoporosis.

Table 7. Risk factors for postmenopausal osteoporosis

Genetic factors
- First-degree relative with osteoporosis or low-trauma fracture
- Caucasian/Asian race
- Slender physical frame (BMI <20)

Lifestyle factors
- Sedentary lifestyle/prolonged immobilization
- Diet low in calcium
- Little exposure to sunlight and no vitamin D supplementation
- Cigarette smoking
- Excessive alcohol consumption (?)
- Excessive consumption of caffeine (?)

Menstrual status
- Premenopausal hypogonadism
- Previous amenorrhea (eg, due to anorexia nervosa, hyperprolactinemia, or exercise-induced amenorrhea)
- Premature menopause

Disease states
- Type I diabetes mellitus
- Hyperthyroidism
- Primary hyperparathyroidism
- Thyrotoxicosis
- Cushing's syndrome
- Multiple myeloma
- Systemic mastocytosis
- Rheumatoid arthritis
- Malabsorption syndromes (eg, celiac disease, Crohn's disease, peptic ulcer)
- Chronic obstructive pulmonary disease
- Anorexia nervosa
- Chronic liver disease (eg, primary biliary cirrhosis)
- Chronic renal disease
- Any disease state that limits mobility (eg, depression)
- Adult nontraumatic fracture

Medications
- Corticosteroids (7.5 mg/day or more of prednisone or equivalent for >6 mo)
- Long-term use of certain anticonvulsants (especially phenytoin and phenobarbital)
- Anticoagulant agents (eg, heparin, warfarin)
- Immunosuppressive drugs (eg, cyclosporine)
- Excessive doses of thyroxine
- Lithium
- Cytotoxic agents
- Gonadotropin-releasing hormone agonists or analogues
- Intramuscular medroxyprogesterone acetate

E.06.b. Evaluation

Risk factors for osteoporosis can often be identified with a simple questionnaire along with the standard physical measurements. Potentially modifiable risk factors should be noted. Risk factors may help explain contributing causes of osteoporosis or help guide therapeutic recommendations but cannot be used to diagnose osteoporosis. A sample evaluation form is found in Table 8.

Table 8. Postmenopausal osteoporosis evaluation form

- Current height, maximum remembered height

- Exercise, type, duration, frequency

- Smoking, ever, amount, duration

- Alcohol consumption, ever, amount, frequency

- History of eating disorders, lowest weight

- Lactose intolerance

- Reproductive status (ie, age at first menstrual period, history of amenorrhea, age of natural/induced menopause, years since menopause)

- Musculoskeletal examination (eg, height loss >1.5 inches or 3.8 cm, fracture after age 34, back pain and location of pain, dorsal kyphosis, scoliosis and location)

- Medical history (eg, maternal history of osteoporosis and/or hip fracture, periodontal gum disease and/or tooth loss, endometriosis, rheumatoid arthritis, overactive thyroid, parathyroid disease, kidney stones/disease)

- Current and past use of medications (eg, oral contraceptive, ERT/HRT, anticonvulsant, glucocorticoid, GnRH agonist, thyroid hormone)

- Mobility, strength, and balance (eg, rise from chair without using arms, rise from floor without difficulty, maintains balance, bend/reach with balance, line walking without hesitation/deviation)

- Miscellaneous signs of alcohol abuse or endocrine disorders

- Laboratory evaluation (eg, complete blood count, erythrocyte sedimentation rate, serum calcium and phosphorus, serum alkaline phosphatase, serum albumin, 24-hr urinary calcium excretion)

- Bone mineral density, absolute value and *T* score of site measured, and method used

---

E.06.c. Bone mineral density measurement

Currently, there is no validated noninvasive technique for assessing bone quality. Bone mineral density testing is the current preferred method to establish the diagnosis of osteoporosis. It is a strong predictor of fracture risk because bone mass accounts for 75% to 85% of the variation in bone strength.

Testing of BMD should be performed based on a woman's risk profile. Testing is not indicated unless the results will influence a treatment or management decision.

Although not all experts agree, NAMS recommends that BMD be measured in all women with medical causes of bone loss and in those who are at least 65 years of age, regardless of additional risk factors.

Testing is also indicated for all postmenopausal women younger than age 65 with one or more of the following risk factors for fracture:

- A nonvertebral fracture after menopause;

- Low body weight (<127 lbs or <58 kg, or BMI <20);

- A history of a first-degree relative who has experienced a hip or vertebral fracture.

Elderly women who have experienced an osteoporotic vertebral fracture may initiate treatment without BMD measurement. A baseline BMD testing may be useful for monitoring the effects of therapy. A nonvertebral fracture in the absence of low BMD is not an indication for treatment. Testing of BMD in early postmenopause may be of value in decision-making about preventive therapy.

Healthy premenopausal women do not require BMD testing because of the low prevalence of osteoporosis in this population. BMD testing is indicated only in premenopausal women who experience a low-trauma fracture or who have known secondary causes of osteoporosis.

Analyses performed by the National Osteoporosis Foundation show that BMD testing is cost-effective for postmenopausal women aged 50 to 60 years with risk factors or for those beyond the age of 60 to 65 with or without risk factors.

Several tests to measure BMD are available, either radiation-based or radiation-free (see Table 9).

Table 9. Tests measuring bone mineral density

Method	Body site
DXA (dual-energy x-ray absorptiometry)	Hip Spine Total body
SXA (single-energy x-ray absorptiometry)	Heel
QUS (quantitative ultrasound)	Heel Shin
QCT (quantitative computed tomography)	Spine
PQTC (peripheral quantitative computed tomography)	Forearm
PDXA (peripheral dual-energy x-ray absorptiometry)	Forearm Finger Heel

---

- *Dual-energy x-ray absorptiometry* (DXA) is the technical standard for measuring BMD. All the recent large, randomized, controlled clinical trials have used DXA of the hip and spine to determine therapeutic efficacy. DXA is the preferred technique because it measures BMD at the important sites of osteoporotic fractures, especially the hip. This radiation-based BMD measurement is based on the principles of x-ray densitometry or absorptiometry — the degree to which tissues absorb radiation. The greater the density, the greater the amount of energy absorbed.

- *Quantitative ultrasound* (QUS) detects the transmission of high-frequency sound waves through or across bone, providing information on bone structure and strength. Ultrasound measurement sites include the heel, finger, tibia, and patella; of all ultrasound measurement sites, the best predictor is the heel (calcaneus). Studies have shown that QUS of the heel predicts hip fracture almost as well as hip DXA.

  The advantages of ultrasound are its low cost, portability of equipment, ease of use, and lack of ionizing radiation. Disadvantages include nonuniform reporting and the measurement of sites unresponsive to therapy.

The cost for BMD testing is covered by Medicare for diagnosing osteoporosis in "estrogen-deficient women who are at risk" (see Table 10). Medicare does not cover BMD testing for premenopausal women or for postmenopausal women under 65 years of age who are receiving ERT/HRT. Medicare will cover a follow-up BMD test every 2 years (in 23 or more months).

Table 10. Medicare coverage for BMD testing

Medicare will cover BMD testing for women who:

- are "estrogen-deficient" and at risk of osteoporosis

- have vertebral abnormalities

- have undergone long-term treatment with systemic glucocorticoids

- have primary hyperparathyroidism

- are undergoing an FDA-approved treatment for osteoporosis (to monitor response)

The total hip is the preferred site for BMD testing, especially in women older than age 60, primarily because of the high prevalence of extraosseous ossification that makes spinal measurements unreliable. The spine, however, is a useful site for BMD measurement in early postmenopausal women, because bone loss tends to be earlier in the spine than in the hip. Although tests at peripheral sites (eg, wrist, calcaneus) can identify women with low bone mass, they may not be as useful as central-site tests (eg, hip, spine) because the results are not as precise. Peripheral site measurements should be limited to the assessment of fracture risk when DXA is not available. They should not be used to diagnose osteoporosis or to follow response to therapy.

E.06.d. Defining osteoporosis

To standardize values from different bone densitometry tests, results are reported as standard deviations, either as a *Z* score or a *T* score.

T scores. A *T* score is based on the mean peak BMD of a normal, young adult population and is expressed in terms of standard deviations from the average value of this reference population. A value above the young normal mean is expressed as a positive *T* score, while a negative *T* score denotes a BMD value below average (but not necessarily below normal) for young women.

Lower BMD T scores indicate more severe osteoporosis and higher risk of fracture. Every decrease of one standard deviation from age-adjusted bone density represents approximately a 10% to 12% change in BMD and an increase in the risk of fracture by a factor of approximately 1.5. The risk of fracture, however, also depends on other factors such as age, frailty, and previous fracture. Older women are at much higher risk of fracture than are younger women with the same T score. A woman who has had at least one vertebral fracture has four times the risk of another vertebral fracture and twice the risk of a hip fracture as a woman with the same age and BMD T score who has not had a fracture. Diseases such as osteomalacia are also associated with low BMD and should be excluded before the diagnosis of osteoporosis is confirmed.

Z scores. A Z score is based on the standard deviation from the mean BMD of a reference population of the same gender, ethnicity, and age. A Z score below minus 2 is generally an unexpectedly low value and suggests that factors other than age may account for the low BMD. Medical causes of bone loss can be present even when Z scores are not low.

DXA testing in *untreated* postmenopausal women should take place at 3- to 5-year intervals. In general, 5-year postmenopausal BMD declines are only about 0.5 in standard deviation from the mean (both T scores and Z scores).

For women receiving osteoporosis therapy, BMD monitoring before 2 years of therapy are completed may not provide clinically useful information. Not observing an increase in BMD is not evidence of treatment failure. In one study, most women who appeared to have lost more than 4% of BMD during the first year of treatment (with either alendronate or raloxifene) showed substantial gains the second year while remaining on the same therapy. However, the decrease could be due to imprecision in the DXA measurement. An apparent decrease in vertebral BMD greater than 4% to 5% would indicate a need to evaluate compliance with therapy and dosing instructions as well as to investigate for secondary causes of bone loss.

In 1994, the World Health Organization (WHO) defined osteoporosis as a BMD T score below -2.5 SD; the skeletal site of measurement was not specified. A revised WHO report published in 2000 stated that a measurement at either the total hip or femoral neck is preferred, but that posterior-anterior (not lateral) vertebral BMD may be used to make the diagnosis (see Table 11). The current industry standard for hip BMD is the total hip, and the accepted reference populations used by all DXA densitometers come from the NHANES III study. NAMS supports use of the revised WHO guidelines.

Table 11. Definition of osteoporosis based on BMD of total hip

Normal	T score above (ie, better than) -1	BMD within 1 SD of a young normal adult
Low bone mass (ie, osteopenia)	T score between -1 and -2.5	BMD between 1 and 2.5 SD below that of a young normal adult
Osteoporosis	T score below (ie, worse than) -2.5	BMD is more than 2.5 SD below that of a young normal adult

Source: World Health Organization 1994.

Interpretation and clinical application of T scores are made after all other pertinent data are evaluated, particularly the age and fracture history of the woman. For example, at the same T score of -2.5, a 75-year-old woman has about 8 to 10 times the hip fracture risk of a 45-year-old woman.

The fracture risk, however, depends on other factors, such as frailty, falls, and previous fractures. For example, a woman who has had a vertebral fracture has a 5-fold increased risk of sustaining another vertebral fracture during the first year after the fracture and twice the risk of a hip fracture as a woman with the same BMD T score who has not had a fracture.

E.06.e. Biochemical bone markers

Biochemical markers of bone turnover cannot diagnose osteoporosis, predict bone density, or predict fracture risk. However, these tests have been studied as a means of assessment to show therapeutic response. Bone turnover changes can provide evidence of osteoporosis therapy efficacy much earlier than BMD changes (sometimes within weeks). The value of such markers in routine clinical practice, however, has not been established.

The rate of bone remodeling affects bone strength, and can be examined by measuring surrogate markers of bone turnover in the blood or urine. Markers examine either bone formation or bone resorption, using serum or urine (see Table 12).

Table 12. Common biochemical bone markers of bone turnover

Formation	Resorption
Serum	*Serum*
Bone alkaline phosphatase (BAP) total and bone specific (Marketed as Alkphase-B, Tandem-R Ostase)	Crosslinked N-telopeptides (NTx) (Marketed as Osteomark)
C-terminal propeptides of type I collagen	*Urine*
	C-telopeptides of type I collagen (CTx) (Marketed as CrossLaps)
N-terminal propeptides of type I collagen	Deoxypyridinoline (Dpd) (Marketed as Pyrilinks-D)
Osteocalcin	Crosslinked N-telopeptides (NTx) (Marketed as Osteomark)
	Pyrindinoline (Pyd) (Marketed as Pyrilinks)

Bone formation markers are serum proteins produced by osteoblast process, and include bone alkaline phosphatase (BAP), osteocalcin (OC), and the C- and N-terminal propeptides of type I collagen.

Bone resorption markers mostly measure breakdown products of type I collagen. These include the modified amino acids (hydroxyproline and galactosyl hydroxylysine), the pyridinium crosslinks (pyridinoline [Pyd] and deoxypyridinoline [Dpd]), and the C-telopeptides (CTx) and N-telopeptides (NTx) of type I collagen associated with the crosslinking site. Collectively, Pyd, Dpd, CTx, and NTx are referred to as collagen crosslinks.

The clinical use of bone turnover markers is not new. Total serum alkaline phosphatase has been used to indicate bone turnover, while alkaline phosphatase and hydroxyproline have been used in the management of Paget's disease. Both tests have been investigated in postmenopausal women.

The biochemical estimates of both bone resorption and formation increase markedly at menopause by 30% to 100% and decrease after treatment with hormones. An increase in bone resorption precedes the increase in formation at menopause so that information on both aspects of remodeling improves estimates of rate of bone loss.

Although biochemical markers of bone turnover have been used in clinical trials of antiresorptive therapies, they have limited use in predicting or assessing the response to antiresorptive therapy in individual patients. Because these markers can vary from day to day by 25% to 30%, it is necessary to take baseline measurements as well as serial measurements during treatment.

In general, the urine crosslinks must be suppressed into the lower quartile of normal range before an adequate antiresorptive effect can be confirmed.

Elevated bone turnover is present in a large number of diseases and conditions as well as resulting from a variety of pharmaceutical therapies (Table 13).

Table 13. Diseases, conditions, and drugs that affect bone turnover markers

- Postmenopausal estrogen deficiency
- Postmenopausal osteoporosis
- Hypogonadism, hyperparathyroidism, and hyperthyroidism
- Paget's disease of the bone
- Renal insufficiency or failure
- Gastrointestinal disease related to nutrition and mineral metabolism
- Rheumatoid arthritis and other connective tissue disorders
- Multiple myeloma, hypercalcemia of malignancy, metastasized neoplasms
- Extended periods of immobilization
- Alcohol or tobacco use
- Recent bone fracture
- Chronic therapy with anticonvulsants, corticosteroids, excess thyroid hormones, gonadotropin-releasing hormone agonists, heparin

Source: Miller et al. *J Clin Densitometry* 1999.

E.06.f. Tests for secondary causes of osteoporosis

Once osteoporosis is diagnosed, any secondary causes of osteoporosis should be identified (see Table 14). Various laboratory tests can identify secondary causes of osteoporosis (see Table 15). Tests that should be performed routinely include a complete blood cell count and serum levels of calcium, alkaline phosphatase, thyroid-stimulating hormone, and albumin, as well as urinary calcium excretion to identify calcium malabsorption or renal calcium leak. Special tests may be appropriate, including measurement of serum protein electrophoresis, parathyroid hormone, and 25-hydroxyvitamin D.

Table 14. Common secondary causes of bone loss

Medications
 Glucocorticoids (eg, prednisone) for >6 mo
 Excessive thyroxine doses
 Long-term use of certain anticonvulsants (eg, phenytoin)
 Anticoagulants (eg, heparin, warfarin)
 Cytotoxic agents
 Gonadotropin-releasing hormone agonists or analogues
 Intramuscular medroxyprogesterone contraceptives
 Immunosuppressives (eg, cyclosporine)

Genetic disorders
 Hemophilia
 Thalessemia
 Hypophosphatasia
 Hemochromatosis

Disorders of calcium balance
 Hypercalciuria
 Vitamin D deficiency

Endocrinopathies
 Cortisol excess
 Cushing's syndrome
 Gonadal insufficiency (primary and secondary)
 Hyperthyroidism
 Type I diabetes mellitus
 Primary hyperparathyroidism

Gastrointestinal diseases
 Chronic liver disease (eg, primary biliary cirrhosis)
 Malabsorption syndromes (eg, celiac disease, Crohn's disease)
 Total gastrectomy
 Billroth I gastroenterostomy

Other disorders and conditions
 Multiple myeloma
 Lymphoma and leukemia
 Systemic mastocytosis
 Nutritional disorders (eg, anorexia nervosa)
 Rheumatoid arthritis
 Chronic renal disease

Table 15. Routine laboratory tests for osteoporosis evaluation

Test	Diagnostic result	Possible secondary cause
Complete blood cell count	Anemia	Multiple myeloma
Serum calcium	Elevated	Hyperparathyroidism
	Low	Vitamin D deficiency, malabsorption
Serum alkaline phosphatase	Elevated	Vitamin D deficiency, malabsorption, hyperparathyroidism
Serum albumin	Used to interpret serum calcium	
Urinary calcium excretion	Elevated	Renal calcium leak, multiple myeloma, metastatic bone cancer, hyperparathyroidism, hyperthyroidism
	Low	Malabsorption, vitamin D deficiency
Thyroid-stimulating hormone	Low	Hyperthyroidism

Bibliography

American Association of Clinical Endocrinologists. American Association of Clinical Endocrinologists 2001 medical guidelines for clinical practice for the prevention and management of postmenopausal osteoporosis. *Endocr Pract* 2001;7:294-311.

Baron JA, Farahmand BY, Weiderpass E, et al. Cigarette smoking, alcohol consumption, and risk for hip fracture in women. *Arch Intern Med* 2001;161:983-988.

Cummings SR, Nevitt MC, Browner WS, et al, for the Study of Osteoporotic Fractures Research Group. Risk factors for hip fracture in white women. *N Engl J Med* 1995;332:767-773.

Cummings SR, Palermo L, Browner W, et al, for the Fracture Intervention Trial Research Group. Monitoring osteoporosis therapy with bone densitometry: misleading changes and regression to the mean. *JAMA* 2000;283:1318-1321.

Eastell R. Forearm fracture. *Bone* 1996;18(suppl 3):S203-S207.

Eastell R. Treatment of postmenopausal osteoporosis. *N Engl J Med* 1998;338:736-746.

Felson DT, Zhang Y, Hannan MT, Kannel WB, Kiel DP. Alcohol intake and bone mineral density in elderly men and women: the Framingham Study. *Am J Epidemiol* 1995;142:485-492.

Gallagher JC, Riggs BL, Eisman J, Hamstra A, Arnaud SB, DeLuca HF. Intestinal calcium absorption and serum vitamin D metabolites in normal subjects and osteoporotic patients: effect of age and dietary calcium. *J Clin Invest* 1979;64:729-736.

Hodgson SF, Johnston CC. AACE clinical practice guidelines for the prevention and treatment of postmenopausal osteoporosis. *Endocr Prac* 1996;2:155-171.

Jergas M, Genant HK. Current methods and recent advances in the diagnosis of osteoporosis. *Arthritis Rheum* 1993;36:1649-1662.

Jensen J, Christiansen C, Rodbro P. Cigarette smoking, serum estrogens, and bone loss during hormone-replacement therapy early after menopause. *N Engl J Med* 1985;313:973-975.

Kanis JA, Johnell O, Oden A, Dawson A, DeLaet C, Johnsson B. Ten-year probabilities of osteoporotic fractures according to BMD and diagnostic thresholds. *Osteoporos Int* 2001;12:989-995.

Kanis JA, Gluer C-C, for the Committee of Scientific Advisors, International Osteoporosis Foundation. An update on the diagnosis and assessment of osteoporosis with densitometry. *Osteoporos Int* 2000;11:192-202.

Kanis J, Melton LJ 3rd, Christiansen C, et al. Perspective: the diagnosis of osteoporosis. *J Bone Miner Res* 1994;9:1137-1141.

Kleerekoper M. Detecting osteoporosis: beyond the history and physical examination. *Postgrad Med* 1998;103:45-68.

Krall EA, Dawson-Hughes B. Smoking and bone loss among postmenopausal women. *J Bone Miner Res* 1991;6:331-338.

Langer RD, Pierce JJ, O'Hanlan DA, et al. Transvaginal ultrasonography compared with endometrial biopsy for the detection of endometrial disease. *N Engl J Med* 1997;337:1792-1798.

Lindsay R, Silverman SL, Cooper C, et al. Risk of new vertebral fracture in the year following a fracture. *JAMA* 2001;285:320-323.

Looker AC, Orwoll ES, Johnston CC Jr, et al. Prevalence of low femoral bone density in older US adults from NHANES III. *J Bone Miner Res* 1995;12:1761-1768.

Marcus R, Hollaway L, Wells B, et al. The relationship of biochemical markers of bone turnover to bone density changes in postmenopausal women: results from the Postmenopausal Estrogen/Progestin Interventions (PEPI) trial. *J Bone Miner Res* 1999;14:1583-1595.

Miller PD, Baran DT, Bilezikian JT, et al. Practical clinical applications of biochemical markers of bone turnover: consensus of an expert panel. *J Clin Densitom* 1999;2:323-342.

National Osteoporosis Foundation. Osteoporosis: *Physician's Guide to Prevention and Treatment of Osteoporosis*. Belle Mead, NJ: Excerpta Medica; 1998.

Nieves JW, Golden AL, Siris E, et al. Teenage and current calcium intake are related to bone mineral density of the hip and forearm in women aged 30-39 years. *Am J Epidemiol* 1995;141:342-351.

Nordin BE, Need AG, Steurer T, Morris MA, Chatterton BE, Horowitz M. Nutrition, osteoporosis, and aging. *Ann NY Acad Sci* 1998;854:336-351.

The North American Menopause Society. Management of postmenopausal osteoporosis: position statement of The North American Menopause Society. *Menopause* 2002;9:84-101.

The North American Menopause Society. The role of calcium in peri- and postmenopausal women: consensus opinion of The North American Menopause Society. *Menopause* 2001;8:84-95.

Rapuri PB, Gallagher JC, Balhorn KE, Ryschon KL. Alcohol intake and bone metabolism in elderly women. *Am J Clin Nutr* 2000; 72:1206-1213.

Russell-Aulet M, Wang J, Thornton JC, et al. Bone mineral density and mass in a cross-sectional study of white and Asian women. *J Bone Miner Res* 1993;8:575-582.

Schneider DL, Barrett-Connor E, Morton DJ. Thyroid hormone use and bone mineral density in elderly women. *JAMA* 1994; 271:1245-1249.

Slemenda CW, Johnston CC Jr. Epidemiology of osteoporosis. In: Lobo RA, ed. *Treatment of the Postmenopausal Woman: Basic and Clinical Aspects*. 2nd ed. Philadelphia, PA: Lippincott Williams & Wilkins; 1999:279-285.

Wasnich RD. Vertebral fracture epidemiology. *Bone* 1996;18:179S-183S.

World Health Organization. *Assessment of Fracture Risk and Its Application to Screening for Postmenopausal Osteoporosis: Report of a WHO Study Group*. Geneva, Switzerland: World Health Organization; 1994. Technical report series 843.

E.07. Abnormal uterine bleeding

Thyroid abnormalities (both hyper- and hypothyroidism), anovulation, hyperprolactinemia, and polycystic ovarian disease may result in abnormal uterine bleeding (AUB). Systemic diseases other than those associated with the endocrine system, such as leukemia, do not frequently present only as AUB. Pregnancy (including miscarriage and ectopic pregnancy) and infection must always be considered as a potential cause. Some therapies (eg, hormone contraceptives, HRT) can also cause uterine bleeding (not abnormal, but irregular). The anatomic causes of AUB include fibroids, cervical and endometrial polyps, endometrial hyperplasia, and cancer (endometrial, cervical, or vaginal).

When perimenopausal women present with AUB, it is important to obtain a history placing emphasis on the clinical features of menstrual flow and restriction of daily activities, intermenstrual uterine bleeding, contraceptive and other medication use, and systemic diseases.

Charting of uterine bleeding may be helpful in assessing menstrual abnormalities. Information should include the days of the menstrual periods, the amount and color of the flow, the presence of clots, and pain associated with the bleeding. These reports are limited by the subjective nature of each woman's assessment. Printed forms often help women to keep reliable records. However, any uterine bleeding in a postmenopausal woman not using HRT warrants further evaluation.

A pelvic examination is essential. The following tests should be ordered selectively: pregnancy, complete blood count (to determine if anemia is present), thyroid-stimulating hormone, coagulation, and serum prolactin.

The following procedures may provide some pertinent information regarding the diagnosis of abnormal uterine bleeding. The advantages and disadvantages of each procedure should be carefully reviewed with the woman.

Endometrial biopsy is a widely used procedure performed in the office setting. It is currently the therapeutic standard for ruling out endometrial hyperplasia or carcinoma, and it may also identify other reasons for the bleeding. During the procedure, a small sample of the uterine lining is removed through the cervix for examination microscopically by a pathologist. The procedure may be uncomfortable and is often painful (particularly if the cervical opening is stenotic). Endometrial biopsy provides a convenient, quick, office-based endometrial evaluation with greater than 90% sensitivity in diagnosing endometrial cancer. The narrow caliber (3-mm outer diameter) biopsy devices, however, may miss some focal benign lesions including polyps and submucous myomata as well as focal malignancies. An annual endometrial biopsy is recommended for any woman with an intact uterus who uses unopposed estrogen.

Transvaginal ultrasonography has been promoted as screening method for asymptomatic disease before or during ERT/HRT, and it has been recommended as a less invasive alternative to biopsy for the detection of endometrial abnormality. Ultrasound evaluation of the pelvis is usually not considered part of routine evaluation of postmenopausal women, but may be useful to rule out pelvic pathology. A probe inserted into the vagina produces sonogram images to measure the thickness of the endometrium and evaluate the adnexa uteri. It is a useful option when biopsy is not acceptable or possible, and some experts are advocates. In a postmenopausal woman experiencing uterine bleeding, an endometrial lining measurement that exceeds a thickness of 5 mm warrants further evaluation, such as biopsy or hysteroscopy, to rule out endometrial hyperplasia or carcinoma.

Sonohysterogram is similar to transvaginal ultrasound, with saline infusion used to better visualize the endometrial cavity. Technological advances and more data have led to increased use of this procedure to evaluate perimenopausal AUB. In one study, unenhanced vaginal sonography was sufficient for evaluating AUB in 65% of 433 women over the age of 39 years who were not clinically menopausal. The remaining 35% underwent saline infusion sonohysterography, which was performed in 71% of the cases for double-wall endometrial thickness greater than 5 mm.

Hysteroscopy is a procedure in which a tiny endoscope is inserted into the vagina and through the cervix to view the uterine lining directly. Hysteroscopy may be useful in identifying and taking biopsies of (or removing) endometrial polyps and submucous fibroids. Hysteroscopy is sometimes performed under anesthesia in an operating room.

Dilation and curettage is a surgical procedure in which the cervix is dilated and the uterine lining is sampled by scraping, or by suction and scraping. Today, this procedure is performed less frequently than endometrial biopsy because it usually requires anesthesia, especially when more than a biopsy is planned. Dilation and curettage can be done in conjunction with hysteroscopy and is used when an endometrial biopsy cannot be performed due to cervical stenosis.

The following strategies represent a prudent approach to endometrial evaluation of the perimenopausal woman presenting with abnormal uterine bleeding:

- Endometrial biopsy should be performed.

- If the histology demonstrates benign endometrium, including hyperplasia without atypia, proceed with medical management.

- If such management does not result in a satisfactory bleeding pattern, unenhanced vaginal sonography should be performed.

- If endometrial measurements are greater than 5 mm, it is appropriate to proceed with sonohysterography or hysteroscopy.

Given the absence of large randomized controlled trials comparing different evaluation strategies, clinicians should use the technique(s) (including endometrial biopsy, sonohysterography, and office diagnostic hysteroscopy) with which they are most technically comfortable and which are most accessible and cost-effective in their practices. In general, it is appropriate to reserve hysteroscopy for women in whom sonohysterography has identified lesions (including focal endometrial thickening) requiring biopsy or excision.

Treatment depends on the cause of the uterine bleeding. Options include medication (eg, adjusting hormone therapy, utilizing low-dose OCs) and surgery (eg, laparoscopy, hysteroscopy, endometrial ablation, dilation and curettage, myomectomy, hysterectomy).

Bibliography

Farquhar CM, Lethaby A. Sowter M, et al. An evaluation of risk factors for endometrial hyperplasia in premenopausal women with abnormal uterine bleeding. *Am J Obstet Gynecol* 1999;181:525-529.

Frazer IS. Changes in the menstrual pattern during the perimenopause. In: Lobo RA, ed. *Treatment of the Postmenopausal Woman: Basic and Clinical Aspects.* 2nd ed. Philadelphia, PA: Lippincott Williams & Wilkins; 1999:69-74.

Seltzer VL, Benjamin F, Deutsch S. Perimenopausal bleeding patterns and pathologic findings. *J Am Med Womens Assoc* 1990;45:132-134.

Weber AM, Belinson JL, Piedmonte MR. Risk factors for endometrial hyperplasia and cancer among women with abnormal bleeding. *Obstet Gynecol* 1999;93:594-598.

E.08. Cancer risk

Cancer is the second leading cause of death for women in the US and Canada, exceeded only by heart disease. In the US, one out of every four deaths is from cancer. Nearly 80% of all cancers are diagnosed at age 55 and older. Women have a 1 in 3 lifetime risk of developing cancer.

Menopause is not associated with increased cancer risk. However, since cancer rates increase with age, women in midlife and beyond should be evaluated for their risk of cancer of the lung, breast, uterus, ovary, colon, rectum, and skin — the most common cancers that affect women.

The causes of various cancers are not known; however, risk factors have been identified. The top cancer risk factors are related to behavior, and include tobacco use, alcohol use, poor nutrition, and lack of exercise. Certain cancers related to viruses can be prevented through lifestyle change or vaccines (HPV, Hep B, HIV). Most skin cancers can be prevented by protecting the skin from the sun's rays.

Table 16. Estimated new cancer cases and deaths in women in 2002

Site	United States		Canada	
	Estimated new cases	*Estimated deaths*	*Estimated new cases*	*Estimated deaths*
Lung and bronchus	79,200	65,700	8,800	7,700
Breast	203,500	39,600	20,500	5,400
Genital system	81,400	26,200	?	?
Ovary	23,300	13,900	2,500	1,550
Endometrium	39,300	6,600	3,600	680
Uterine cervix	13,000	4,100	1,400	410
Vulva	3,800	800	?	?
Vagina and other genital	2,000	800	?	?
Colorectal	75,700	28,800	8,100	3,000
Colon	57,300	25,000	?	?
Rectum	18,400	3,800	?	?
Urinary/bladder	15,000	4,000	1,300	470
Melanoma of the skin	23,500	2,700	1,850	330
Thyroid	15,800	800	1,450	120
Pancreas	15,600	15,200	1,700	1,700

Sources: *Cancer Facts & Figures 2002; Canadian Cancer Statistics 2002.*

An estimated 30% of all US cancer deaths and 70% of US lung cancer deaths are attributed to smoking. The number of newly diagnosed cases is continuing to rise, which parallels the increasing number of women who smoke cigarettes. Second-hand smoke (ie, nonsmokers' exposure to tobacco smoke) also poses health risks. One study showed that the risk of lung cancer is about 30% higher for wives of smokers than for wives of nonsmokers. Smoking is also related to an increased risk of cancer of the mouth and throat as well as cervical cancer. New screening techniques for lung cancer being evaluated include low-dose helical CT scans and molecular markers found in sputum samples.

An estimated 30% of all US cancer deaths are attributed to diet and obesity. Excessive alcohol consumption and physical inactivity also increase cancer risk. Healthy nutrition, increased physical activity, smoking cessation, and decreased alcohol intake may decrease cancer risk.

In US and Canadian women, breast cancer has the highest incidence, whereas lung cancer has the highest mortality (see Table 16). If all cancers were diagnosed at a localized stage, 5-year survival could be 95%.

Overall, African Americans are more likely to develop cancer than any other US racial or ethnic group. Breast cancer incident rates are highest among Caucasians and lowest in American Indians. African Americans have the highest incidence of colon and rectal cancer plus lung and bronchial cancer, followed by Caucasians, Asian/Pacific Islanders, Hispanic Americans, and American Indians.

E.08.a. Breast cancer

Breast cancer is the second major cause of cancer mortality in North American women. For many women, breast cancer is their primary health concern.

A woman's lifetime risk of developing breast cancer is about 1 in 8, and the risk changes as she ages. Nearly half of all breast cancer cases occur in women 65 years and older. In the United States and Canada, fewer than 10% of cases occur in women under age 40 and about 15% occur in women under age 50. Current estimates are that by age 50, 2% of US and Canadian women will have developed breast cancer. By age 60, between 4% and 5% will have the disease; by age 70, about 7%; and by age 80, between 9% and 10%.

Among racial/cultural groups in the United States, white non-Hispanic women have the highest incidence of breast cancer although African American women have the highest mortality from the disease, possibly related to later stages of diagnosis, more estrogen-receptor negative tumors, and more aggressive tumors. The 5-year survival for African Americans is 71% versus 86% for US Caucasians. The 5-year survival rate is 82% for Canadian women.

Although the incidence of breast cancer has increased in recent years, mortality rates have not increased, perhaps due to earlier intervention. Smaller, less-advanced tumors that would have been missed without mammography can now be detected. According to US statistics, if breast cancer is detected while it is still localized, the 5-year survival rate is 97%, up from 72% in the 1940s.

In Canada, following three decades of small, annual increases, breast cancer incidence in women has leveled off since 1993. Mortality rates have declined steadily since 1986. These trends are attributed to screening programs and improved treatments.

Medical research has identified several potential cancer-causing genes, including BRCA1 (linked to both breast and ovarian cancers) and BRCA2 (associated with breast cancer only). Although the genes have been identified, more research is needed to identify which women to test, how to protect from gene discrimination, and what to do if the test results are positive.

Several potential risk factors for breast cancer have been identified (see Table 17).

Table 17. Potential risk factors for breast cancer

- Personal history of breast, endometrial, ovarian, or (possibly) colon carcinoma
- History of breast cancer in a mother or sister, especially while premenopausal
- Menarche before age 12
- Late menopause (10-year delay)
- Nulliparity or having the first child after age 30
- Obesity after menopause ($\geq$20 kg [44 lbs] weight gain)
- Alcohol consumption (>2 drinks/day)
- Lack of exercise (<4 hr/wk)
- Diet low in vegetables and fruits
- Exposure to intense radiation
- Long-term use (>5 years ?) of continuous-combined HRT
- Long-term use of other HRT regimens and unopposed ERT (?)

Many women overestimate the importance of a positive family history as a risk factor for breast cancer. Most breast cancers occur in women without a positive family history.

Diet also affects breast cancer risk. Consumption of well-done meats and exposure to heterocyclic amines (or other compounds) formed during high-temperature cooking may increase breast cancer risk. The evidence linking dietary fat intake to breast cancer risk has been conflicting, but current studies do not show an increased risk. Alcohol consumption has been associated with breast cancer in many studies, although there is some evidence that excess risk from alcohol consumption may be reduced by adequate folate intake. The role of phytoestrogens on breast cancer risk is being explored, but with mixed early results. Tomato and tomato-based products contain lycopenes that may play a protective role in breast and cervical cancer.

A positive association between adiposity and breast cancer risk has been documented. One report found that avoiding adult weight gain may contribute importantly to the prevention of breast cancer after menopause, particularly among women who do not use postmenopausal hormones. Physical activity appears to reduce the risk of breast cancer, but more research is needed to determine the level of activity necessary. A lifetime of physical activity may be the key.

Benign breast masses (eg, fibroadenomas, cysts) become much less common after menopause for women not using hormones. Any new growth observed after menopause is suspicious for breast cancer, and biopsy should be considered.

ERT/HRT may stimulate the growth of benign breast masses, although findings have been conflicting regarding a possible link between ERT/HRT and breast cancer, particularly after long-term use (>5 yr). Some data link greater occurrence of lobular breast cancers with progestogen use. The Women's Health Initiative, a large study of postmenopausal women aged 50 to 79 years, found that continuous-combined HRT with oral conjugated equine estrogens (0.625 mg/day) and oral medroxyprogesterone acetate (2.5 mg/day) increased the risk of invasive breast cancer by 26%, which translates to 38 cases among HRT users versus 30 cases among placebo users per 10,000 person-years; no significant difference was observed for in situ breast cancers. This increased risk was a contributing factor in terminating the trial early (after 5.2 years of a planned 8-year study), as risks outweighed benefits. Several studies report decreased mortality rates in hormone users who develop breast cancer. All women should have a breast exam and mammogram prior to beginning ERT/HRT and at regular intervals thereafter.

One model available to predict breast cancer risk is the Gail Model Risk Assessment Tool, developed and verified by the National Cancer Institute. This model is based on a woman's age, age at first delivery, age at menarche, number of biopsies, and presence of atypia.

Table 18. Recommendations for mammograms in peri- and postmenopausal women

The American Cancer Society recommends annual mammograms beginning at age 40, in the absence of unusual findings.

The National Cancer Institute recommends mammograms every 1 or 2 years between ages 40 and 50, then annually thereafter.

The Canadian Cancer Society recommends a mammogram every 2 years between the ages 50 and 69, with more frequent mammograms or more detailed testing when abnormalities are found.

The US Preventive Services Task Force recommends screening mammography, with or without clinical breast examination, every 1 to 2 years for women aged 40 and older.

The North American Menopause Society recommends annual mammograms beginning at age 40 (in the absence of unusual findings) and a mammogram before initiating ERT/HRT.

Because many breast cancer risk factors are nonmodifiable and some risks are unknown, early detection is the best strategy. Monthly self-examination should be encouraged, as most breast cancers are detected by women themselves. Mammography recommendations for peri- and postmenopausal women are presented in Table 18.

A clinical breast exam should be performed annually (close to the scheduled mammogram). The best time for a breast exam or mammogram is immediately following menses or HRT-induced bleeding.

The following physical signs and symptoms should be investigated by mammography:

- Breast lump, thickening, swelling, distortion, or tenderness;

- Skin irritation or dimpling;

- Nipple pain, scaliness, or retraction.

Mammography is a screening tool and does not provide an accurate diagnosis. The false-negative rate for screening mammography is at least 10% to 15%.

Mammography sensitivity depends on a number of factors, including the size of the lesion, the woman's age, current use of any hormone therapy, and the extent of follow-up. In the 5-year Breast Cancer Detection Demonstration Project, the estimated sensitivity of the combined clinical examination and mammography was 75%; mammography alone was 71%. The specificity was 94% to 99%.

The appearance of breast tissue on a mammogram changes according to its composition. Fat is radiolucent and appears dark on a mammogram, while stromal and epithelial tissue have greater optical density and appear light. The data are conflicting regarding an association with radiologically dense breast tissue and an increased risk of breast cancer.

The mammographic appearance of the breasts becomes increasingly radiolucent after menopause, in response to decreased estrogen and progesterone levels. For example, 76% of women aged 75 to 79 and not using ERT/HRT have radiolucent breasts compared with 38% of women aged 25 to 29.

Hormone therapy increases breast density. Sensitivity of mammography may be reduced by 15% in women using ERT/HRT. Former hormone users have the same mammographic sensitivity as never users. Because of this hormonal effect, some clinicians discontinue ERT/HRT for 2 weeks before a mammogram to allow breast density to decrease.

In the PEPI trial, almost all increases in breast density occurred within the first year of ERT/HRT therapy. In other trials, women who use estrogen plus progestin, especially continuous-combined HRT, have shown the greatest increase in breast density. ERT and cyclic HRT have not produced as much of an effect. ERT/HRT use may also contribute to more homogeneous breast tissue, which may result in breast enlargement.

Women with breast implants and those older than age 40 with fibrocystic changes also have more dense breasts.

Ultrasound is being used more frequently to evaluate developing focal asymmetric densities and any palpable masses of the breast. New methods for detection include digital mammography, which is similar to regular mammograms but images are digitized and can be stored on film. This may improve the sensitivity of mammography in women with dense breasts, but clinical trials are needed to confirm this. Ductal lavage is a recently approved minimally invasive technique in which a small flexible catheter is inserted into a periareolar duct to collect cells for examination.

E.08.b. Endometrial cancer

Endometrial cancer affects cells that line the inside of the uterus (the endometrium). Fewer than 3 in 100 US women who live to age 50 will develop cancer of the endometrium in their remaining lifetime, and far fewer will die from the disease. Endometrial cancer is the sixth leading cause of cancer death in US and Canadian women.

The 1-year relative survival rate for endometrial cancer is 93%. The 5-year relative survival rate is 95%, if diagnosed at an early stage, but 64% if diagnosed at a regional metastasized stage. At every stage, relative survival rates for whites exceed those for blacks by at least 18%.

Various risk factors for endometrial cancer have been identified (see Table 19).

Table 19. Risk factors for developing endometrial cancer

- Obesity
- Diabetes
- Gallbladder disease
- Infertility
- Early menarche
- Late menopause
- Nulliparity
- History of anovulation
- Prolonged episodes of amenorrhea (except during pregnancy)
- Use of unopposed estrogen (in women with a uterus)
- Use of tamoxifen
- Hypertension (?)

Previous pregnancy and oral contraceptive use appear to provide some protection against endometrial cancer. Hereditary colon cancer has been associated with endometrial cancer. Signs and symptoms of endometrial cancer include abnormal uterine bleeding or spotting.

Long-term ERT (ie, unopposed estrogen) is associated with a dramatic increase in endometrial hyperplasia and in the incidence of low-grade endometrial cancer. Although most endometrial cancer attributed to unopposed estrogen use does not reduce lifespan, a hysterectomy is necessary to cure the condition. Adding progestogen to ERT (ie, HRT) reduces the risk for endometrial cancer almost to the level of taking no estrogen at all. NAMS has developed screening parameters for endometrial cancer for women using ERT/HRT (see Table 20).

The American Cancer Society and NAMS recommend that all women over age 40 should have an annual pelvic examination. Although a pelvic examination does not uncover uterine cancers, the examination is valuable for detecting other cancers as well as other adverse health conditions.

Table 20. NAMS screening parameters for endometrial cancer for women using ERT/HRT

- Women prescribed *continuous-cyclic* HRT (ie, estrogen every day plus cycled progestogen) should undergo a baseline pelvic examination. Endometrial evaluation should be considered if uterine bleeding occurs at any time other than the expected time of withdrawal uterine bleeding, or when heavier or more prolonged withdrawal uterine bleeding occurs.

- Women administered *continuous-combined* HRT (ie, estrogen and progestogen every day) should undergo a baseline pelvic examination. Endometrial evaluation must be considered when irregular uterine bleeding persists more than 6 months after beginning therapy. Early biopsy can be considered on the basis of individual circumstances.

- Women with a uterus generally should not take unopposed ERT. When such a regimen is used despite this recommendation, women should undergo routine pelvic examinations and endometrial evaluations at baseline and annually thereafter. Endometrial evaluation should be performed after any episode of uterine bleeding; re-evaluation is necessary when uterine bleeding is persistent.

E.08.c. Cervical cancer

The mortality rate from cervical cancer has dropped sharply over the years but remains a serious concern. In 1998, 25% of new cancer cases and more than 40% of cancer deaths from cervical cancer occurred in US women over age 60. In Canada in 1993, about 29% of new cancer cases occurred in women over age 60, and cervical cancer accounted for 64% of cancer deaths in women over age 55. The 1-year survival rate is 89%, with a 5-year survival rate of 70%. When detected at an early stage, the 5-year survival rate improves to 91%.

As screening with the Papanicolaou test (Pap smear) has become more prevalent, preinvasive lesions are detected more frequently than invasive cancer. Survival with preinvasive lesions is nearly 100%. Unfortunately, many women who develop invasive cervical cancer have never had a Pap smear.

Incident rates are higher in African Americans; however, Caucasians are more likely than African Americans to have cancers detected at an early stage.

Several risk factors for cervical cancer have been identified (see Table 21).

Studies have shown that virtually all cervical cancers are related to infection by the sexually transmitted infection human papilloma virus (HPV). HPV is characterized by benign growths in the genital area (ie, genital warts) of both men and women, but it can be asymptomatic. Spread of HPV can be reduced considerably by the use of condoms.

Symptoms of cervical cancer include abnormal bleeding and spotting, and abnormal vaginal discharge.

A pelvic examination and Pap test are key elements of a comprehensive physical examination for women older than age 40. However, about half of US women diagnosed with cervical cancer have never had a Pap test. In addition, many women stop getting pelvic exams and Pap tests when their menstrual periods stop at menopause.

The Pap test is used primarily for diagnosis of precancerous and cancerous conditions of the cervix and vagina. Virtually all deaths from cervical cancer could be prevented by having routine Pap tests and by adhering to safer sex practices.

The Pap smear is a simple office procedure in which samples for cytologic evaluation are obtained from the cervix and endocervix. In addition to checking for precancerous changes, cells can be evaluated for hormonal effect and microorganisms using smears obtained from the lateral vaginal wall.

New tests and methods are being developed to increase the accuracy of Pap smear analysis. A computer-based evaluation technique is being evaluated in which a computer screens and identifies the most abnormal cells to be reviewed. Thin-prep Pap testing is a procedure in which cells are washed into a fluid, spun into a pellet, and then sliced and stained results in a thin even preparation where abnormal cells are more easily detected by reducing preparation variables and decreasing ambiguous atypical cells. These techniques may improve Pap smear accuracy by as much as 30%. Currently there is no "best" method. Thin-prep Pap smears also can be used for detection of HPV and other viruses.

Table 21. Risk factors for cervical cancer

Human papilloma virus

Sexual intercourse at an early age

Multiple sexual partners

Sexual partners who have had multiple partners

HIV-positive status

Smoking

The single most important determinant of the success of the Pap smear is regular screening intervals. The American College of Obstetricians and Gynecologists, American Cancer Society, Canadian Cancer Society, and NAMS recommend an annual Pap test and pelvic examination for peri- and postmenopausal women. Women who do not have any risk factors for developing cervical cancer and who have had three consecutive normal Pap tests may be tested less often than annually. However, these women should continue to have an annual pelvic exam. In the United States, Medicare covers annual Pap tests for women at high risk and every 2 years for women not at high risk.

Women with abnormal Pap test results and those who have had cancer may need to be tested more often or undergo additional testing, such as colposcopy (magnified visual examination of the cervix) and biopsy.

After hysterectomy, depending on the reason for the surgery, a Pap test may still be appropriate for some women to detect cytologic changes in the vaginal vault. Annual pelvic exams are recommended even if the uterus and both ovaries have been removed.

Pap tests are especially important in women who

- smoke cigarettes,

- have unprotected sexual intercourse,

- have had human papilloma virus detected in their Pap test or have had genital warts,

- have HIV infection (or AIDS).

Women who are HIV-positive are more likely to progress from precancer to cancer and may need more frequent screening.

E.08.d. Ovarian cancer

Cancer of the ovaries causes more deaths than any other cancer of the reproductive system, primarily because it usually is detected in an advanced stage. In the United States, the 1-year survival rate is 78%, 50% for 5 years. If ovarian cancer is detected and treated early, 95% of women survive at least 5 years; however, only 25% of cases are detected at the localized stage. It accounts for 4% of all cancers among US women and is the fifth leading cause of cancer deaths among US and Canadian women.

The risk for ovarian cancer increases with age, particularly in nulliparous women, and peaks in the 8th decade. Women with a family or personal history of breast or ovarian cancer, including those positive with BRCA1 and BRCA2 are at increased risk. An association has been seen between hereditary nonpolyposis colon cancer and endometrial and ovarian cancer.

Some epidemiologic studies have reported an association between perineal talc exposure and ovarian cancer; however, this association remains controversial. The Nurses' Health Study provided little support for any substantial association, although the investigators reported that perineal talc use may modestly increase the risk of ovarian cancer. A review of the epidemiologic literature revealed that the application of perineal powder containing only cornstarch is not a risk factor for ovarian cancer.

Published data on the role of ERT/HRT and risk of ovarian cancer are conflicting. Most epidemiologic studies have shown no association or a modest increase.

Use of tamoxifen may result in ovarian cysts, but an increase in ovarian cancer risk has not been found.

Previous pregnancy, past use of oral contraceptives, and bilateral tubal ligation help protect against this disease.

The most common sign of ovarian cancer is enlargement of the abdomen, caused by accumulation of fluid. However, many women have bloating or weight gain in the abdominal area, making this sign less definitive. In women over 40, digestive disturbances (eg, stomach discomfort, gas, distention) that persist and cannot be explained by any other cause indicate the need for a thorough evaluation for ovarian cancer, including a carefully performed pelvic examination and/or ultrasound. Abnormal uterine bleeding is rarely associated with ovarian cancer.

The American Cancer Society recommends that all women over age 40 should have an annual pelvic examination for potential ovarian cancer.

No satisfactory screening tests are available for ovarian cancer. Although the blood test CA 125 is neither specific nor sensitive enough, some experts recommend that women at high risk (defined as having several family members with breast or ovarian cancer) have both a pelvic ultrasound and a CA 125 test. The CA 125 test becomes slightly more accurate after menopause, although its cost-effectiveness has not been determined. The addition of pelvic ultrasound as a second screen increases the specificity but detects only about one-half of the early stage tumors.

E.08.e. Colorectal cancer

Although fewer North American women are being diagnosed with cancer of the colon or rectum compared with the recent past, nearly 29,000 are expected to die from colorectal cancer during 2001. Colorectal cancer is the third leading cause of cancer death in US and Canadian women. The overall 1-year survival rate is 82%, with a 5-year survival rate of 61% (but 8% for distant metastasized carcinoma). If detected in an early, localized stage, the 5-year survival rate increases to 90%; however, only 37% of colorectal cancers are discovered early. The decline in incident rates is attributed to increased screening and removal of adenomatous polyps, which prevents the progression to invasive cancer.

Various risk factors for colorectal cancer have been identified (see Table 22).

Table 22. Risk factors for colorectal cancer

- Age (the incidence significantly rises with age between 40 and 45 and peaks at age 75)
- Family or personal history of colorectal cancer or adenomatous polyps
- Colorectal adenomatous polyps
- Inflammatory bowel disease
- Diet low in fruits and vegetables
- Smoking
- Physical inactivity (?)
- High-fat, low-fiber diet (?)

Colorectal cancer risk may be lowered by exercise, healthy eating habits, and not smoking. Colorectal cancer risk may also be reduced with aspirin or other nonsteroidal anti-inflammatory drug, calcium, or ERT/HRT.

Rectal bleeding, blood in the stool, and a change in bowel habits may be a sign of colon or rectal malignant tumors. Other causes of the symptoms can include diverticulitis, ileitis, colitis, and polyps.

The principal screening tests for detecting colorectal cancer are fecal occult blood testing, digital rectal examination, sigmoidoscopy, colonoscopy, and barium enema.

Fecal occult blood testing is the standard of care for annual screening. The most common fecal occult blood test is the guaiac-impregnated card. The positive predictive value for cancer is only about 5% to 10%, however, which can result in discomfort, cost, and occasional complications from unnecessary follow-up tests. The best way to conduct this test is to have the woman obtain a stool sample on three consecutive days.

Digital rectal examination is of limited value as a screening test for colorectal cancer as it can only evaluate 7 to 8 cm of the 11-cm rectal mucosa. It should be performed prior to sigmoidoscopy, colonoscopy, or double-contrast barium enema and during a pelvic exam.

Sigmoidoscopy uses a flexible procotosigmoidoscope to examine up to 50 cm of the rectum and sigmoid colon. Its primary use is to detect cancers of and other abnormalities in the gastrointestinal tract, such as hemorrhoids, polyps, or ulcers that could cause blood in the stool, because it only evaluates the lower colon. Its value, as compared to colonoscopy, has been questioned.

Colonoscopy is the examination of the large intestine with a flexible fiberoptic colonoscope. Air introduced through the colonoscope distends the intestinal walls to enhance visualization. Colonoscopy is also used to evaluate polypoid lesions that are beyond the reach of a sigmoidoscope. During colonoscopy, polyps are removed for biopsy and photographs of visualized lesions can be taken. Colonoscopy can be used to follow women with previous polyps, colon cancer, or high-risk factors.

Barium enema with air contrast increases the contrast and quality of x-rays of the rectum.

Screening recommendations are presented in Table 23.

Table 23. Colorectal screening recommendations for women aged 50 and older

Choose from one of the following screening options:

- Yearly fecal occult blood test (FOBT);
- Flexible sigmoidoscopy every 5 years; or
- Yearly FOBT plus flexible sigmoidoscopy every 5 years (preferred by ACS).

Plus:

- Double-contrast barium enema every 5 years and
- Colonoscopy every 10 years.

Women with family history of colon cancer, polyps, or symptoms or those at high risk for colorectal cancer should be considered for a more frequent and possibly earlier testing schedule.

Source: American Cancer Society 2002.

E.08.f. Pancreatic cancer

Pancreatic cancer is the fourth leading cause of cancer death in US and Canadian women. Cancer of the pancreas is generally asymptomatic until advanced stages. Jaundice may be the first symptom if the cancer develops near the common bile duct. Risk of pancreatic cancer increases with age, smoking, diet high in fat, and, possibly, alcohol intake. The 1-year survival is 20% and 5-year survival is 4%. Average survival is 6 months or less from date of diagnosis. No effective screening strategy exists.

E.08.g. Skin cancer

The most common skin cancers are basal cell and squamous cancer, which have a high cure rate. Melanoma is more serious because of its tendency to metastasize quickly. The 5-year survival rate for malignant melanoma is 88%. If diagnosed at a localized stage, the 5-year survival rate is 96%.

Signs and symptoms of melanoma include any change in the skin or mole or other dark pigmented growths or spots, scaliness, oozing, bleeding, change in appearance of a bump or a nodule, spread of pigmentation beyond the border, change in sensation, itchiness, tenderness, or pain. Moles should be evaluated for asymmetry, border irregularities, variability in color, diameter greater than 6 mm, or a sudden or progressive increase in size.

Risk factors include excessive exposure to ultraviolet radiation, coal tar, pitch, creosote, arsenic, or radon. Having severe sunburns during childhood greatly increases the risk for melanoma later in life. Additional risk factors include a fair complexion, family history of melanoma, and multiple nevi or atypical nevi. Measures to lower risk for melanoma are found in Table 24.

**Table 24. Risk reduction measures
for melanoma**

Limit exposure to sun between 10 AM and 4 PM

Cover skin when outdoors

Wear sunglasses to protect the skin around the eyes

Use sunscreen with sun protection factor (SPF) of 15 or higher

Avoid severe sunburns in children

Bibliography

American Cancer Society guidelines for early detection of breast cancer. Accessible at http://www.cancer.org/cancerinfo.

American College of Obstetricians and Gynecologists. Management of anovulatory bleeding. *ACOG Practice Bulletin No. 14.* Washington, DC: ACOG; 2000.

American College of Obstetricians and Gynecologists. The use of hormonal contraception in women with coexisting medical conditions. *Practice Bulletin 18.* Washington, DC: American College of Obstetrics and Gynecologists; July 2000.

Andersson K, Mattson L-A, Rybo G, et al. Intrauterine release of levonorgestrel: a new way of adding progestogen in hormone replacement therapy. *Obstet Gynecol* 1992;79:963-967.

Archer DF. Hormone replacement therapy and reinitiation of uterine bleeding: mechanisms and management. In: Cameron IT, Frazer IS, Smith SK, eds. *Clinical Disorders of the Endometrium and Menstrual Cycle.* Oxford, Eng: University Press; 1997:415-429.

Archer DF, Dorin MH, Heine W, et al. Uterine bleeding in postmenopausal women on continuous therapy with estradiol and norethindrone acetate. *Obstet Gynecol* 1999;94:323-329.

Armstrong K, Eisen A, Weber B. Assessing the risk of breast cancer. *N Engl J Med* 2000;342:564-571.

Baines CJ, McFarlane DV, Miller AB. Sensitivity and specificity of first screen mammography in 15 NBSS centres. *Can Assoc Radiol J* 1988;39:273-276.

Beresford SA, Weiss NS, Voigt LF, McKnight B. Risk of endometrial cancer in relation to use of oestrogen combined with cyclic progestogen therapy in postmenopausal women. *Lancet* 1997; 349:458-461.

Boyd NF, Byng JW, Jong RA, Fishell EK, et al. Quantitative classification of mammographic densities and breast cancer risk: results from the Canadian National Breast Cancer Screening Study. *J Nat Cancer Inst* 1995;87:670-675.

Boyd NF, Martin LJ, Noffel M, Lockwood GA, Trichler DL. A meta-analysis of studies of dietary fat and breast cancer risk. *Br J Cancer* 1993;68:627-636.

Breast Cancer in Canada. Population and Public Health Branch; 2001. Accessible at http://www.hc-sc.gc.ca/hpb/lcdc/bc/updates/breast_e.html.

Burger HG, Dudley EC, Hopper JL, et al. The endocrinology of the menopausal transition: a cross-sectional study of a population-based sample. *J Clin Endocrinol Metab* 1995;80:3537-3545.

Bush TL, Whiteman M, Flaws JA. Hormone replacement therapy: a qualitative review. *Obstet Gynecol* 2001;98:498-508.

Byers T, Levin B, Rothenberger D, Dodd GD, Smith RA, for the American Cancer Society Detection and Treatment Advisory Group on Colorectal Cancer. American Cancer Society guidelines for screening and surveillance for early detection of colorectal polyps and cancer: update 1997. *CA Cancer J Clin* 1997;47:154-160.

Byrne C, Schairer C, Wolfe J, et al. Mammographic features and breast cancer risk: effects with time, age, and menopause status. *J Natl Cancer Inst* 1995;87:1622-1629.

Canadian Cancer Statistics 2002. Toronto, ON, Canada: National Cancer Institute of Canada; 2002. Accessible at http://www.ncic.cancer.ca.

Cancer Facts & Figures 2002. Atlanta, GA: American Cancer Society; 2001. Accessible at http://www.cancer.org/eprise/main/docroot/stt/stt_0.

Cancer Facts & Figures for African Americans 2000-2001. Atlanta, GA: American Cancer Society; 2001. Accessible at http://www.cancer.org/eprise/main/docroot/stt/stt_0_2001.

Cancer Facts & Figures for Hispanics 2000-2001. Atlanta, GA: American Cancer Society; 2001. Accessible at http://www.cancer.org/eprise/main/docroot/stt/stt_0_2001.

Cancer Prevention & Early Detection: Facts & Figures 2002. Atlanta, GA: American Cancer Society; 2002. Accessible at http://www.cancer.org/eprise/main/docroot/stt/stt_0.

Chen C-L, Weiss NS, Newcomb P, Barlow W, White E. Hormone replacement therapy in relation to breast cancer. *JAMA* 2002; 287:734-741.

Clevenger-Hoeft M, Syrop CH, Stovall DW, et al. Sonohysterography in premenopausal women with and without abnormal bleeding. *Obstet Gynecol* 1999;94:516-520.

Col NF, Hirota LK, Orr RK, Erban JK, Wong JB, Lau J. Hormone replacement therapy after breast cancer: a systemic review and quantitative assessment of risk. *J Clin Oncol* 2001;19:2357-2363.

Colditz GA, Hankinson SE, Hunter DJ, et al. The use of estrogens and progestins and the risk of breast cancer in postmenopausal women. *N Engl J Med* 1995;332:1589-1593.

Davis A, Godwin A, Lippman J, et al. Triphasic norgestimate-ethinyl estradiol for treating dysfunctional uterine bleeding. *Obstet Gynecol* 2000;96:913-920.

Dennis LK. Analysis of the melanoma epidemic, both apparent and real: data from the 1973 through 1994 surveillance, epidemiology, and end results program registry. *Arch Dermatol* 1999;135:275-280.

Dijkhuizen FP, Mol BW, Brolmann HA, et al. The accuracy of endometrial sampling in the diagnosis of patients with endometrial carcinoma and hyperplasia: a meta-analysis. *Cancer* 2000; 89: 1765-1772.

Fabian CJ, Kimler BF, Zalles CM, et al. Short term breast cancer prediction by random periareolar fine-needle aspiration cytology and the Gail risk model. *J Nat Cancer Inst* 2000;92:1217-1227.

Farquhar CM, Lethaby A, Sowter M, et al. An evaluation of risk factors for endometrial hyperplasia in premenopausal women with abnormal menstrual bleeding. *Am J Obstet Gynecol* 1999;181:525-529.

Fisher B, Constantino JP, Wickerham DL, et al. Tamoxifen for the prevention of breast cancer: Report of the NSABP Project P-1. *J Natl Cancer Inst* 1998;90:1371-1388.

Friedenreich CM, Bryant HE, Courneya KS. Case-control study of lifetime physical activity and breast cancer. *Am J Epidemiol* 2001;154:336-347.

Friedenreich CM, Rohan TE. A review of physical activity and breast cancer. *Epidemiology* 1995;6:311-317.

Gail MH, Brinton LA, Byar DP, et al. Projecting individualized probabilities of developing breast cancer for white females examined annually. *J Natl Cancer Inst* 1989;81:1879-1886.

Gertig DM, Hunter DJ, Cramer DW, et al. Prospective study of talc use and ovarian cancer. *J Natl Cancer Inst* 2000;92:249-252.

Glazier MG, Bowman MA. A review of the evidence for the use of phytoestrogens as a replacement for traditional ERT. *Arch Intern Med* 2001;161:1161-1172.

Goldstein RB, Bree RL, Benson CB, et al. Evaluation of the woman with postmenopausal bleeding. *J Ultrasound Med* 2001;20:1025-1036.

Goldstein SR, Zeltser I, Horan CK, Snyder JR, Schwartz LB. Ultrasonography-based triage for perimenopausal patients with abnormal uterine bleeding. *Am J Obstet Gynecol* 1997;177:102-108.

Greendale GA, Reboussin BA, Sie A, et al. Effects of estrogen and estrogen-progestin on mammographic parenchymal density. Postmenopausal Estrogen/Progestin Interventions (PEPI) Investigators. *Ann Intern Med* 1999;130:262-269.

Hankinson SE, Willett WC, Manson JE, et al. Alcohol, height, and adiposity in relation to estrogen and prolactin levels in postmenopausal women. *J Natl Cancer Inst* 1995;87:1297-1302.

Harvard report on cancer prevention. Causes of human cancer: obesity. *Cancer Causes Control* 1996;7(suppl 1):S11-S13.

Harvey JA, Pinkerton JV, Herman CR. Short-term cessation of hormone replacement therapy and improvement of mammographic specificity. *J Natl Cancer Inst* 1997;89:1623-1625.

Huang Z, Hankinson SE, Colditz GA, et al. Dual effects of weight and weight gain on breast cancer risk. *JAMA* 1997;278:1407-1411.

Hurskainen R, Teperi J, Rissanen P, et al. Quality of life and cost-effectiveness of levonorgestrel-releasing intrauterine system versus hysterectomy for treatment of menorrhagia: a randomised trial. *Lancet* 2001;357:273-277.

Imperiale TF, Wagner DR, Lin CY, Larkin GN, Rogge JD, Ransohoff DF. Risk of advanced proximal neoplasms in asymptomatic adults according to the distal colorectal findings. *N Engl J Med* 2000;343:169-174.

Kaunitz AM. Injectable contraception: new and existing options. *Obstet Gynecol Clin North Am* 2000;27:741-780.

Kaunitz AM, Masciello A, Ostrowski M, et al. Comparison of endometrial biopsy with the endometrial Pipelle and Vabra aspirator. *J Reprod Med* 1988;33:427-431.

Kavanagh AM, Mitchell H, Giles GG. Hormone replacement therapy and accuracy of mammographic screening. *Lancet* 2000; 355:270-274.

Knekt P, Jarvinen R, Seppanen R, Pukkala E, Aromaa A. Intake of dairy products and the risk of breast cancer. *Br J Cancer* 1996; 73:687-691.

Knight JA, Martin LJ, Greenberg CV, et al. Macronutrient intake and change in mammographic density at menopause: results from a randomized trial. *Cancer Epidemiol Biomarkers Prev* 1999; 8:123-128.

Kurman RJ, Kaminski PF, Norris HJ. The behavior of endometrial hyperplasia. A long term study of "untreated" hyperplasia in 170 patients. *Cancer* 1985;56:403-412.

Langer RD, Pierce JJ, O'Hanlon KA, et al. Transvaginal ultrasonography compared with endometrial biopsy for the detection of endometrial disease. *N Engl J Med* 1997;337:1792-1798.

Laya MB, Larson EB, Taplin SH, White E. Effect of estrogen replacement therapy on the specificity and sensitivity of screening mammography. *J Natl Cancer Inst* 1996;88:643-649.

Lieberman DA, Weiss DG, Bond JH, et al. Use of colonoscopy to screen asymptomatic adults for colorectal cancer. Veterans Affairs Cooperative Study Group 380. *N Engl J Med* 2000;343:162-168.

Longnecker MP, Newcomb PA, Mittendorf R, et al. Risk of breast cancer in relation to lifetime alcohol consumption. *J Natl Cancer Inst* 1995;87:923-929.

McNicholas MM, Heneghan JP, Milner MH, Tunney T, Hourihane JB, MacErlaine DP. Pain and increased mammographic density in women receiving hormone replacement therapy: a prospective study. *AJR* 1994;163:311-315.

National Cancer Institute. Statement from the National Cancer Institute on the National Caner Advisory Board recommendations on mammography. Accessible at http://www.cancernet.nci.nih.gov/news/pdq.html.

The North American Menopause Society. Clinical challenges of perimenopause: consensus opinion of The North American Menopause Society. *Menopause* 2000;7:5-13.

O'Connor H, Magos A. Endometrial resection for the treatment of menorrhagia. *N Engl J Med* 1996; 335:151-156.

O'Malley MS, Fletcher SW. US Preventative Services Task Force. Screening for breast cancer with breast self-examination: a critical review. *JAMA* 1987;257:2196-2203.

Olsen O, Gøtzsche PC. Cochrane review on screening for breast cancer with mammography. *Lancet* 2001;358:1340-1342.

Papillo JL, Zarka MA, St. John TL. Evaluation of the ThinPrep Pap test in clinical practice: a seven-month 16,314-case experience in northern Vermont. *Acta Cytol* 1998;42:203-208

Parsons AK, Londono JL. Detection and surveillance of endometrial hyperplasia and carcinoma. In: Lobo RA, ed. *Treatment of the Postmenopausal Woman: Basic and Clinical Aspects.* Philadelphia, PA: Lippincott Williams & Wilkins; 1999:513-538.

Persson I, Thurfjell E, Holmberg L. Effect of estrogen and estrogen-progestin replacement therapies on mammographic breast parenchymal density. *J Clin Oncol* 1997;15:3201-3207.

Reid RL. Progestins in hormone replacement therapy: impact on endometrial and breast cancer. *J SOGC* 2000;22:677-681.

Riman T, Persson I, Nilsson S. Hormonal aspects of epithelial ovarian cancer: review of epidemiologic evidence. *Clin Endocrinol* 1998;49:695-707.

Risch HA, Marrett LD, Jain M, Howe GR. Differences in risk factors for epithelial ovarian cancer by histologic type. Results of a case-control study. *Am J Epidemiol* 1996;144:363-372.

Rodriguez C, Calle EE, Coates RJ, Miracle-McMahill HL, Thun MJ, Heath CW Jr. Estrogen replacement therapy and fatal ovarian cancer. *Am J Epidemiol* 1995;141:828-835.

Rosenberg RD, Hunt WC, Williamson MR, et al. Effects of age, breast density, ethnicity, and estrogen replacement therapy on screening mammographic sensitivity and cancer stage at diagnosis: review of 183,134 screening mammograms in Albuquerque, New Mexico. *Radiology* 1998;209:511-518.

Roubidoux MA, Wilson TE, Orange RJ, Fitzgerald JT, Helvie MA, Packer SA. Breast cancer in women who undergo screening mammography: relationship of hormone replacement therapy to stage and detection method. *Radiology* 1998;208:725-728.

Schairer C, Gail M, Byrne C, et al. Estrogen replacement therapy and breast cancer survival in a large screening study. *J Natl Cancer Inst* 1999;91:264-270.

Sellers TA, Mink PJ, Cerhan JR, et al. The role of hormone replacement therapy in the risk for breast cancer and total mortality in women with a family history of breast cancer. *Ann Intern Med* 1997;127:973-980.

Seltzer VL, Benjamin F, Deutsch S. Perimenopausal bleeding patterns and pathologic findings. *J Am Med Womens Assoc* 1990; 45:132-134.

Shushan A, Peretz T, Uziely B, Lewis A, Mor-Yosef S. Ovarian cysts in premenopausal and postmenopausal tamoxifen-treated women with breast cancer. *Am J Obstet Gynecol* 1996;174:141-144.

Smith B, Lee M, Leader S, Wertlake P. Economic impact of automated primary care screening for cervical cancer. *J Reprod Med* 1999:44:518-528.

Smith-Bindman R, Kerlikowske K, Feldstein VA, et al. Endovaginal ultrasound to exclude endometrial cancer and other endometrial abnormalities. *JAMA* 1998;280:1510-1517.

Spencer CP, Whitehead MI. Endometrial assessment re-visited. *Br J Obstet Gynaecol* 1999;106:623-632.

Speroff L. Management of the perimenopausal transition. *Contemp OB/GYN* 2000;45:16-37.

Stomper PC, D'Souza DJ, DiNitto PA, Arrendondo MA. Analysis of parenchymal density on mammograms in 1353 women 25-79 years old. *AJR* 1996;167:1261-1265.

Stomper PC, Van Voorhis BJ, Ravnikar VA, Meyer JE. Mammographic changes associated with post menopausal hormone replacement therapy: a longitudinal study. *Radiology* 1990;174:487-490.

Stratton J, Pharoah P, Smith S, Easton D, Ponder B. A systematic review and meta-analysis of family history and risk of ovarian cancer. *Br J Obstet Gynaecol* 1998;105:493-499.

Sturdee DW, Barlow DH, Ulrich LG, et al. Is the timing of withdrawal bleeding a guide to endometrial safety during sequential oestrogen-progestagen replacement therapy? UK Continuous Combined HRT Study Investigators. *Lancet* 1994;344:979-982.

Treolar AE, Boynton RE, Behn BG, et al. Variation of the human menstrual cycle through reproductive life. *Int J Fertil* 1967; 12(1 part 2):77-126.

US Department of Health and Human Services. *Physical Activity and Health: A Report of the Surgeon General.* Atlanta, GA: Centers for Disease Control and Prevention, National Center for Chronic Disease Prevention and Health Promotion, 1996.

US Preventive Services Task Force. Screening for breast cancer: recommendations and rationale. 2002. Accessible at http://www.ahcpr.gov/clinic/3rduspstf/breastcancer/.

Vogel VG. Reducing the risk of breast cancer with tamoxifen in women at increased risk. *J Clin Oncol* 2001;19(18S):87S-92S.

Weber AM, Belinson JL, Piedmonte MR. Risk factors for endometrial hyperplasia and cancer among women with abnormal bleeding. *Obstet Gynecol* 1999;93:594-598.

Weiss M, Loprinzi CL, Creagan ET, Dalton RJ, Novotny P, O'Fallon JR. Utility of follow-up tests for detecting recurrent disease in patients with malignant melanomas. *JAMA* 1995;274: 1703-1705.

Whysner J, Mohan M. Perineal application of talc and cornstarch powders: evaluation of ovarian cancer risk. *Am J Obstet Gynecol* 2000;182:720-724.

Williams SR, Frenchek B, Speroff T, et al. A study of combined continuous ethinyl estradiol and norethindrone acetate for postmenopausal hormone replacement. *Am J Obstet Gynecol* 1990;162:438-446.

Wong C, Hempling RE, Piver MS, Natarajan N, Mettlin CJ. Perineal talc exposure and subsequent epithelial ovarian cancer: a case-control study. *Obstet Gynecol* 1999;93:372-376.

The Writing Group for the PEPI Trial. Effects of hormone replacement therapy on endometrial histology in postmenopausal women. The Postmenopausal Estrogen/Progestin Interventions (PEPI) Trial. *JAMA* 1996;275:370-375.

Zhang S, Hunter DJ, Hankinson SE, et al. A prospective study of folate intake and the risk of breast cancer. *JAMA* 1999; 281:1632-1637.

Zheng W, Gustafson DR, Sinha R, et al. Well-done meat intake and the risk of breast cancer. *J Natl Cancer Inst* 1998;90:1724-1729.

E.09. Vulvovaginal health

Before menopause, vulvovaginal problems usually indicate infectious disease. In peri- and postmenopausal women, most complaints are due to vaginal atrophy caused by a loss of estrogen. Other causes should always be ruled out. Often, a comprehensive medical history provides the best clue. If the reported complaint includes a gradual reduction in vaginal secretions during sexual activity, the cause is probably atrophic vaginitis. If the problem is acute, especially associated with vaginal discharge, pelvic pain, and/or following sexual activity with a new partner, the cause is more likely to be a sexually transmitted infection. Infections of the sebaceous, Bartholin's, or Skene's glands are possible, along with vulvar and vaginal cancers. Any suspicious growths or color changes should be biopsied.

One common vaginal pathogen is monilia (yeast). Women often recognize recurrent infections and treat them empirically with over-the-counter medications. Clinicians should question women about these symptoms and be prepared to investigate the cause(s), as other conditions can imitate yeast infections.

Vulvar irritation, erythema, and pruritus may also be due to vulvar skin disease or an increase in vulvar sensitivity to cleaning agents or allergy. Sometimes a biopsy is required to make the correct diagnosis.

The pelvic examination should include assessment for vaginal atrophy, whether or not vulvovaginal problems have been disclosed. Friability and pallor of the vaginal epithelium should be noted, along with bleeding from minimal trauma (eg, speculum insertion). Biopsy may be indicated for persistent symptoms.

Vaginal fluid should also be examined, noting the amount, character, and pH. Loss of the healthy acidic vaginal pH is a reliable sign of estrogen loss and atrophic changes.

A vaginal health index, taken over the years, provides valuable clinical guidance regarding treatment and individual response to ERT (see Table 25). However, recording this information is not the standard of care for most providers.

Bibliography

Bachmann GA, Ebert GA, Burd ID. Vulvovaginal complaints. In: Lobo, RA, ed. *Treatment of the Postmenopausal Woman: Basic and Clinical Aspects.* 2nd ed. Philadelphia, PA: Lippincott Williams & Wilkins; 1999:195-202.

Bachmann GA, Notelovitz M, Gonzalez SJ, Thompson C, Morecraft BA. Vaginal dryness in menopausal women: clinical characteristics and nonhormonal treatment. *Clin Prac Sexual* 1991;7:25-32.

Table 25. Vaginal health index

Condition	1	2	3	4	5
Overall elasticity	None	Poor	Fair	Good	Excellent
Fluid secretion, type, and consistency	None	Scant, thin, yellow	Superficial layer of thin white	Moderate level of thin white	Normal (white flocculent)
pH	6.1 or above	5.6-6.0	5.1-5.5	4.7-5.0	4.6 or below
Epithelial integrity	Petechiae noted before contact	Petechiae noted after contact	Bleeds with scraping	Not friable, thin epithelium	Not friable, normal
Moisture	None, epithelium inflamed	None, epithelium not inflamed	Minimal	Moderate	Normal

Source: Bachmann et al. *Clin Prac Sexual* 1991.

E.10. Sexual function

A sexual history focuses on the conditions or circumstances that affect sexual function. A sexual history should be confidential, nonjudgmental, and sensitive to the woman's specific conditions (see Table 26).

Table 26. Areas of focus for a sexual history

Menstrual history	Substance abuse and alcohol history
Obstetric history	Psychosocial issues
Gynecologic history	Age-related issues
Drug-related side effects	Sexual satisfaction
Relationship history	

Epidemiologic data indicate that between one-third and one-half of peri- and postmenopausal women may experience a problem with one or more aspects of sexual functioning. These include hypoactive sexual desire disorder, sexual arousal disorder, orgasmic disorder, and sexual pain disorders.

Various questionnaires have been used to assess sexual function. The Watts Sexual Function Questionnaire (used in the PEPI trial) focuses on four subscales: desire, arousal, orgasm, and satisfaction. The Personal Experiences Questionnaire (PEQ) collects data on six factors: feelings for the partner, sexual responsivity, frequency of sexual activities, libido, partner problems, and vaginal dryness/dyspareunia. The Sexual Energy Scale (SES) has been designed to objectively measure the effect of androgen on a woman's subjective experience of vitality/sexual energy.

A newer model is the Female Sexual Function Index (FSFI), a brief, self-report measure. Six domains are included: desire, subjective arousal, lubrication, orgasm, satisfaction, and pain associated with intercourse. It is designed to address the gender differences in patterns of female sexual function.

A variety of psychological, sociocultural, interpersonal, and biologic factors may contribute to sexual dysfunction. Healthcare providers should encourage women to discuss any concerns they may have. The Melbourne Women's Midlife Health Project reported that the major factors affecting women's sexuality in midlife are their feelings for their partner and sexual performance difficulties experienced by their partner. Other social variables, such as stress at work or interpersonal stress, and educational level affect sexual functioning indirectly via effects on symptoms and well-being. Other studies have illustrated that for early

postmenopausal women, dyspareunia plays an important role. As menopause progresses, delayed orgasm and reduced libido begin to become more significant factors. During peri- and postmenopause, an untreated anxiety disorder or depression, whether new or chronic, may impact sexual function.

Clinicians should use a validated instrument, such as the FSFI, to assess female sexual function. In addition, clinicians should be sensitive to issues related to sexual orientation and should not assume that all women are heterosexual.

An assessment of all potential physical, psychological, or social factors amenable to intervention should be the primary therapeutic consideration for women who express a specific complaint of loss of libido.

Often, the first noticeable vulvovaginal change associated with menopause is reduced vaginal lubrication during sexual arousal. All women of perimenopausal age onward should have a thorough evaluation of vaginal health, regardless of symptoms or sexual activity. Some women on ERT/HRT may have sexual problems related to decreased estrogenization of the vulvar-vaginal tissues despite estrogen therapy.

The role of androgen insufficiency in female sexual dysfunction is receiving increased attention.

Women with sexual dysfunction of extended duration or who do not respond to medical intervention and simple counseling should be referred to a specialist in the treatment of sexual problems.

Bibliography

Bachmann G, Bancroft J, Braunstein, et al. Female androgen insufficiency: the Princeton consensus statement on definition, classification, and assessment. *Fertil Steril* 2002;77:660-665.

Dennerstein L, Dudley EC, Hopper JL, Burger H. Sexuality, hormones and the menopausal transition. *Maturitas* 1997;26:83-93.

Dennerstein L, Lehert P, Burger H, Dudley E. Factors affecting sexual functioning of women in the mid-life years. *Climacteric* 1999;2:254-262.

Gassman A, Santoro N. The influence of menopausal hormone changes on sexuality; current knowledge and recommendations for practice. *Menopause* 1994;1:91-98.

Lucisano A, Acampora MG, Russo N, Maniccia E, Montemurro A, Dell'Acqua S. Ovarian and peripheral plasma levels of progestogens, androgens and oestrogens in post-menopausal women. *Maturitas* 1984;6:45-53.

Pugeat M, Crave JC, Tourniaire J, Forest MG. Clinical utility of sex hormone-binding globulin measurement. *Horm Res* 1996; 45:148-155.

Rosen R, Brown C, Heiman J, et al. The female sexual function index (FSFI): a multidimensional self-report instrument for the assessment of female sexual function. *J Sex Marital Ther* 2000;26:191-208.

Sarrel PM. Sexuality and menopause. *Obstet Gynecol* 1990;75 (4 suppl):26S-30S.

Simon J, Klaiber E, Witta B, Bowen A, Yang HM. Differential effects of estrogen-androgen and estrogen-only therapy on vasomotor symptoms, gonadotropin secretion, and endogenous androgen bioavailability in postmenopausal women. *Menopause* 1999;6:138-146.

Slater CC, Hodis HN, Mack WJ, Shoupe D, Paulson RJ, Stanczyk FZ. Markedly elevated levels of estrone sulfate after long-term oral, but not transdermal, administration of estradiol in postmenopausal women. *Menopause* 2001;8:200-203.

Tuiten A, Van Honk J, Koppeschaar H, Bernaards C, Thijssen J, Verbaten R. Time course of effects of testosterone administration on sexual arousal in women [published erratum in *Arch Gen Psychiatry* 2002;59:136]. *Arch Gen Psychiatry* 2000;57:149-153.

Warnock JK, Bundren JC, Morris DW. Female hypoactive sexual desire disorder due to androgen deficiency: clinical and psychometric issues. *Psychopharmacol Bull* 1997;33:761-766.

E.11. Urinary incontinence

Although as many as 30% of women aged 45 to 64 experience urinary incontinence, fewer than half of these women seek help.

Diagnosis of the exact cause(s) of a woman's incontinence requires a complete physical examination (including a pelvic exam), medical history (including medications), sexual history, and urinalysis. Additional specialized studies of the bladder are warranted, in some cases.

The medical history should include specific questions about urinary incontinence (see Table 27). Bowel function is also important, including the number of bowel movements per week, the use of laxatives, and any difficulty controlling the bowel (fecal incontinence).

To determine the extent of any incontinence, it may be helpful for women to keep a urinary diary for 1 week, providing a day-by-day account of information related to incontinence (see Table 28). Other useful information includes proximity to toilet facilities both during the day and at night.

Table 27. Standard questions regarding urinary incontinence

- How long have you had problems with your bladder?

- How many times do you urinate during the day? (frequency)

- How often do you get up during sleeping at night to urinate? (nocturia)

- Do you worry that you can't get to the bathroom in time? (urgency)

- Can you stop the flow of urine? (tests strength of pelvic floor muscles)

- Do you ever lose your urine before you reach the toilet? (urge incontinence)

- Do you leak urine with coughing, sneezing, walking, or lifting? (stress incontinence)

Table 28. Data to include in a urinary diary

- Type and amount of fluid intake and time of day

- Amount of urine voided and time of day (normal total 24-hour urine volume is 1-1.5 liters)

- Any urge sensed before voiding

- Amount of urine leaked (eg, a few drops, wet underwear, soaked clothing) plus the time of day and type of activity when leakage occurred

- Use of external protection (pads), quantity used, and how wet the pad is when changed

---

The following observations should be included in the physical examination:

- hydration state,

- presence of edema,

- assessment of mobility (with immobility possibly contributing to a woman's inability to reach the toilet),

- abdominal distension,

- surgical scars and hernias,

- pelvic organ prolapse,

- muscle tone and grip of the circumvaginal and anal sphincter muscles,

- perineum (when the bladder is full) in both the standing and supine positions (with an attempt to provoke leakage by coughing),

- neurologic exam including perineal sensation and a bulbocavernosus reflex test.

Measuring a postvoid residual is recommended to determine whether the bladder is completely emptied. A standard urinalysis will exclude other causes, such as diabetes mellitus and proteinuria, that might reflect renal disease, infection, or hematuria. Urine cytology might be obtained depending on the woman's smoking and history of irritative voiding symptoms.

Bibliography

DeMarco EF. Urinary tract disorders in perimenopausal and postmenopausal women. In Lobo RA, ed. *Treatment of the Postmenopausal Woman: Basic and Clinical Aspects.* 2nd ed. Philadelphia, PA: Lippincott Williams & Wilkins; 1999:213-227.

E.12. Psychological health

A detailed psychosocial history is the first step in identifying mental health problems. Most women present to their healthcare providers with symptoms of psychological problems before they consult a mental health professional. Therefore, it is the responsibility of the clinician to conduct an initial assessment of psychological health.

Assessment of psychological health includes asking about changes in mood, appetite, sleep, energy, sexual function, concentration, memory, and suicidal thoughts. Symptoms such as prolonged tiredness, loss of interest in normal activities, sadness, or irritability may result from depression. Use of alcohol or other illegal substances may mask mood problems. Information on family or past history of depression or other psychiatric disorders, as well as previous responses to psychopharmacologic medication and psychotherapy, must also be obtained.

The most common psychiatric disorder in women is depression. Depressive disorders are common in many countries and present a major public health problem. The World Health Organization (WHO) has predicted that, by 2020, major depression will be second only to ischemic heart disease as a cause of disability. One in eight Americans will experience an episode of depression in their lifetime. The rate of depression in US and Canadian women is twice the rate for men. The most predictive factor for depression during midlife and beyond is a prior history.

If a perimenopausal woman does not have a history of depression and has recently developed mood changes or depressive symptoms (ie, not clinical depression) after experiencing menopausal symptoms (eg, hot flashes), her primary problem may be what some have proposed as the "domino effect" of menopausal symptoms. According to this model, estrogen fluctuations result in hot flashes and night sweats, leading to sleep disturbance, which, in turn, precipitates psychological and cognitive symptoms of depression. Women experiencing induced menopause may be especially susceptible to this sort of emotional distress.

A number of clinical findings may indicate that a woman requires further psychiatric or psychosocial evaluation. The American Psychiatric Association has developed valid and reliable criteria for diagnosing psychological disorders. Table 29 presents the symptoms of a major depressive disorder (ie, clinical depression).

Women exhibiting relevant symptoms should be screened for clinical depression using tools such as the Beck Depression Inventory or the Zung Self-Rating Depression Scale.

A second form of depression, dysthymic disorder, is also a prevalent condition. This chronic (ie, has persisted for >2 years) mood disorder is in contrast to the more acute and more severe symptomatology of a major depressive disorder, and is generally more difficult to treat.

A medical history, physical examination, and routine laboratory tests can rule out illnesses that are often associated with depression. Depression also may be a side effect of medications (see Table 30).

In addition, an evaluation of anxiety is needed to differentiate normal day-to-day anxiety from pathological responses that require pharmacological intervention and/or psychotherapy, such as obsessive-compulsive and posttraumatic stress disorders. Anxiety may also be a warning symptom of a panic disorder (distinguished by shortness of breast, chest pain, dizziness, heart palpitations, and/or feelings of "going crazy" or being "out of control") or depression.

Depressive and anxiety disorders should be diagnosed and treated with appropriate counseling and psychotropic medications, when needed. In many cases, referral to a healthcare professional with psychiatric training is appropriate.

Table 29. DSM-IV criteria for major depressive episode

Five or more of the following symptoms have been present during the same 2-week period and represent a change from previous functioning; at least one of the symptoms is either (1) depressed mood or (2) loss of interest or pleasure. (Do not include symptoms that are clearly due to a general medical condition, or mood-incongruent delusions or hallucinations.)

1. Depressed mood most of the day, nearly every day as indicated by either subjective report (eg, feels sad or empty) or observation made by others (eg, appears tearful).

2. Markedly diminished interest or pleasure in all, or almost all, activities most of the day, nearly every day (as indicated by either subjective account or observation made by others).

3. Significant weight loss when not dieting or weight gain (eg, a change of more than 5% of body weight in a month) or decrease or increase in appetite nearly every day.

4. Insomnia or hypersomnia nearly every day.

5. Psychomotor agitation or retardation nearly every day (observable by others, not merely subjective feelings of restlessness or being slowed down).

6. Fatigue or loss of energy nearly every day.

7. Feelings of worthlessness or excessive or inappropriate guilt (which may be delusional) nearly every day (not merely self-reproach or guilt about being sick).

8. Diminished ability to think or concentrate or indecisiveness nearly every day (either by subjective account or as observed by others).

9. Recurrent thoughts of death (not just fear of dying), recurrent suicidal ideation without a specific plan, or a suicide attempt or a specific plan for committing suicide.

Source: American Psychiatric Association 1995.

Bibliography

American Psychiatric Association. *Diagnostic and Statistical Manual of Mental Disorders. Primary Care Version.* 4th ed. Washington, DC: American Psychiatric Association; 1995.

Landau C, Milan FB. Assessment and treatment of depression during the menopause: a preliminary report. *Menopause* 1996;3:210-207.

The North American Menopause Society. Clinical challenges of perimenopause: consensus opinion of The North American Menopause Society. *Menopause* 2000;7:5-13.

Parikh SV, Lam RW, for the CANMAT Depression Work Group. Clinical guidelines for the treatment of depressive disorders: I. Definitions, prevalence, and health burden. *Can J Psychiatry* 2001;46(suppl 1):13S-20S.

Rosenthal MB. Psychiatric disorders and the menopause: evaluation and treatment. *Menopause Management* 1993;2(1):35-39.

Schmidt PJ, Rubinow DR. Menopause-related affective disorders: a justification for further study. *Am J Psychiatry* 1991;148:844-852.

Sherwin BB. Impact of the changing hormonal milieu on psychologic functioning. In: Lobo RA, ed. *Treatment of the Postmenopausal Woman: Basic and Clinical Aspects.* 2nd ed. Philadelphia, PA: Lippincott Williams & Wilkins; 1999:179-188.

Table 30. Medications associated with depression

- Antihypertensives (eg, clonidine, thiazides, beta blockers, hydralazine)

- Sedatives (eg, alcohol, barbiturates, benzodiazepines, chloral hydrate)

- Steroids (eg, corticosteroids, oral contraceptives, prednisone)

- Dopamine agonists (eg, levodopa, bromocriptine, amantadine)

- Anticonvulsants (eg, phenytoin, carbamazepine)

- Analgesics (eg, ibuprofen, indomethacin, opiates)

- H_2-receptor antagonists (eg, cimetidine, ranitidine)

- Stimulant withdrawal (eg, amphetamines, cocaine)

Source: Landau. *Menopause* 1996.

E.13. Domestic abuse risk

Domestic violence includes physical, sexual, and mental abuse. Clinicians must be alert for signs of abuse. Direct questioning should be a routine part of all evaluations (see Table 31).

A case-control study of domestic violence found that women at greatest risk for injury from domestic violence are those with a male partner who has any of the following characteristics, listed in the order of importance:

- abuses alcohol,

- is a former or estranged husband or a former boyfriend,

- uses illegal drugs,

- is intermittently employed,

- was recently unemployed,

- has less than a high school education.

Controlled studies from primary care settings have consistently found abused women to have a significantly higher prevalence of the following physical and mental health problems: injury, gastrointestinal problems (especially chronic irritable bowel syndrome), chronic pain (head, neck, fibromyalgia), gynecological problems (especially pelvic pain, urinary tract infections, sexually transmitted infections), and mental health problems (especially depression). Assessment for abuse is especially important in women presenting with these symptoms.

Table 31. Questions for detecting abuse

- Have you ever been emotionally or physically abused by your partner or someone important to you?

- Within the last year, have you been pushed or shoved, hit, slapped, kicked, or otherwise physically hurt by someone?

- Within the past year, has anyone forced you to have sexual activities?

- Are you afraid of your partner or anyone else?

Bibliography

Coker AL, Smith PH, Bethea L, King MR, McKeown RE. Physical health consequences of physical and psychological intimate partner violence. *Arch Fam Med* 2000;9:451-457.

Dutton MA, Mitchell B, Haywood Y. The emergency department as a violence prevention center. *J Am Med Womens Assoc* 1996;51:92-95.

Gielen AC, O'Campo PJ, Campbell JC, et al. Women's opinions about domestic violence screening and mandatory reporting. *Am J Prev Med* 2000;19:279-85.

Humphreys J, Parker B, Campbell JC. Intimate partner violence against women. In: Taylor D, Fugate-Woods N, eds. *Annual Review of Nursing Research*. New York, NY: Springer Publishing Co; 2001:275-306.

Kyriacou DN, Anglin D, Taliaferro E, et al. Risk factors for injury to women from domestic violence. *N Engl J Med* 1999;341:1892-1898.

Leserman J, Li Z, Drossman DA, Hu YJ. Selected symptoms associated with sexual and physical abuse history among female patients with gastrointestinal disorders: the impact on subsequent health care visits. *Psychol Med* 1998;28:417-425.

E.14. Sexually transmitted infections

A number of tests are available to screen for sexually transmitted infection (STI), when indicated. Clinicians should not assume that older women are not at risk. Vaginal atrophy increases risk for contracting an STI. In addition, older women may not be as knowledgeable about infection risks or willing to take steps to minimize these risks as younger women who have lived with the threat of AIDS their entire sexual lives.

STI testing could include screening for the following pathogens (listed alphabetically):

Chlamydia. Most chlamydial infections occur in women under age 25. In peri- and postmenopausal women, testing is recommended only for those at high risk for sexually transmitted diseases. These include women with multiple sex partners, a sex partner who has had multiple sexual contacts, or a sex partner with a chlamydial infection. All women with purulent cervical discharge should be screened. Until recently, direct culture testing has been recognized as the most specific test for chlamydia. Newer technologies, such as antigen-detection and direct nucleic acid probe assays, may provide improved sensitivity, availability, and lower cost options for testing. Urine screening and self-administered swabs are being studied as possible alternatives.

Gonorrhea. The highest incidence of gonorrhea infection occurs in women under age 25. Because gonorrhea infection is relative uncommon in the general population of peri- and postmenopausal women, testing is recommended only in women at high risk for infection. These include women with multiple sex partners, a sex partner who has had multiple sexual contacts, a sex partner with culture-proven gonorrhea, and women with a history of repeated episodes of gonorrhea.

For gonococcal infections, direct culture testing is the most sensitive and reproducible diagnostic method. Other tests, such as Gram's stained urethral smears, serology, and fluorescent antibody microscopy, lack the speed, accuracy, and low cost of culture testing.

Human immunodeficiency virus (HIV). For peri- and postmenopausal women, routine screening for HIV (the AIDS virus) is recommended only in women seeking treatment for sexually transmitted disease; past or present intravenous (IV) drug users; women with multiple sex partners; women having sexual contact with partners who were HIV-infected, bisexual, or IV drug users; women born or living in an area with a high prevalence of HIV infection; and women who received a blood transfusion between 1978 and 1985.

The initial screening test to detect antibodies to HIV is the ELISA test. This test has high sensitivity and specificity; however, false-negative results can occur in the first 6 to 12 weeks after infection, before antibodies develop. Some immunologic disorders may cause a false-positive test result; thus, a second test is warranted in women with a positive HIV result on an ELISA test.

Other tests to validate results include the Western blot test, radioimmunoprecipitation assays, and indirect immunofluorescence assays. The Western blot test is the most common test and has a false-positive rate of less than 0.001%.

Women being screened for HIV should sign a consent form and be provided pre- and posttest counseling.

Human papilloma virus (HPV). There is a substantial body of evidence that indicates all cervical cancers are related to infection with HPV. The 2001 consensus guidelines for the m management of women with cervical cytological abnormalities now include recommendations for HPV testing in the evaluation of atypical squamous cells of undetermined significance (ASC-US). Some laboratories are equipped to evaluate abnormal Pap results with high-risk HPV testing.

Syphilis. Routine screening of women is not recommended, based on the low incidence of syphilis in the general population. However, screening is justified in women who engage in sex with multiple partners, who live in areas where syphilis is prevalent, or who had sexual contact with persons with syphilis.

Bibliography

Centers for Disease Control and Prevention. Chlamydia in the United States; April 2001. Accessible at http://www.cdc.gov/nchstp/dstd/Fact_Sheets/chlamydia_facts.htm.

Centers for Disease Control and Prevention. 1998 guidelines for treatment of sexually transmitted diseases. *MMWR Recomm Rep* 1998;47(RR-1):1-111.

Department of Health, United Kingdom. Cervical screening: launch of test for human papilloma virus (HPV) status; Jan 30, 1998. Accessible at http://www.doh.gov.uk/cmo/cmo983.htm.

Gilson RJ, Mindel A. Recent advances: sexually transmitted infections. *BMJ* 2001;322:1160-1164.

Report of the US Prevention Services Task Force. *Guide to Clinical Preventive Services.* 2nd ed. Philadelphia, PA: Lippincott Williams & Wilkins; 1998.

US Preventive Services Task Force. Screening for chlamydial infection: recommendations and rationale. *Am J Prev Med* 2001;20:90-94.

Wright TC, Jr, Cox JT, Massad LS, Twiggs LB, Wilkinson EJ, for the 2001 ASCCP-sponsored consensus conference. 2001 consensus guidelines for the management of women with cervical cytological abnormalities. *JAMA* 2002;287:2120-2129.

The menopause transition is an appropriate time for a complete review of a woman's risk for diseases in later years, including osteoporosis and cardiovascular disease. It is also an opportunity for counseling on risk status and reduction.

Menopause is a natural biologic event. Perhaps 15% to 25% of women reach menopause virtually free of any menopause-related complaint. Others have symptoms that may need treatment, although many women need to be reminded that receiving no treatment is an option. Treatment can include lifestyle modification, nonprescription remedies, prescription therapies, and/or complementary and alternative medicine (CAM) therapies.

The clinician should ask each woman what outcomes she expects from the therapeutic intervention. Women differ in their expectations, and not all treatments can provide the outcomes they desire. By better understanding the potential outcomes, a treatment plan can be devised that is acceptable for both the clinician and the woman.

Perhaps the most important element of a comprehensive menopause-related therapeutic plan is lifestyle modification. Modifiable lifestyle areas include substance use, exercise, stress reduction, nutrition, and weight management. Clinicians need to encourage all women to adopt the principles of a healthy lifestyle.

F.01. Substance use

Use of substances such as tobacco, alcohol, caffeine, and illegal drugs contribute to poor health. Clinicians are challenged to assist women at midlife and beyond to adopt healthier habits regarding substance use.

F.01.a. Smoking

Smoking is the single greatest preventable cause of illness and premature death. Smoking is responsible for more than 142,000 deaths annually in women in the United States alone (36,000 from lung cancer) and 15,000 deaths per year in Canadian women (5,400 from lung cancer). Smoking cessation is the single most important change a woman can make to reduce her risk of disease.

Smokers tend to reach menopause up to 2 years earlier than nonsmokers, placing smokers at increased risk for diseases associated with diminished levels of estrogen. Nevertheless, plasma levels of estradiol and estrone have not been associated with smoking in either pre- or postmenopausal women. However, among postmenopausal women who take oral estrogen replacement therapy (ERT), smokers have lower serum estrone and estradiol levels than nonsmokers.

Smoking significantly increases the risk for coronary heart disease (CHD) and cancer. Stopping smoking can be beneficial in reducing that risk. The Nurses' Health Study found that, after women stopped smoking, one-third of the excess risk of CHD was eliminated within 2 years. After 10 to 14 years, the excess risks for total mortality, as well as that for both CHD and total cancer mortality, approached that of women who never smoked.

This same study also found that among current smokers, a younger age at natural menopause was associated with a higher risk of CHD. However, among those who did not smoke or who were past smokers, CHD risk was not affected. These same observations may also be true for women following induced menopause.

The rise in lung cancer risk is almost entirely related to smoking. Risk of cervical and vulvar cancer also increases with smoking.

Smoking is associated with more rapid bone loss in women. Smoking during adolescence and early adulthood may impede the achievement of optimal peak bone mass. Also, women who smoke have higher fracture rates than nonsmoking women. In the Nurses' Health Study, hip fracture risk increased linearly with greater cigarette consumption. Risk declined after quitting, but the benefit was not observed until 10 years after cessation. In this study, both the increase in risk among current smokers and the decline in risk after smoking cessation were, in part, accounted for by differences in body weight. The mechanisms by which smoking might affect bone mass are not known, although some evidence suggests that some component of cigarette smoke interferes with estrogen metabolism.

Smoking jeopardizes dental health for several reasons. It has a direct influence on gingival tissues caused by the heat and chemical constituents of tobacco smoke. It contributes to the development of osteoporosis and has antiestrogenic effects. It may also potentiate the development of periodontitis by inhibiting tissue oxygen levels, by limiting gingival blood supply, and by impairing antibacterial immune responses, thereby increasing the likelihood of infection.

Nearly all smokers acknowledge that tobacco use is harmful to their health, but they underestimate the magnitude of their risk. Some women may stop smoking when their healthcare providers discuss their health risks, particularly if they already show some signs of disease, such as osteoporosis. For many smokers, the risk of future disease does not outweigh the current perceived benefits of smoking or barriers to stopping. Despite the health risks of smoking, some women are more encouraged to stop by realizing the adverse effect that smoking has on facial wrinkles.

Approximately one-third of smokers try to stop smoking each year, but only 20% of them seek help. Those who do are more successful; less than 10% who try to stop on their own are successful over the long term. Several attempts are typically required before a smoker truly quits.

The addictive nature of nicotine is the primary physiological obstacle to quitting. Established patterns must also be broken to break through the psychological barriers (eg, smoking is part of the daily routine, such as ending a meal; using smoking to handle stress).

Even brief interventions by the healthcare professional during an office visit promote smoking cessation. Women who need assistance to stop smoking may benefit from smoking cessation therapies. Most successful is a combination of behavior modification techniques, group support, and drug therapy. Several prescription therapies are FDA-approved for smoking cessation: slow-release bupropion and nicotine-replacement products in gum, transdermal patch, nasal spray, and vapor inhaler formulations. Most experts consider these products to be equivalent in efficacy. The majority of US states have funded programs to assist with smoking cessation.

F.01.b. Alcohol

Drinking alcohol (even a small amount) can trigger hot flashes in some women. Although some studies have suggested that alcohol consumption may lower endogenous estrogen levels, one study in postmenopausal women using HRT found that acute alcohol consumption was associated with significant, sustained elevations in circulating estradiol to levels 300% higher than those used clinically.

Moderate alcohol consumption appears to lower the risk of hip fractures in women 65 years of age and older, possibly because moderate consumption increases endogenous estradiol concentrations and calcitonin excretion, which may inhibit bone resorption. In the Nurses' Health Study, women who consumed 75 g or more of alcohol per week had significantly higher bone densities at the lumbar spine compared with nondrinkers, although alcohol intakes less than 75 g/wk were also of benefit. This positive association was observed among both current users and never users of ERT/HRT. However, alcohol consumption was not associated with a higher femoral bone density.

In addition, there is evidence that light to moderate alcohol use may lower the cardiovascular mortality rate in women. In one study, the survival benefit associated with light to moderate drinking appeared to be largely confined to women at greater risk for coronary heart disease and those 50 years of age or older.

Women are more affected by alcohol than men due to many factors, including having less water in their bodies to dilute the alcohol, less enzyme to digest the alcohol, and hormonal differences that may affect absorption. Death rates from alcohol abuse are 50% to 100% higher for women than they are for men.

Both women and men who drink have a higher risk of cancer. Women who consume 1 to 2 drinks daily may be at increased risk for breast cancer. The mechanism of this effect is not known, but the association may be due to carcinogenic actions of alcohol or its metabolites, or to alcohol-induced changes in levels of hormones such as estrogen.

Alcoholic beverages, along with cigarette smoking and use of snuff and chewing tobacco, can also cause cancers of the oral cavity, esophagus, and larynx. The combined use of tobacco and alcohol leads to a greatly increased risk of oral and esophageal cancers. The effect of tobacco and alcohol combined is greater than the sum of their individual effects.

Compared with men, women who drink experience greater damage to the liver and a higher risk of stroke. Higher levels of alcohol use (defined as more than 7 drinks per week; 1 drink equals 12 oz beer, 4 oz wine, or 1 oz liquor) may increase certain cardiovascular risks, such as hypertension, stroke, and coronary artery disease. Heavy alcohol consumption has also been shown to increase the risk of falls and hip fractures. Excessive alcohol consumption may have detrimental effects on bone, the liver, and other body systems. Heavy drinkers who stop may have withdrawal symptoms.

Drinking moderate amounts of alcohol can cause hair and skin to appear dull and can worsen acne and dandruff. Alcohol can lead to weight gain through its "empty" calories (ie, low nutritional content). Those who abuse alcohol can suffer from malnutrition. Moderate alcohol consumption is also associated with insomnia, even when consumed hours before bedtime.

One method for determining if a woman is abusing alcohol is to use the "TACE" questions. Total scores from the four questions of two or more suggest alcohol abuse.

T (tolerance)
How many drinks does it take to make you feel high? (If the answer is more than 2 drinks, give a score of 2.)

A (annoyed)
Have people annoyed you by criticizing your drinking? (Score 1 for yes.)

C (cut down)
Have you felt you ought to cut down on your drinking? (Score 1 for yes.)

E (eye opener)
Have you ever had a drink first thing in the morning to steady your nerves or get rid of a hangover? (Score 1 for yes.)

Because of the health risks associated with heavy alcohol consumption, women should be counseled to limit themselves to 1 drink per day and a maximum of 7 per week. For women who do not drink, the potential benefits of moderate drinking do not outweigh the potential risks.

F.01.c. Caffeine

All caffeine-containing drinks (eg, coffee, tea, colas, "energy" drinks) can have a negative effect on health. Caffeine ingestion may trigger hot flashes and can contribute to insomnia, even when consumed hours before bedtime. Also, caffeine is a natural diuretic, which increases dehydration.

Caffeine has been proposed as a risk factor for bone loss in postmenopausal women, but many of the studies linking caffeine to bone loss have been confounded by covariates, and study findings are inconsistent. Brewed coffee (2-3 cups/day) has been associated with accelerated bone loss from the spine and total body in women with elemental calcium intakes below 800 mg/day; whether this effect is from caffeine has not been determined. Increasing dietary calcium intake can counteract the increased urinary calcium excretion associated with caffeinated beverages.

F.02. Exercise

Physical inactivity is a risk factor for many diseases, including heart disease and diabetes. Recent national surveys report that over one-third of US women aged 45 and over participate in no leisure-time physical activity; less than 20% participate in regular, sustained physical activity at the recommended level of at least 30 minutes for at least 5 times per week.

In Canada, the National Population Health Survey (1996/97) reported similar results. Only 15% of Canadian women aged 40 to 54 were classified as sufficiently active. Another 54% reported regular participation in physical activity, 18% were occasionally active, and 23% were inactive.

When performed regularly, activities such as brisk walking, running, aerobics, dancing, tennis, and strength training can help the heart, muscles, bones, balance, and weight management. New guidelines suggest that 30 minutes of moderate exercise (which can be divided into 10-minute sessions) on most, preferably all, days of the week has marked health benefits.

Exercises can be divided into three basic types:

- *Strength training* (or resistance exercises) — Exercise that provides muscle resistance, such as free weights or weight machines. These exercises increase bone density, increase lean muscle mass, and improve caloric metabolism. Older women, in particular, need these exercises to build strength to prevent falls.

- *Aerobic* — Exercising the cardiovascular and respiratory system. Examples include brisk walking, jogging, rowing, and cycling. Low-impact aerobics are easier on the joints than high-impact aerobics and, thus, may be a better choice for women at midlife.

- *Flexibility* — Stretching exercises help maintain flexibility and reduce stiffness with aging. Improving flexibility and balance also helps protect against falls.

Clinicians should provide guidance to women regarding which type(s) and level of exercise are appropriate and encouragement to work exercise into their routine for the rest of their lives. If a woman has been sedentary, she should be advised to start slowly and progress gradually. She should begin with strength exercises that engage all muscle groups, perform these exercises 3 times per week on alternate days for a minimum of 10 to 12 weeks, then reduce strength exercises to 2 times per week and add aerobic exercise to the program.

Exercise can have a positive effect on many menopause-related complaints. Some women report fewer hot flashes when they exercise regularly. In addition, exercise promotes better, more restorative sleep and stimulates endorphin production, a neuropeptide with analgesic activity.

Exercise is clearly linked to reducing osteoporosis risk. A meta-analysis of controlled trials published from 1966 to 1996 showed that exercise training programs prevented or reversed almost 1% of bone loss per year in the lumbar spine and femoral neck for both pre- and postmenopausal women. The effects of exercise on bone mass are attributed to a stimulation of osteoblast activity.

The type of exercise is important. Most experts agree that weight-bearing and strength-training exercises provide the most bone benefits.

Weight-bearing exercises are those in which a woman's bones and muscles work against gravity. These include any exercises in which the feet and legs bear one's body weight, such as jogging/running, brisk walking/hiking, climbing stairs, dancing, and racquet sports.

Strength-training exercises are those activities that improve muscle mass through muscle resistance. Some evidence shows that strength training curbs bone loss in women who do not use ERT/HRT. Strength training can be performed as few as two times a week and need not involve special equipment other than simple weights.

Physical activity plays an important role in reducing the risk of falls, and thus fractures, in elderly women with osteoporosis. Exercise programs for the elderly reduce risk of falling by 10%, and programs that include training for balance reduce the risk by nearly 20%. Exercise for women with established osteoporosis should not include heavy weight bearing or activity so vigorous that it may trigger fracture.

Programs that may be useful adjuncts to office counseling include the "Choose to Move" program offered by the American Heart Association. In a randomized clinical trial, participants in this 12-wk intervention not only increased their weekly exercise activity but also their knowledge of cardiovascular risk factors, leading to diet modification to reduce consumption of high-fat foods.

Canada's "Physical Activity Guide to Healthy Active Living" is a similar resource that provides recommendations for the types and amounts of activity necessary to maintain or improve health.

F.03. Stress reduction

Although menopause has not been shown to raise stress levels, women at midlife may face many new stressors. Stress negatively affects quality of life, produces a variety of symptoms, and may aggravate some medical conditions.

Many women can benefit from stress-reducing strategies, such as exercise, meditation, yoga, massage, paced respiration (deep, slow abdominal breathing), biofeedback, and behavior-modification techniques. Research supports the benefit of paced respiration in reducing hot flashes in some women. Although not proven in controlled clinical trials, some women report fewer hot flashes when they engage in activities to enhance relaxation, such as meditation, yoga, massage, or even just a leisurely bath. Women should be encouraged to recognize their own life stressors, to find stress-relieving strategies that work for them, and to take time to relax every day.

F.04. Nutrition

Nutritional guidelines recommend consuming a variety of foods. Diets should be high in grain products, vegetables, and fruits as well as low in saturated fats and cholesterol. The current recommendations include at least five fruit and vegetable servings daily. Low to moderate use of sugar, salt, and alcohol is recommended along with adequate physical activity to balance energy intake.

Women of peri- or postmenopausal age may benefit from added calcium, vitamin D, and some B-vitamins: folic acid, vitamin B_{12}, and vitamin B_6. There should be an emphasis on nutrient-dense foods so that, even at reduced caloric intake, women maintain adequate protein and essential micronutrients. Whole grain or enriched breads and cereals that provide more folic acid should be chosen. Regular consumptions of dietary supplements containing folic acid should be balanced with supplemental B_{12}.

It is important to maintain fluid intake, even when food intake is declining. Water is the best choice for the eight glasses of fluid intake per day that are recommended. Relying on thirst as a trigger for fluid intake may result in too low of an intake, since the sensation of thirst may decline with age.

The potential benefits of reducing total dietary fat intake have not been conclusively established. The influence of fat intake on endogenous estrogen levels is controversial. The Nurses' Health Study found higher fat intake to be associated with lower serum estradiol levels. However, a meta-analysis of estrogen and dietary fat studies in pre- and postmenopausal women found that, on average, dietary fat reduction was associated with lower serum estradiol levels.

F.04.a. Heart disease and diet

There has been consistent evidence from observational studies that elevated serum cholesterol is a major risk factor for heart disease, the incidence of which increases in women after menopause. Studies have consistently shown that changes in saturated fat intake and the relative contribution of polyunsaturated to saturated fat are closely associated with serum cholesterol levels.

Dietary guidelines from the *Healthy People 2010* that apply to heart disease prevention are as follows:

- Include at least two servings of fruit daily;

- Include at least three servings of vegetables daily, with at least one-third of these as dark green or orange vegetables;

- Limit salt intake to less than 2,400 mg/day;

- Limit saturated fat intake to less than 10% of total calories;

- Limit total fat intake to less than 30% of total calories;

- Reduce the consumption of alcohol.

In addition, the American Heart Association (AHA) eating plan also recommends the following for women:

- Limit polyunsaturated fat to 10% of calories and make up the remaining fat intake with monounsaturated fat, such as olive oil or canola oil;

- Limit cholesterol intake to 300 mg daily.

The Mediterranean-style step I diet is the most recent recommendation from the AHA. It is a modification of the AHA step 1 diet and emphasizes more root vegetables and fish, replacing beef, lamb, and pork with poultry, eating fruit every day, and replacing butter and cream with margarine high in α-linolenic acid. Exclusive use of rapeseed oil and olive oil are recommended for salads and food preparation. Moderate consumption of wine is allowed.

The diet is based on results from the Lyon Diet Heart Study, a randomized, controlled trial of prevention after a first myocardial infarction. During nearly 4 years of follow-up, the group assigned to the Mediterranean-style step 1 diet experienced a significantly lower risk of recurrent heart disease than the control group. Further research is needed to verify these findings in other populations and to better understand which specific constituents confer the protective effect.

The relationship between dietary intake of specific types of fat, particularly trans-fatty acids, and the risk of coronary heart disease (CHD) remains unclear. Trans-fatty acids are formed when liquid oils are hydrogenated for use as stick margarines or shortening. Saturated fatty acids are the major dietary factors that raise serum levels of low-density lipoprotein cholesterol. Findings from the Nurses' Health Study suggest that replacing saturated fat and trans-fatty acids with unhydrogenated monounsaturated and polyunsaturated fats is more effective than reducing overall fat intake in preventing CHD in women. A diet high in cold-water fish (eg, salmon, tuna, halibut) provides omega-3 fatty acids, which are linked to prevention of CHD. Flaxseeds and flaxseed oil are other sources of omega-3 fatty acids.

Reducing egg consumption, because of high cholesterol content, has been widely recommended in the past. However, studies of egg consumption and risk of CHD have failed to demonstrate an association once other dietary factors are taken into account.

Flavonoids found in fruits and vegetables have antioxidant properties. Studies in men have found inconsistent effects for dietary flavonoids, while studies in women support a protective effect. In the Iowa Women's Health Study, flavonoids were associated with lower death rates from heart disease, and the source of flavonoid intake most associated with low heart disease death rate was broccoli. In the Finnish mobile clinic health cohort, more than 20 years of follow-up found that flavonoids were associated with a lower risk of mortality from heart disease in women. It should be noted that tea is a major source of flavonoids in some cultures, and two studies have suggested that tea drinking has a protective effect in women against the risk of heart disease.

Fruits and vegetables rich in antioxidant vitamins appear to be associated with a lower risk of heart disease. Observational epidemiological studies have found associations between vitamin C-rich fruits and vegetables and lower risk of heart disease, but evidence in favor of vitamin C supplements is less convincing. The evidence that vitamin E in either foods or supplements may be associated with lower risk of heart disease comes from animal, observational, and some randomized trial studies, but more results are needed to clarify the association.

Fruits and vegetables are a good source of dietary folate. This form of folate differs from the synthetic form, commonly known as folic acid, in that it has lower bioavailability. Folic acid is the form found in supplements, fortified cereals, and enriched and whole wheat flour and whole grain products. Folic acid is one of the key vitamins that regulate homocysteine (a by-product of protein metabolism). The others are vitamin B_{12} and vitamin B_6. A recent meta-analysis showed that higher homocysteine levels are associated with increased risk of heart disease in women. The Nurses' Health Study demonstrated that higher intake of folic acid is associated with lower risk of CHD in that cohort of women. It is therefore considered prudent to increase consumption of folic acid, and, perhaps, vitamin B_{12} and B_6, while awaiting the results of secondary CHD prevention trials that are in progress.

Whole grains have consistently been associated with a lower risk of CHD in women. In 1999, the FDA allowed this health claim for whole-grain foods that are low in fat, and many breakfast cereals, breads, and grains.

The Dietary Approaches to Stop Hypertension (DASH) study, in which all participants had mild hypertension, demonstrated that a combination diet high in fruits and vegetables (8 to 10 servings daily) with added low-fat dairy products (two servings daily) achieved reduction in blood pressure of a similar order of magnitude to that obtained by drug treatment. The DASH diet appeared to have added benefit beyond a diet high in fruit and vegetables, which may be due to increased calcium intake. A subsequent study demonstrated further benefit with restricted salt intake.

Soy products have potential effects on reducing heart disease risk. In 1999, the FDA advised that consuming 25 g/day of soy protein as part of a diet low in saturated fat and cholesterol may reduce the risk of heart disease. A recent randomized trial of postmenopausal women showed a small beneficial effect on plasma lipid levels of 60 g/day isolated soy protein. More research is needed to clarify the health effects of soy foods, isoflavones, and isoflavone-fortified foods.

F.04.b. Osteoporosis and diet

A balanced diet plays a crucial role in bone development and maintenance of bone health throughout life. Adequate intakes of calories, protein, and calcium are required to achieve genetically determined peak bone mass. After peak bone mass is attained, proper nutrition remains important for maintaining bone mass and strength. Calcium and vitamin D have well-known roles in bone metabolism, especially in maintaining bone mass in women older than 65 years. It has been suggested that a diet low in dairy products (which might be followed to reduce cholesterol) might severely limit calcium intake, thereby significantly increasing the risk for postmenopausal osteoporosis. Adequate calcium intake should be maintained through use of low-fat dairy products or calcium supplements.

F.04.c. Cancer and diet

To decrease cancer risk, the American Cancer Society recommends the following.

Select most foods from plant sources. Eat five or more servings of fruits and vegetables each day. Eat several servings each day of other foods from plant sources, such as breads, cereals, grain products, rice, pasta, or beans. Many scientific studies (but not all) show that eating fruits and vegetables (especially green and dark yellow vegetables, and those in the cabbage family, soy products, and legumes) protect against colon cancer and lung cancer. The recommendation applies to foods in their fresh, frozen, canned, dried, or juice forms, but not to specific nutrients or other substances that might be extracted from them.

Grains such as wheat, rice, oats, barley, and the foods made from them are recommended at the level of 6 to 11 servings daily. Because of their vitamin and mineral content, it is best to obtain fiber from fruits, vegetables, and whole grains rather than from fiber supplements. Whole grains contain folate, calcium, and selenium, for example, which have been associated with a lower risk of colon cancer. Legumes, such as dried beans, pinto beans, lentils, and soybeans, are also rich in nutrients that may protect against cancer.

Limit intake of high-fat foods, particularly from animal sources. Choose foods low in fat. Limit consumption of meats, especially high-fat meats. High-fat diets have been associated with an increased risk of colon and rectal cancer, prostate cancer, and endometrial cancer.

Controversy still remains regarding the association between dietary fat intake and risk of breast cancer. A review of dietary fat intervention studies concluded that dietary modification (reducing fat consumption below 20% calories from fat) may offer an approach to breast cancer prevention. Results from the Women's Health Initiative, a large study of postmenopausal women, may provide more specific data.

A recent meta-analysis of eight cohort studies investigated the independent associations between intakes of specific types of fat and breast cancer risk. Only a weak positive association between substitution of saturated fat for carbohydrates was found with increased breast cancer risk. The results, although not statistically significant, were also consistent with the findings from southern European countries that high intakes of olive oil, a rich source of monounsaturated fat, are associated with a reduced risk of breast cancer.

Alcohol consumption also has been associated with breast cancer. Reducing alcohol intake to one drink or less per day is a good option for women who drink regularly to reduce their risk for breast cancer.

Although there have been suggestions of a possible beneficial effect of tea, especially green tea, on cancer risk, the evidence is far from conclusive. Research on the role of soy foods, isoflavones, and other phytoestrogens on breast and other female-related cancers also is continuing, without definitive results to date.

F.05. Weight management

Many women gain weight during the menopause transition. However, neither menopause nor ERT/HRT is responsible for this weight gain.

In the United States, nearly two-thirds of women aged 50 and older are overweight, half of whom are obese, and the incidence has risen in the past few decades. More than 40% of Canadian women are estimated to be overweight or obese.

Regardless of gender, higher levels of body weight and body fat are associated with increased risk for numerous adverse health consequences, such as cardiovascular disease, diabetes mellitus, and arthritis. Obese postmenopausal women also have a higher rate of breast cancer than nonobese postmenopausal women. One study found that gaining 15 to 20 pounds after age 18 increases the risk of myocardial infarction later in life. Conversely, overweight women who lose just 10% of their body weight can reap many health benefits, including a significant lowering of blood pressure.

Moderating factors — including age, sex, family history, body fat distribution, diet, and physical activity — can affect an individual's risk of becoming overweight.

Being underweight can also be unhealthy. Very thin women are at increased risk for osteoporosis. Premenopausal women who over-diet or over-exercise can become so thin that their menstrual cycles stop temporarily, placing them at higher risk for osteoporosis later in life.

Efforts to manage weight in peri- and postmenopausal women are essential. The advice to eat a healthful diet, increase physical activity, and avoid further weight gain is appropriate for almost all women at or above a healthy weight. For those who are overweight or obese, weight loss is indicated.

Physical activity can help balance caloric intake with energy expenditure. Both physical activity and controlled caloric intake are necessary to achieve or maintain a healthy body weight. In the Women's Healthy Lifestyle Project, a 54-month controlled clinical trial, women prevented weight gain (and minimized LDL-cholesterol elevations) during the menopause transition by increasing physical activity and consuming a low-fat diet with moderate caloric restrictions.

No single diet or eating regimen is right for all women. In counseling regarding weight loss, women should be encouraged to set realistic goals achieved through long-term lifestyle change. Emphasis should be placed on changing eating habits rather than relying on diets, especially faddish diets. Support can be obtained from family members, coworkers, and friends. The benefits of eating at regular intervals (ie, every 4-5 hours) and engaging in a regular exercise program — perhaps the most important element — should be emphasized.

Regular exercise appears to have the most beneficial effect on minimizing weight gain in midlife women. Although both aerobic and resistance exercises will consume calories and eventually decrease weight, evidence suggests that peri- and postmenopausal women looking for a lower body-fat ratio will benefit more from resistance-type exercise. This type of exercise builds more lean body muscle tissue and creates a more slender phenotype. Since lean muscle mass is more metabolically active, muscle building allows women to lose weight without excessively decreasing food consumption. This is important because with aging, calorie restriction seems to become less effective in achieving weight loss.

Adequate calcium intake may not be obtained in a low-calorie diet. Calcium supplements may be necessary.

For overweight women, the initial goal should be to reduce body weight by approximately 10% over 6 to 12 months. This can be accomplished through a management program that includes a controlled diet with a deficit of 500 to 1,000 calories per day, reducing dietary fat intake to less than 30% of total energy intake, and participating in regular physical activity.

When diet and exercise are not enough to control weight, various organization and support groups (eg, Weight Watchers, Overeaters Anonymous) may be helpful. Prescription drugs for weight loss are also available, but should be prescribed with caution.

The level of intervention required depends on the BMI category and the presence of comorbidities (see Table 1). The benefits and risks of obesity treatment must be assessed on an individual basis, as recommended in the NIH Guidelines on the Identification, Evaluation, and Treatment of Overweight and Obesity in Adults.

Table 1. Intervention by BMI category

BMI	Intervention
<18.5	lifestyle changes
18.5-24.9	no treatment needed
25-26.9	lifestyle changes, if comorbidities present
27-29.9	lifestyle changes plus drug therapy, if comorbidities present
30-35	lifestyle changes plus drug therapy
35-39.9	lifestyle changes plus drug therapy; surgery needed if comorbidities present
>40	lifestyle changes, drug therapy, and surgery indicated

Lifestyle changes are diet, exercise, and behavior therapy. Comorbidities include hypertension, diabetes mellitus, hyperlipidemia.

Drug therapies indicated for the treatment of obesity include sibutramine (Meridia), orlistat (Xenical), and phentermine HCl (Adipex-P). These are recommended only when lifestyle changes have not controlled weight in women with elevated BMIs, as indicated on the table. For the very obese, surgical stomach stapling may be indicated. The benefits and risks of such procedures must be thoroughly addressed by clinicians.

Various herbal remedies and nutritional supplements are advertised to promote weight loss by boosting the metabolic rate; however, controlled clinical studies have not been conducted. Chromium picolinate is touted to help burn fat and build muscle. Studies are conflicting regarding chromium's effect on weight, although at least one study found that, when combined with a diet and exercise program, chromium produced favorable changes in body composition (more lean tissue and less fat). However, toxic effects are not well known. Remedies containing ephedra should be avoided. This plant contains the stimulant ephedrine, which can cause adverse effects on the central nervous system, heart rate, and blood pressure.

Bibliography

AACE/ACE obesity statement. *Endocr Prac* 1997;3:164-188.

American Cancer Society. Cancer Prevention & Early detection: Facts & Figures 2002. Atlanta, GA: American Cancer Society; 2002. Accessible at http://www.cancer.org/eprise/main/docroot/stt/stt_0.

Beresford SA, Boushey CJ. Homocysteine, folic acid and cardiovascular disease risk. In: Bendich A, Deckelbaum R, eds. *Preventive Nutrition.* 2nd ed. Totowa, NJ: Humana Press; 2001:191-219.

Bolton-Smith C, Woodward M, Fenton S, Brown CA. Does dietary trans fatty acid intake relate to the prevalence of coronary heart disease in Scotland? *Eur Heart J* 1996;17:837-845.

Calle EE, Thun MJ, Petrelli JM, Rodriguez C, Heath CW. Body mass index and mortality in a prospective cohort of U.S. adults. *N Engl J Med* 1999;341:1097-1105.

Canadian Society for Exercise Physiology. *Canada's Physical Activity Guide to Healthy Active Living.* Accessible at http://www.hc-sc.gc.ca/ hppb/paguide/intro.html.

Cassidenti DL, Vijod AG, Vijod MA, Stanczyk FZ, Lobo RA. Short-term effects of smoking on the pharmacokinetic profiles of micronized estradiol in postmenopausal women. *Am J Obstet Gynecol* 1990;163:1953-1960.

Cornuz J, Feskanich D, Willett WC, Colditz GA. Smoking, smoking cessation, and risk of hip fracture in women. *Am J Med* 1999; 106:311-314.

Cummings SR, Nevitz MC, Browner WS, et al, for the Study of Osteoporotic Fractures Research Group. Risk factors for hip fracture in white women. *N Engl J Med* 1995;332:767-773.

Drewnowski A, Warren-Mears VA. Does aging change nutrition requirements? *J Nutr Health Aging* 2001;5:70-74.

Emmert DH, Kirchner JT. The role of vitamin E in the prevention of heart disease. *Arch Fam Med* 1999;8:537-542.

Feskanich D, Korrick SA, Greenspan SL, Rosen HN, Colditz GA. Moderate alcohol consumption and bone density among postmenopausal women. *J Womens Health* 1999;8:65-73.

Fuchs CS, Stampfer MJ, Colditz GA, et al. Alcohol consumption and mortality among women. *N Engl J Med* 1995;332:1245-1250.

Geleijnse JM, Launer LJ, Hofman A, Pols HA, Witteman JC. Tea flavonoids may protect against atherosclerosis: the Rotterdam Study. *Arch Intern Med* 1999;159:2170-2174.

Ginsburg ES, Mello NK, Mendelson JH, et al. Effects of alcohol ingestion on estrogens in postmenopausal women. *JAMA* 1996;276:1747-1751.

Harris SS, Dawson-Hughes B. Caffeine and bone loss in healthy postmenopausal women. *Am J Clin Nutr* 1994;60:573-578.

Health Canada. *Physical Activity of Canadians: Baby Boomers Aged 40 to 54.* Ottawa, ON, Canada: National Population Health Survey Highlights; 1999.

Hu FB, Stampfer MJ, Manson JE, et al. Dietary fat intake and the risk of coronary heart disease in women. *N Engl J Med* 1997; 337:1491-1499.

Jensen J, Christiansen C, Rodbro P. Cigarette smoking, serum estrogens, and bone loss during hormone-replacement therapy early after menopause. *N Engl J Med* 1985;313:973-975.

Jacobs DR Jr, Meyer KA, Kushi LH, Folsom AR. Whole-grain intake may reduce the risk of ischemic heart disease death in postmenopausal women: the Iowa Women's Health Study. *Am J Clin Nutr* 1998;68:248-257.

Joshipura KJ, Hu FB, Manson JE, et al. The effect of fruit and vegetable intake on risk for coronary heart disease. *Ann Intern Med* 2001;134:1106-1114.

Kato I, Toniolo P, Akhmedkhanov A, et al. Prospective study of factors influencing the onset of natural menopause. *J Clin Epidemiol* 1998;51:1271-1276.

Kawachi I, Colditz GA, Stampfer MJ, et al. Smoking cessation and time course of decreased risks of coronary heart disease in middle-aged women. *Arch Intern Med* 1994;154:169-175.

Knekt P, Jarvinen R, Reunanen A, Maatela J. Flavonoid intake and coronary mortality in Finland: a cohort study. *BMJ* 1996;312:478-481.

Koffman DM, Bazzarre T, Mosca L, Redberg R, Schmid T, Wattigney WA. An evaluation of Choose to Move 1999: an American Heart Association physical activity program for women. *Arch Intern Med* 2001;161:2193-2199.

Kohlmeier L, Kark JD, Gomez-Gracia E, et al. Lycopene and myocardial infarction risk in the EURAMIC Study. *Am J Epidemiol* 1997;146:618-626.

Krall EA, Dawson-Hughes B. Smoking and bone loss among postmenopausal women. *J Bone Miner Res* 1991;6:331-338.

Kris-Etherton P, Eckel RH, Howard BV, St. Jeor S, Bazzarre TL, for the Nutrition Committee, Population Science Committee, and Clinical Science Committee of the American Heart Association. AHA science advisory: Lyon Diet Heart Study. Benefits of a Mediterranean-style diet. National Cholesterol Education Program/American Heart Association step I dietary pattern on cardiovascular disease. *Circulation* 2001;103:1823-1825.

Kritckevsky SB, Kritchevsky D. Egg consumption and coronary heart disease: an epidemiologic overview. *J Am Coll Nutr* 2000; 19(5 suppl):549S-555S.

Kuller LH, Simkin-Silverman LR, Wing RR, Meilahn EN, Ives DG. Women's Healthy Lifestyle Project: a randomized clinical trial. *Circulation* 2001;103:32-37.

Kushi LH, Meyer KA, Jacobs DR Jr. Cereals, legumes, and chronic disease risk reduction: evidence from epidemiologic studies. *Am J Clin Nutr* 1999;70(3 suppl):451S-458S.

Landolt HP, Roth C, Dijk DJ, Borbely AA. Late-afternoon ethanol intake affects nocturnal sleep and the sleep EEG in middle-aged men. *J Clin Psychopharmacol* 1996;16:428-436.

Liu S, Stampfer MJ, Hu FB, et al. Whole-grain consumption and risk of coronary heart disease: results from the Nurses' Health Study. *Am J Clin Nutr* 1999;70:412-419.

Lloyd T, Johnson-Rollings N, Eggli DF, Kieselhorst K, Mauger EA, Cusatis DC. Bone status among postmenopausal women with different habitual caffeine intakes: a longitudinal investigation. *J Am Coll Nutr* 2000;19:256-261.

Longnecker MP, Newcomb PA, Mittendorf R, et al. Risk of breast cancer in relation to lifetime alcohol consumption. *J Natl Cancer Inst* 1995;87:923-929.

Makomaski Illing EM, Kaiserman M. Mortality attributable to tobacco use in Canada and its regions,1994-1996. *Health Canada* 1999;20:111-117.

Montemuro S, Fluker M, Rogers J, Derzko C. Menopause: healthy living. Canadian consensus on menopause and osteoporosis. *J SOGC* 2001;23:842-848.

Moore T, Conlin P, Ard J, Svetky L. DASH diet is effective treatment for stage 1 isolated systolic hypertension. *Hypertension* 2001; 38:155-158.

National Cholesterol Education Program/American Heart Association step I dietary pattern on cardiovascular disease. *Circulation* 2001;103:1823-1825.

National Institutes of Health Consensus Development Panel on Osteoporosis Prevention, Diagnosis, and Therapy. Osteoporosis prevention, diagnosis, and therapy. *JAMA* 2001;285:785-795.

Nelson ME, Fiatarone MA, Morganti CM, et al. Effects of high-intensity strength training on multiple risk factors for osteoporotic fractures: a randomized controlled trial. *JAMA* 1994;272:1909-1914.

The North American Menopause Society. Management of postmenopausal osteoporosis: position statement of The North American Menopause Society. *Menopause* 2002;9:84-101.

The North American Menopause Society. The role of isoflavones in menopausal health: consensus opinion of The North American Menopause Society. *Menopause* 2000;7:215-229.

Notelovitz M, Martin D, Tesar R, et al. Estrogen therapy and variable-resistance weight training increase bone mineral in surgically menopausal women. *J Bone Miner Res* 1991;6:583-590.

Potter JD. Nutrition and colorectal cancer. *Cancer Causes Control* 1996;7:127-146.

Province MA, Hadley EC, Hornbrook MC, et al. The effects of exercise on falls in elderly patients: a preplanned meta-analysis of the FICSIT trials. Frailty and injuries: cooperative studies of intervention techniques. *JAMA* 1995;273:1341-1347.

Reubinoff BE, Wurtman J, Rojansky N, et al. Effects of hormone replacement therapy on weight, body composition, fat distribution, and food intake in early postmenopausal women: a prospective study. *Fertil Steril* 1995;64:963-968.

Rexrode KM, Carey VJ, Hennekens CH, Walters EE, et al. Abdominal adiposity and coronary heart disease in women. *JAMA* 1998; 280:1843-1848.

Ricci TA, Chowdhury HA, Heymsfield SB, Stahl T, Pierson RN Jr, Shapses SA. Calcium supplementation suppresses bone turnover during weight reduction in postmenopausal women. *J Bone Miner Res* 1998;13:1045-1050.

Rigotti NA. Treatment of tobacco use and dependence. *N Engl J Med* 2002;346:506-512.

Rimm EB, Willett WC, Hu FB, et al. Folate and vitamin B_6 from diet and supplements in relation to risk of coronary heart disease among women. *JAMA* 1998;279:359-364.

Russell RM, Rasmussen H, Lichtenstein AH. Modified food guide pyramid for people over seventy years of age. *J Nutr* 1999; 129:751-753.

Sacks FM, Svetkey LP, Vollmer WM, et al, for the DASH-Sodium Collaborative Research Group. Effects on blood pressure of reduced dietary sodium and the Dietary Approaches to Stop Hypertension (DASH) diet. *N Engl J Med* 2001;344:3-10.

Schatzkin A, Lanza E, Corle D, et al for the Polyp Prevention Trial Study Group. Lack of effect of a low-fat, high-fiber diet on the recurrence of colorectal adenomas. *N Engl J Med* 2000; 342:1149-1155.

Slavin JL, Jacobs D, Marquart L, Wiemer K. The role of whole grains in disease prevention. *J Am Diet Assoc* 2001;101:780-785.

Slemenda CW, Hui SL, Longcope C, et al. Cigarette smoking, obesity, and bone mass. *J Bone Miner Res* 1989;4:737-741.

Smith-Warner SA, Spiegelman D, Adami HO, et al. Types of dietary fat and breast cancer: a pooled analysis of cohort studies. *Int J Cancer* 2001;92:767-774.

Smith-Warner SA, Spiegelman D, Yaun S, et al. Alcohol and breast cancer in women: a pooled analysis of cohort studies. *JAMA* 1998;279:535-540.

Sokol RJ, Martier SS, Ager JW. The T-ACE questions: practical prenatal detection of risk-drinking. *Am J Obstet Gynecol* 1989;160:863-868.

Stampfer MJ, Hennekens CH, Manson JE, Colditz GA, Rosner B, Willett WC. Vitamin E consumption and the risk of coronary disease in women. *N Engl J Med* 1993;328:1444-1449.

Stampfer MJ, Hu FB, Manson JE, Rimm EB, Willett WC. Primary prevention of coronary heart disease in women through diet and lifestyle. *N Engl J Med* 2000;343:16-22.

Stephens NG, Parsons A, Schofield PM, et al. Randomized controlled trial of vitamin E in patients with coronary disease: Cambridge Heart Antioxidant Study (CHAOS). *Lancet* 1996;347:781-786.

US Department of Health and Human Services. *Healthy People 2010.* Washington, DC: US Department of Health and Human Services; 2000. Accessible at www.health.gov/healthypeople/document/.

Varenna M, Binelli L, Zucchi F, Ghiringhelli D, Sinigaglia L. Unbalanced diet to lower serum cholesterol level is a risk factor for postmenopausal osteoporosis and distal forearm fracture. *Osteoporos Int* 2001;12:296-301.

Velie E, Kulldorff M, Schairer C, Block G, Albanes D, Schatzkin A. Dietary fat, fat subtypes, and breast cancer in postmenopausal women: a prospective cohort study. *J Natl Cancer Inst* 2000; 92:833-839.

Verhoef P, Stampfer MJ, Buring JE, et al. Homocysteine metabolism and risk of myocardial infarction: relation with vitamins B_6, B_{12}, and folate. *Am J Epidemiol* 1996;143:845-859.

Warren MP, Artacho CA. Role of exercise and nutrition. In Lobo, RA, ed. *Treatment of the Postmenopausal Woman: Basic and Clinical Aspects.* 2nd ed. Philadelphia, PA: Lippincott Williams & Wilkins; 1999:417-436.

Wing RR, Matthews KA, Kuller LH, Meilahn EN, Plantinga PL. Weight gain at the time of menopause. *Arch Intern Med* 1991; 151:97-102.

Wolff I, van Croonenborg JJ, Kemper HC, Kostense PJ, Twisk JW. The effects of exercise training programs on bone mass: a meta-analysis of published controlled trials in pre- and postmenopausal women. *Osteoporos Int* 1999;9:1-12.

Wu AH, Pike MC, Stram DO. Meta-analysis: dietary fat intake, serum estrogen levels, and the risk of breast cancer. *J Natl Cancer Inst* 1999;91:529-534.

Wurtman JJ. Depression and weight gain: the serotonin connection. *J Affect Disord* 1993;29:183-192.

Yochum L, Kushi LH, Meyer K, Folsom AR. Dietary flavonoid intake and risk of cardiovascular disease in postmenopausal women [published erratum in *Am J Epidemiol* 1999;150:432]. *Am J Epidemiol* 1999;149:943-949.

Yong LC, Brown CC, Schatzkin A, Schairer C. Prospective study of relative weight and risk of breast cancer: the Breast Cancer Detection Demonstration Project follow-up study, 1979 to 1987-1989. *Am J Epidemiol* 1996;143:985-995.

Yusuf S, Dagenais G, Pogue J, Bosch J, Sleight P, for the Heart Outcomes Prevention Evaluation Study Investigators. Vitamin E supplementation and cardiovascular events in high-risk patients. *N Engl J Med* 2000;342:154-160.

Zeigler RG, Mayne ST, Swanson CA. Nutrition and lung cancer. *Cancer Causes Control* 1996;7:157-177.

Zemel MB. Calcium modulation of hypertension and obesity: mechanisms and implications. *J Am Coll Nutr* 2001; 20(5 suppl):428S-435S.

Many nonprescription (ie, over-the-counter) therapies are available to treat menopause-related symptoms. Women should be questioned about all therapies they are using, including those available over the counter (OTC). Nonprescription products are not without risk and can result in misuse (eg, taking higher than the recommended dose or combining them with other therapies with which they may adversely interact).

Some nonprescription products for menopause-related symptoms and other conditions of midlife and beyond are promoted as "natural." Because this term is defined inconsistently and it is associated with misinformation and misunderstanding, NAMS avoids its use except when distinguishing (natural) progesterone from synthetic progestins (available by prescription).

Many of these products are marketed as dietary supplements. Among the nonprescription products are vitamin E, soy products, and a variety of herbal products. Scientific data supporting the use of these products are limited. For information about complementary and alternative medicine (CAM) approaches (including soy and herbal products), see Section I.

G.01. Government regulations for dietary supplements

Until recently, US marketers of dietary supplements could make "structure and function" health claims (eg, enhances muscles) without prior FDA review, but they could not claim that a product prevents, treats, or cures a disease (eg, prevents heart attacks, cures depression) unless the FDA had approved the claim. In February 2000, the FDA announced its decision to permit dietary supplement marketers to make health claims for "natural conditions" (eg, hot flashes, age-related memory loss) without providing documentation for efficacy or safety. Serious medical conditions (eg, prevents heart attacks, prevents osteoporosis) remain in the disease category under the new ruling.

Most dietary supplements, composed of essential nutrients such as vitamins and minerals, were first classified as food. In 1990, the Nutrition Labeling and Education Act added "herbs or similar nutritional substances" to its definition of dietary supplements. In 1994, Congress passed the Dietary Supplement Health and Education Act (DSHEA), which created a dietary supplement category that is neither drug nor food. It defines a dietary supplement as a pill, capsule, tablet, or liquid that contains a "dietary ingredient." These include vitamins, minerals, amino acids, enzymes, organ tissues, herbs, and plants in various forms (such as extracts) and combinations.

Under the current law, the marketer is responsible for ensuring that the labels are truthful and not misleading, that labels contain enough information for consumers to make an informed choice, that the serving size ("dosage") is appropriate, and that all the dietary ingredients in the product are accurately listed and safe. The label must identify the product as a dietary supplement. If a product is suspected of causing harm, the FDA can halt sales and have it analyzed.

In Canada, the regulations are similar to those in the United States. Although Health Canada's Office of Natural Health Products was created in 1999 to oversee regulation, labeling, monitoring, and research of natural health products, there is no routine surveillance for product quality. Several hundred herbal product brands have been reviewed and issued Drug Identification Numbers (DIN) or General Public numbers (GP) by the Therapeutic Products Program of Health Canada; however, this review confirms a product's formulation, labeling, and instructions, not bioactivity or clinical efficacy. The Society of Obstetricians and Gynaecologists of Canada advise Canadian women to purchase only those brands with a DIN or GP.

Bibliography

Chandler F, ed. *Herbs: Everyday Reference for Health Professionals.* Ottawa, ON, Canada: Canadian Pharmacists Association and the Canadian Medical Association; 2000.

Fluker MR, Montemuro S. Complementary approaches. *J SOGC* 2001;23:1204-1213.

US Food and Drug Administration Center for Food Safety and Applied Nutrition. *Dietary Supplement Health and Education Act of 1994.* Accessible at http://vm.cfsan.fda.gov/~dms/dietsupp.html.

G.02. Vitamins and minerals

The human body requires more than 45 vitamins and minerals to maintain health. Since 1994, the National Academy of Sciences has been involved in revising dietary reference standards known as Dietary Reference Intakes (DRIs). This provides a set of four nutrient-based reference values designed to replace the Recommended Dietary Allowances (RDA) in the United States and the Recommended Nutrient Intakes (RNI) in Canada. The DRIs include Recommended Dietary Allowances (RDA), Estimated Average Requirements (EAR), Adequate Intake (AI), and Tolerable Upper Intake Levels (UL). Table 1 lists selected RDAs and ULs for women aged 50 and older.

Table 1. Selected dietary intake recommendations for women aged 50 and older

Nutrient	Recommended Dietary Allowances (RDA)	Tolerable Upper Intake Level (UL)
Vitamins		
Vitamin A	3,300 IU	10,000 IU
Vitamin C	—	>2,000 mg/day
— nonsmokers	75 mg	—
— smokers	110 mg	—
Vitamin D	—	50 µg/day
— age 50-70	400 IU	—
— age 70+	600 IU	—
Vitamin E	15 mg	1,000 mg/day
Folate	400 µg	1,000 mg/day
Vitamin B_6 (pyridoxine)	1.5 mg	100 mg
Vitamin B_{12}	2.4 µg	No UL established
Minerals		
Calcium	1,200 mg	2,500 mg/day
Magnesium	320 mg	350 mg/day
Phosphorus	700 mg	1 g/day (age 19-70 yr); 3 g/day (>70 yr)

G.02.a. Calcium

Calcium is the body's most abundant mineral. Almost all (99%) of the total calcium stores are contained in the skeletal structure, with the remainder in the cells of soft tissue, the bloodstream, and extracellular fluid, where it exerts an effect on the cardiovascular system, nervous system, and muscles.

The importance of an adequate calcium intake for skeletal health is well-established. In addition, calcium is associated with beneficial effects in several nonskeletal disorders, primarily hypertension, colorectal cancer, obesity, and nephrolithiasis, although the extent of those effects and mechanisms involved have not been fully explored. Low calcium intake may also be associated with premenstrual syndrome.

Calcium requirements for skeletal maintenance fluctuate throughout a woman's life. During the teen years, calcium requirements are high because of the demands of a rapidly growing skeleton. During a woman's 20s, less calcium is required as bone turnover stabilizes and peak adult bone mass is achieved. Calcium requirements remain stable until menopause when the bone resorption rate increases and bone mass declines, associated with the fall in ovarian estrogen production. Calcium needs rise at that time because of a decrease in the efficiency of utilization of dietary calcium, which is also associated with the fall in ovarian estrogen production. The amount of calcium needed is also affected by the age-related decrease in intestinal absorption.

Most experts and clinicians follow published guidelines from either the National Institutes of Health (NIH) or the National Academy of Sciences (NAS). Optimally, food sources should provide the required calcium intake, with additional calcium supplementation added, as needed. United States and Canadian postmenopausal women have low calcium intakes, with median intakes of approximately 600 mg/day.

Current guidelines from the NIH (established in 1994) regarding osteoporosis prevention recommend the following daily amounts of elemental calcium:

- Premenopausal women aged 25 to 50   1,000 mg

- Postmenopausal women younger than age 65 and using ERT   1,000 mg

- Postmenopausal women not on ERT   1,500 mg

- All women older than age 65   1,500 mg

In 1997, the NAS published its revised recommendations for daily elemental calcium consumption. Although the amounts for older women are less than those recommended by the NIH, the NAS guidelines call for more calcium during the teen years.

- Age 19-30   1,000 mg

- Age 31-50   1,000 mg

- Age 51 and older   1,200 mg

Adults absorb only 30% to 50% of a calcium load, and the absorption decreases with age. By age 65, intestinal calcium absorption typically has declined to below 50% of peak adolescent absorption, which affects the amount of calcium needed in the gut. The renal enzymatic activity that produces vitamin D metabolites (which control calcium absorption) decreases with age. Dietary factors that limit calcium absorption include the following:

- lack of vitamin D (as a result of age-related declines in intake, dermal synthesis, renal enzymatic activity, and intestinal responsiveness),

- consuming excessive amounts of oxalic acid (found in spinach and some other greens),

- consuming large amounts of phytates (a type of fiber found in wheat bran and some other grains),

- possibly, consuming tannins (found in tea).

Evidence indicates that other dietary components, such as fat, phosphorus, magnesium, and caffeine, have negligible effects on calcium absorption at generally applicable intake levels. Calcium, on the other hand, has been shown to lower the rate of iron absorption in single-meal tests; however, in general, the body up-regulates iron absorption to compensate. Nevertheless, it is generally advised that iron supplements not be taken with calcium.

Dairy products are the most common source of dietary calcium. They have a high calcium content and are reasonably priced. A glass of milk will provide about 300 mg of calcium. Leafy green vegetables, nuts, and dried beans also contain calcium. Various calcium-fortified foods are available, such as special soy products and fruit juices.

An estimated 25% of the US population and 70% of the world's population may have some degree of lactase nonpersistence (ie, inability to metabolize lactose in dairy products), leading to diarrhea, bloating, and gas. Lactase nonpersistence is more common among people of Asian, African, and South American descent. Other gastrointestinal problems (eg, celiac disease, irritable bowel syndrome, Crohn's disease, gastrointestinal infection) can cause lactose intolerance — either temporary or permanent. However, many women with lactase nonpersistence may condition their intestinal flora to produce lactase by gradually increasing their dairy intake.

Women who find it difficult to meet their calcium goals include those who are lactose intolerant, follow a vegetarian diet, or have poor eating habits. Many clinicians recommend calcium supplements for all women to ensure that adequate levels are achieved. Supplements should be taken in small doses (250-500 mg) throughout the day, usually with meals. Consuming calcium supplements with meals also can minimize the potential for gastrointestinal side effects.

The total dosage of a calcium supplement is based on the amount of elemental calcium contained in a supplement. For example, 1,250 mg of calcium carbonate (40% elemental calcium) provides 500 mg of calcium. Most products list the available calcium per serving. Recommended calcium levels (either reference values or dietary recommended intakes) refer to elemental calcium.

Clinicians should advise women to consider the amount of calcium consumed in their diets before determining the amount necessary to take in supplements. The use of higher than recommended calcium intakes produces no currently recognized health benefits to women, and side effects can occur. Intakes greater than 2,500 mg/day (the upper limit for healthy adults set by the National Academy of Sciences) can increase the risk for hypercalciuria and, possibly, hypercalcemia which, in extreme cases, can lead to kidney damage.

Not all experts agree on what kind of calcium is best. The two most common types of calcium supplements consist of calcium carbonate or calcium citrate.

- Calcium carbonate (eg, Tums) provides 40% elemental calcium. Calcium carbonate products are typically less expensive than most other types of calcium supplements and are the most widely used calcium supplement.

- Calcium citrate supplements (eg, Citracal) contain the tetrahydrated form, providing 21% of elemental calcium. In healthy individuals, most experts agree that absorption of calcium citrate and calcium carbonate appears to be about the same, if taken with meals.

Other calcium products on the market include the following:

- Effervescent calcium supplements are calcium products (typically calcium carbonate) combined with materials that facilitate dissolving in water or orange juice to aid swallowing and improve absorption. Liquid forms are also available.

- Calcium citrate malate, which usually costs more than calcium carbonate.

- Calcium chelates are supplements containing calcium that is chelated (ie, bound) to an amino acid (eg, bisglycinocalcium) in an attempt to make calcium more readily absorbed. These exhibit superior absorbability, although at a higher cost.

- Bone meal, dolomite, or oyster shell calcium supplements. In the past, some of these contained toxic contaminants, especially lead; however, a more recent analysis of the most commonly used brands did not reveal toxic levels of contaminants.

Data from more than 20 studies indicate that calcium monotherapy results in bone losses of 0.014% per year compared with 1.0% per year in untreated women, and longer-term trials have shown this sustained benefit for up to 4 years. The most pronounced effect is seen in women 5 or more years postmenopause, although all peri- and early postmenopausal women need to maintain adequate calcium intake for their general health and to prevent additional loss of bone mineral density (BMD) associated with lower estrogen levels. More importantly, in the presence of adequate vitamin D, calcium has been found to reduce the incidence of spine, hip, and other fractures. Also, in controlled clinical trials of calcium supplementation without additional vitamin D, a mean dose of 1,050 mg/day reduced spinal fracture rates from 25% to 70%.

In a review of 17 trials looking at the benefits of exercise, including resistance training and low- to high-impact exercise, calcium supplementation significantly improved BMD.

The NAMS Consensus Opinion on the role of calcium in peri- and postmenopausal women states that calcium alone or with vitamin D (especially in women ≤5 years postmenopause) is not as effective in reducing menopause-related bone loss as are ERT/HRT, selective estrogen-receptor modulators (SERMs), or bisphosphonates.

Calcium supplementation, however, did improve the efficacy of both ERT/HRT and nasal calcitonin.

In the key trials with selective estrogen-receptor modulators (SERMs) and bisphosphonates, all participants have received calcium. Therefore, true placebo controls have not been used. This is because of the well-established need for adequate calcium intake.

A meta-analysis of the relation between dietary calcium intake and blood pressure concluded that supplemental calcium intake significantly lowers blood pressure (systolic –0.15 mm Hg per 100 mg/day of calcium; diastolic –0.051 mm Hg per 100 mg/day of calcium) for some, but not all, treatment cohorts. These data are not sufficient to support a general recommendation that women take calcium solely to prevent or treat hypertension.

High calcium intake may provide protection against colorectal cancer. In the largest controlled trial (930 men and women), 1,200 mg/day of calcium significantly reduced the risk of recurrent colorectal adenomas (RR, 0.85). Again, these data are not sufficient to support a general recommendation that women take calcium solely to prevent colorectal cancer.

The third National Health and Nutrition Examination Survey (NHANES III) found an inverse correlation between dietary calcium intake and the risk of obesity. Other investigators found a similar inverse relationship between BMI and calcium intake in two studies of perimenopausal women as well as a significant weight loss in a controlled trial of calcium supplementation in older women. This may be due to the fact that low calcium intake increases parathyroid hormone and 1,25-dihydroxyvitamin D levels and stimulates adipose cell metabolism to switch from lipolysis to lipogenesis, which results in fat storage. The NAMS Consensus Opinion on calcium agrees that the limited data suggest a statistically strong, inverse correlation, but that calcium intake explains only a part of the variability in body weight in postmenopausal women.

Several studies have indicated that calcium intakes up to 1,500 mg/day do not appear to increase the risk of developing renal calculi and probably reduce the risk. In the Nurses' Health Study, women with dietary calcium intakes above 1,000 mg/day had a significantly reduced relative risk of 0.65 of developing an initial renal calculus compared with women with lower calcium intakes.

Finally, 1,000 mg/day of supplemental calcium plus vitamin D reduced tooth loss over a 5-year period in a study of 145 healthy individuals aged 65 years or older.

G.02.b. Vitamin D

Vitamin D primarily affects the bones, kidneys, and intestines. It raises calcium blood levels through several pathways, helping to maintain blood calcium levels in the normal range. If vitamin D is lacking, calcium is not well absorbed, no matter how much calcium is consumed. Without adequate vitamin D, a woman is at increased risk for osteoporosis. Vitamin D deficiency is also a cause of chronic fatigue.

Vitamin D is synthesized from the skin's exposure to ultraviolet rays in sunlight. The liver converts the vitamin to its active form (25-hydroxyvitamin D_3). In general, approximately 15 minutes of sun exposure daily is considered adequate, although clinical trial data have not confirmed this. Risk factors for inadequate sun exposure include long work hours, living in northern latitudes, being homebound or institutionalized, using high SPF sunscreens, or avoiding the sun. There is some evidence that dark skin pigmentation partially inhibits conversion of sunlight to useable vitamin D.

For women at risk of inadequate sun exposure, vitamin D will need to be obtained through meals or supplements. The current RDA for vitamin D is 400 International Units (IU) daily for women aged 51 to 70 years and 600 IU/day for women over age 70. The National Osteoporosis Foundation recommends 400 to 800 IU/day for women at risk of suboptimal intake, such as women who are elderly, chronically ill, or institutionalized. Some research suggests that vitamin D deficiency may be more common than had been thought among adults living in northern latitudes and that optimum intakes for vitamin D, like calcium, may be higher than the RDA.

Vitamin D can be toxic in high amounts; one possible outcome is hypercalciuria. The tolerable upper limit is 2,000 IU/day, and most people should avoid daily amounts over 1,000 IU.

Good food sources of vitamin D include egg yolks, liver, and oily fish (eg, herring, salmon). Fish oil (one teaspoon of cod liver oil provides 1,100 IU) is another option. Caution is needed with fish oil or fish oil capsules, however, since these also contain vitamin A; both vitamins D and A are fat-soluble and can be stored in the body at levels high enough to be toxic.

Milk (fortified with vitamin D) is an excellent source of vitamin D; however, one would have to drink a quart of milk (4 cups) each day to obtain 400 IU of vitamin D. Not many people consume that much milk on a regular basis nor is that amount of milk recommended daily. Use of low-fat (1%) or skim milk avoids unneeded calories and fat.

Dietary requirements can usually be met with a daily multivitamin/mineral supplement. The standard recommendation for most clinicians involved in the prevention and treatment of osteoporosis is a multivitamin/mineral supplement for all individuals over age 65, unless contraindicated by specific medical conditions. Nearly all multivitamins provide the necessary 400 IU. The ability to convert vitamin D to its active form to facilitate calcium absorption is less efficient with aging. A multivitamin containing vitamin D enhances optimal calcium absorption in older individuals.

Many calcium supplements contain vitamin D (usually 125-200 IU/tablet). Women in midlife may also find this a convenient way to obtain adequate levels of both nutrients. It is not necessary, however, for all women to take a combined supplement of vitamin D and calcium.

In studies of women over age 65, those receiving 700 to 800 IU of vitamin D daily (along with calcium) had fewer hip and other nonvertebral fractures. In addition, findings of the Nurses' Health Study suggested an inverse association between total intake of vitamin D (food and supplements) and colorectal cancer.

G.02.c. Vitamin E

Vitamin E acts as an antioxidant in the blood and tissues. It enhances the immune system and is needed for iron metabolism.

The recommended vitamin E daily intake has been increased to 15 mg for both women and men. Food sources include nuts, seeds, whole grains, vegetable oil, and wheat germ.

The equivalent from supplements is 22 IU of d-alpha-tocopherol (natural source) or 33 IU of dl-alpha-tocopherol (synthetic form). The natural form is the only type of vitamin E that human blood can maintain and transfer to cells when needed. For easiest digestion, vitamin E supplements should be taken with a meal containing fats. Since vitamin E is a fat-soluble vitamin, overdoses can cause toxic effects.

There is anecdotal evidence that vitamin E (400-800 IU/day) relieves hot flashes, although this is not supported by controlled clinical trials. A placebo-controlled, randomized crossover trial evaluated vitamin E supplements (800 IU/day for 4 weeks) for relief of hot flashes in 120 women who were breast cancer survivors. Vitamin E therapy was associated with only a marginal (not statistically significant) decrease in hot flashes.

Data investigating the role of vitamin E in preventing low-density lipoprotein oxidation are inconclusive. In the Nurses' Health Study, women taking vitamin E supplements for more than 2 years had a lower relative risk of a major coronary event compared with those not using this supplement. The Cambridge Heart Antioxidant Study reported a significant reduction in the risk of nonfatal myocardial infarction in patients taking high doses of vitamin E (400 or 800 IU).

There is no strong evidence that vitamin E prevents cancers in women.

Women taking anticoagulants, such as warfarin (Coumadin), should be cautioned against taking vitamin E supplements because of potential synergistic effects.

G.02.d. B vitamins

The B-complex vitamins are sometimes used by women in midlife and beyond to help relieve dry skin and dry hair.

Elevated plasma homocysteine levels, which vitamin B_6, B_{12}, and folate have been shown to lower, have been linked to an increased risk of vascular disease. Data from the Nurses' Health Study showed that after controlling for cardiovascular risk factors, women with the highest folate and vitamin B_6 intake had a lower relative risk for fatal and nonfatal heart attacks than women with low intake.

In 2002, the FDA agreed to allow manufacturers of B vitamins to make the following claim regarding reduction of cardiovascular disease risk: "As part of a well-balanced diet that is low in saturated fat and cholesterol, folic acid, vitamin B_6, and vitamin B_{12} may reduce the risk of vascular disease."

Virtually all multivitamins contain the recommended amounts of B vitamins. Vitamin B supplements can cause the urine to turn bright yellow-orange and to have an unusual odor.

Vitamin B_{12} is needed to make red blood cells and help maintain nerve function. Vitamin B_{12} is found in all animal foods. Older adults who develop atrophic gastritis lack the stomach acid that separates vitamin B_{12} from protein foods. They can become vitamin B_{12} deficient and at risk for pernicious anemia. However, vitamin B_{12} is absorbed from supplements even in the presence of gastric atrophy.

The RDA for women for vitamin B_{12} is 2.4 mcg. Vitamin B_{12} is not toxic in high doses.

Vitamin B_6 (pyridoxine) is needed for metabolism of protein and fat, plays an important role in the development of red blood cells, and supports the production of serotonin in the brain. Low vitamin B_6 levels have been observed among depressed women and some women using hormones (eg, oral contraceptives). An insufficiency of vitamin B_6 has been associated with insomnia and irritability.

Food sources of vitamin B_6 include whole grains, green vegetables, bananas, beans, nuts, and meat. The RDA for women is 1.5 mg. It is generally not advisable to take more than 100 mg of vitamin B_6 daily because of neurologic problems seen with high daily doses taken long term.

Folate supports cell division and growth as well as the development of red blood cells. Folate works with vitamin B_{12} to synthesize DNA.

Folate is the main form in food; folic acid is the primary form of the vitamin in supplements. Good sources of folate include oranges and green leafy vegetables. In addition, some foods (eg, breakfast cereals) have been fortified with folic acid. It may be necessary to take a folic acid supplement to get the RDA of 400 mcg. The synthetic folic acid in supplements and fortified foods can raise blood folate more effectively than can folate derived from food. Adequate vitamin B_{12} is needed for folate efficacy (taking extra vitamin B_{12} may be necessary).

Folic acid in multivitamins was associated with a reduced risk of colon cancer in the Nurses' Health Study. Folate from dietary sources was related to a modest reduction in risk. However, long-term use of multivitamins containing folate (>15 years) was associated with a significant risk reduction (RR, 0.25; 95% CI, 0.13-0.51), although use for less than 15 years did not offer a significant benefit. The same study suggested that the increased risk of breast cancer associated with heavy alcohol consumption may be reduced with 600 mcg/day of total folate intake.

G.02.e. Vitamin A

Vitamin A is a regulator of cell differentiation, protects cells from injury by free radicals, and is necessary for the health of skin, mucous membranes, eyes, and the immune system.

The RDA for vitamin A is 3,300 IU. The best food sources include liver, oily fish, egg yolks, milk, cheese, and butter. Because vitamin A is fat-soluble, overdoses can cause toxic effects.

There is no consensus on the efficacy of vitamin A supplements in cancer prevention. In the Nurses' Health Study, women with the highest total vitamin A intake (from food and supplements) had a significantly decreased incidence of breast cancer compared with women with lower intakes. Only women with a low intake of vitamin A from food were found to benefit from vitamin A supplements.

A Swedish study linked a high intake of vitamin A with low bone density and an increased risk of hip fractures among women. This study corroborates findings from animal studies showing that hypervitaminosis A leads to bone fragility and spontaneous fracture.

G.02.f. Vitamin C

Vitamin C (ascorbic acid) is an antioxidant with many roles in the human body, including wound healing, enhancing the immune system, and helping iron absorption. Food sources include citrus fruits, broccoli, and tomatoes.

The RDA calls for an increase from 60 mg to 75 mg for women (90 mg for men) to achieve maximum saturation in the body. Smokers require an extra 35 mg daily because of greater exposure to oxidative damage. Nonsmokers regularly exposed to tobacco smoke will also need to increase their vitamin C intake. When more than 500 mg is taken daily, there is increased urinary excretion of oxalate and urate. Daily doses below 2,000 mg avoid gastrointestinal problems.

Increased serum ascorbic acid levels have been associated with a decreased prevalence of coronary heart disease and stroke. Vitamin C has also normalized vascular function in individuals with coronary artery disease and associated risk factors, including hypercholesterolemia, hypertension, diabetes, and smoking. However, the American Heart Association and the American Cancer Society, while supporting the increased consumption of fruits and vegetables, do not endorse the use of vitamin C or other antioxidant supplements to reduce the risk of disease.

Supplementary vitamin C may provide a protective effect with respect to cataract formation. Women in the Nurses' Health Study who consumed vitamin C supplements (average dose 500 mg) for at least 10 years were significantly less likely to develop cataracts than women who did not take vitamin C supplements (average dietary intake 130 mg/day).

Vitamin C supplements have been associated with a significantly decreased prevalence of gallbladder disease in alcohol drinkers, but not in nondrinkers.

G.02.g. Chromium

Chromium helps insulin regulate blood glucose levels. No RDA has been established; the adequate intake established by the National Academy of Sciences for women aged 50 and older is 20 mcg/day. Good food sources include cereals, meats, poultry, fish, and beer.

Promotion of high doses of chromium for weight loss has become popular in recent years, but valid trials are lacking. The presumed safety of chromium picolinate and picolinic acid has been questioned. In a 1995 article, chromosomal damage was induced both by the chromium picolinate salt and the ligand in hamster ovary egg germ cells, raising the possibility of mutagenesis and carcinogenesis. The effects were seen with concentrations that were achievable in the serum of humans who take the recommended doses.

The role of chromium supplements in individuals with chromium deficiency or glucose intolerance has not been defined.

G.02.h. Iron

The RDA of elemental iron for menstruating women is 18 mg/day. After menopause, the amount is 8 mg/day. Women who use multivitamin/mineral supplements should be advised to use the appropriate formulation.

Iron is readily available in food. Supplements should not be used without documented iron deficiency. Iron excess is damaging to the cardiovascular system.

Women experiencing heavy uterine bleeding may need additional iron. Iron deficiency is also a cause of chronic fatigue.

G.02.i. Magnesium

Magnesium effects include regulating bone building, increasing gastrointestinal motility, and softening stool, and, possibly, improving mood and providing headache relief. Magnesium deficiency impairs secretion of parathyroid hormone, an action that may reduce calcium absorption and retention, leading to abnormal bone calcification. However, one study found that taking 789 to 826 mg/day (more than double the average daily intake of 280 mg for postmenopausal women) did not affect calcium absorption.

The RDA for women aged 50 and older is 320 mg. The best dietary sources include wheat products, whole grain breads and cereals, pasta, nuts, leafy green vegetables, meats, and milk. Whole grain products contain more magnesium than do refined starches (eg, white bread, white pasta).

Magnesium deficiency can result from diuretic use, diabetes, chronic diarrhea, and alcohol abuse.

Some clinicians support the use of magnesium supplements, not only to counteract any constipating effect of some calcium supplements but also for its bone effects. There is no agreement on what ratio of calcium to magnesium is best (1:1 or 2:1). There is no definitive evidence on the need for magnesium supplements in women who do not have a deficiency. Magnesium deficiency is rare and can be diagnosed only with small intestine biopsy. With adequate calcium intake, many clinicians do not believe that supplementation with magnesium is necessary. Overdoses from magnesium supplements can cause diarrhea, although there is no evidence of adverse effects from consuming naturally occurring magnesium in foods.

G.02.j. Others

The minerals boron, phosphorus, manganese, zinc, and copper are promoted as essential supplemental nutrients in midlife and beyond.

Boron acts as a cofactor in magnesium metabolism and, thus, helps in bone regulation. There is no daily recommended intake for boron, but obtaining 1.5 to 3.0 mg daily is probably adequate — an amount obtainable from eating 5 portions of fruits and vegetables (depending on the boron content of the soil they were grown in). Boron deficiency will exacerbate magnesium deficiency, but boron deficiency is rare, except in alcoholics. A daily multivitamin/mineral with 3 to 9 mg is safe; overdoses can cause nausea, vomiting, and diarrhea.

Phosphorus is an important mineral for bones, with too much or too little resulting in bone loss. One symptom of phosphorus deficiency is bone pain. Low phosphorus levels can result from poor eating habits, intestinal malabsorption, and excessive use of antacids that bind to phosphorus. The RDA for women aged 50 and older is 700 mg, with upper limits set at 3,000 mg/day for women older than 70 and 4,000 mg/day for those aged 50 to 70. Most phosphorus comes from additives in foods such as soft drinks. Other food sources include milk, yogurt, cheese, peas, meat, eggs, and some cereals and bread.

Manganese, zinc, and *copper* may also be related to bone health, among other effects. A multivitamin/mineral supplement will provide a safe amount.

Bibliography

Alaimo K, McDowell MA, Briefel RR. Dietary intake of vitamins, minerals, and fiber of persons ages 2 months and over in the United States: third National Health and Nutrition Examination survey, phase 1, 1988-91. *Adv Data* 1994;259:1-28.

Aloia JF, Vaswani A, Yeh JK, Ross PL, Flaster E, Dilmanian FA. Calcium supplementation with and without hormone replacement therapy to prevent postmenopausal bone loss. *Ann Intern Med* 1994;120:97-103.

Baron JA, Beach M, Mandel JS, et al. Calcium supplements for the prevention of colorectal cancer. *N Engl J Med* 1999;340:101-107.

Barton DL, Loprinzi CL, Quella SK, et al. Prospective evaluation of vitamin E for hot flashes in breast cancer survivors. *J Clin Oncol* 1998;16:495-500.

Birkett NJ. Comments on a meta-analysis of the relation between dietary calcium intake and blood pressure. *Am J Epidemiol* 1998; 148:223-228.

Blatt MHG, Weisbader H, Kupperman HS. Vitamin E and climacteric syndrome. *Arch Intern Med* 1953;91:792-799.

Chapuy MC, Arlot ME, Duboeuf F, et al. Vitamin D and calcium to prevent hip fractures in elderly women. *N Engl J Med* 1992; 327:1637-1642.

Chevalley T, Rizzoli R, Nydeggar V, et al. Effects of calcium supplements on femoral bone mineral density and vertebral fracture rate in vitamin-D-replete elderly patients. *Osteoporos Int* 1994;4:245-252.

Clemens TL, Adams JS, Henderson SL, Holick MF. Increased skin pigment reduces the capacity of the skin to synthesize vitamin D_3. *Lancet* 1982;1:74-76.

Combs GF Jr. *The Vitamins: Fundamental Aspects in Nutrition and Health.* Orlando, FL: Academic Press; 1991:179-204.

Cummings RG. Calcium intake and bone mass: a quantitative review of the evidence. *Calcif Tissue Int* 1990;47:194-201.

Cummings SR, Black DM, Thompson DE, et al. Effect of alendronate on risk of fracture in women with low bone density but without vertebral fractures: results from the Fracture Intervention Trial. *JAMA* 1998;280;2077-2082.

Cummings SR, Nevitt MC, Browner WS, et al. Risk factors for hip fracture in white women. *N Engl J Med* 1995;332:767-773.

Curhan GC, Willett WC, Speizer FE, Spiegelman D, Stampfer MJ. Comparison of dietary calcium with supplemental calcium and other nutrients as factors affecting the risk for kidney stones in women. *Ann Intern Med* 1997;126:497-504.

Davies KM, Heaney RP, Recker RR, et al. Calcium intake and body weight. *J Clin Endocrinol Metab* 2000;85:4635-4638.

Dawson-Hughes B, Dallal GE, Krall EA, et al. A controlled trial of the effect of calcium supplementation on bone density in postmenopausal women. *N Engl J Med* 1990;323;878-883.

Dawson-Hughes B, Harris SS, Krall EA, et al. Effect of calcium and vitamin D supplementation on bone density in men and women 65 years of age or older. *N Engl J Med* 1997;337:670-676.

Deehr MS, Dallal GE, Smith KT, Taulbee JD, Dawson-Hughes B. Effects of different calcium sources on iron absorption in postmenopausal women. *Am J Clin Nutr* 1990;51:95-99.

Elders PJ, Lips P, Netelenbos JC, et al. Long-term effect of calcium supplementation on bone loss in perimenopausal women. *J Bone Min Res* 1994;9:963-970.

Ettinger B, Genant HK, Cann CE. Postmenopausal bone loss is prevented by treatment with low-dosage estrogen with calcium. *Ann Intern Med* 1987;106:40-45.

Gallagher JC, Riggs BL, Eisman J, Hamstra A, Arnaud SB, DeLuca HF. Intestinal calcium absorption and serum vitamin D metabolites in normal subjects and osteoporotic patients: effects of age and dietary calcium. *J Clin Invest* 1979;64:729-736.

Giovannucci E, Stampfer MJ, Colditz GA, et al. Multivitamin use, folate, and colon cancer in women in the Nurses' Health Study. *Ann Intern Med* 1998;129:517-524.

Gloth FM III, Gundberg CM, Hollis BW, Haddad JG Jr, Tobin JD. Vitamin D deficiency in homebound elderly persons. *JAMA* 1995;274:1683-1686.

Hansen C, Werner E, Erbes HJ, Larrat V, Kaltwasser JP. Intestinal calcium absorption from different calcium preparations: influence of anion and solubility. *Osteoporosis Int* 1996;6:386-393.

Heaney RP, Dowell S, Bierman J, Hale C, Bendich A. Absorbability and cost-effectiveness in calcium supplementation. *J Am Coll Nutr* 2001;20:239-246.

Heaney RP, Recker RR, Stegman MR, Moy AJ. Calcium absorption in women: relationships to calcium intake, estrogen status, and age. *J Bone Miner Res* 1989;4:469-475.

Hoeger WW, Harris C, Long EM, Hopkins DR. Four-week supplementation with a natural dietary compound produces favorable changes in body composition. *Adv Ther* 1998;15:305-314.

Holick MF. Vitamin D and bone health. *J Nutr* 1996;126(suppl 4): S1159-S1164.

Holick MF, Matsuoka LY, Wortsman J. Age, vitamin D, and solar ultraviolet [letter]. *Lancet* 1989;2(8671):1104-1105.

Hudson T. *Women's Encyclopedia of Natural Medicine: Alternative Therapies and Integrative Medicine.* Los Angeles, CA: Keats Publishing; 1999.

Hunter DJ, Manson JE, Colditz GA, et al. A prospective study of the intake of vitamins C, E and A and the risk of breast cancer. *N Engl J Med* 1993;329:234-240.

Ilich-Ernst JZ, McKenna AA, Badenhop NE, et al. Iron status, menarche, and calcium supplementation in adolescent girls. *Am J Clin Nutr* 1998;68:880-887.

Jacques PF, Taylor A, Hankinson SE, et al. Long-term vitamin C supplement use and prevalence of early age-related lens opacities. *Am J Clin Nutr* 1997;66:911-916.

Kass-Annese B. Alternative therapies for menopause. *Clin Obstet Gynecol* 2000;43:162-183.

Kuczmarski RJ, Flegal KM, Campbell SM, Johnson CL. Increasing prevalence of overweight among US adults. The National Health and Nutrition Examination Surveys, 1960 to 1991. *JAMA* 1994; 272:205-211.

Krall EA, Dawson-Hughes B. Smoking increases bone loss and decreases intestinal calcium absorption. *J Bone Miner Res* 1999;14:215-220.

Krall EA, Wehler C, Garcia RI, et al. Calcium and vitamin D supplements reduce tooth loss in the elderly. *Am J Med* 2001;111:452-56.

Laitinen K, Valimaki M. Alcohol and bone. *Calcif Tissue Int* 1991;49(suppl):S70-S73.

Levine M, Conry-Cantilena C, Wang Y, et al. Vitamin C pharmacokinetics in healthy volunteers: evidence for a recommended dietary allowance. *Proc Natl Acad Sci USA* 1996;93:3704-3709.

Martinez ME, Giovannucci EL, Colditz GA, et al. Calcium, vitamin D and the occurrence of colorectal cancer among women. *J Natl Cancer Inst* 1996;88:1375-1382.

MacLean D. Nova Scotia Heart Health Program, Health and Welfare Canada, Nova Scotia Department of Health. *The Report of the Nova Scotia Nutrition Survey.* Halifax, NS, Canada; 1993.

McLaren HC. Vitamin E in the menopause. *Br Med J* 1949;2:1378-1382.

Melhus H, Michaelsson K, Kindmark A, et al. Excessive dietary intake of vitamin A is associated with reduced bone mineral density and increased risk for hip fracture. *Ann Intern Med* 1998;129:770-778.

Meydani SN, Meydani M, Blumberg JB, et al. Vitamin E supplementation and in vivo immune response in healthy elderly subjects. *JAMA* 1997;277:1380-1386.

National Institutes of Health. NIH Consensus Development Panel on Optimal Calcium Intake. Optimal calcium intake. *JAMA* 1994; 272:1942-1948.

Nielsen FH. Studies on the relationship between boron and magnesium which possibly affects the formation and maintenance of bones. *Magnes Trace Elem* 1990;9:61-69.

Nieves JW, Komar L, Cosman F, Lindsay R. Calcium potentiates the effect of estrogen and calcitonin on bone mass: review and analysis. *Am J Clin Nutr* 1998;67:18-24.

Nordin BE. Calcium and osteoporosis. *Nutrition* 1997;13:664-686.

Nordin BE, Need AG, Steurer T, et al. Nutrition, osteoporosis, and aging. *Ann NY Acad Sci* 1998;854:336-351.

The North American Menopause Society. Management of postmenopausal osteoporosis: position statement of The North American Menopause Society. *Menopause* 2002;1:84-101.

The North American Menopause Society. The role of calcium in peri- and postmenopausal women: consensus opinion of The North American Menopause Society. *Menopause* 2001;8:84-95.

Recker RR. Calcium absorption and achlorhydria. *N Engl J Med* 1985;313:70-73.

Recker RR, Hinders S, Davies KM, et al. Correcting calcium nutritional deficiency prevents spine fractures in elderly women. *J Bone Miner Res* 1996;11:1961-1966.

Reid JR, Ames RW, Evans MC, Gamble GD, Sharpe SJ. Effect of calcium supplementation on bone loss in postmenopausal women [published erratum appears in *N Engl J Med* 1993;329:1281]. *N Engl J Med* 1993;328:460-464.

Reid JR, Ames RW, Evans MC, Gamble GD, Sharpe SJ. Long-term effects of calcium supplementation on bone loss and fractures in postmenopausal women: a randomized controlled trial. *Am J Med* 1995;98:331-335.

Riggs BL, O'Fallon WM, Muhs J, O'Connor MK, Kumar R, Melton LJ 3rd. Long-term effects of calcium supplementation on serum parathyroid hormone level, bone turnover, and bone loss in elderly women. *J Bone Miner Res* 1998;13:168-174.

Rimm EB, Willett WC, Hu FB, et al. Folate and vitamin B_6 from diet and supplements in relation to risk of coronary heart disease among women. *JAMA* 1998;279:359-364.

Seidl MM, Stewart DE. Alternative treatments for menopausal symptoms: systematic review of scientific and lay literature. *Can Fam Physician* 1998;44:1299-1308.

Simon JA, Grady D, Snabes MC, et al. Ascorbic acid supplement use and the prevalence of gallbladder disease. *J Clin Epidemiol* 1998;5:257-265.

Simon JA, Hudes ES, Browner WS. Serum ascorbic acid and cardiovascular disease prevalence in US adults. *Epidemiology* 1998;9:316-321.

Specker BL. Evidence for an interaction between calcium intake and physical activity on changes in bone mineral density. *J Bone Miner Res* 1996;11:1539-1544.

Stampfer MJ, Hennekens CH, Manson JE, et al. Vitamin E consumption and the risk of coronary disease in women. *N Engl J Med* 1993;328:1444-1449.

Standing Committee on the Scientific Evaluation of Dietary Reference Intakes. *Dietary Reference Intakes for Calcium, Phosphorus, Magnesium, Vitamin D, and Fluoride.* National Academy of Sciences, Institute of Medicine. Washington, DC: National Academy Press; 1999. Accessible at http://www.books.nap.edu/books/0309063507/html/index.html.

Standing Committee on the Scientific Evaluation of Dietary Reference Intakes. *Dietary Reference Intakes for Thiamin, Riboflavin, Niacin, Vitamin B_6, Folate, Vitamin B_{12}, Pantothenic Acid, Biotin, and Choline.* National Academy of Sciences, Institute of Medicine. Washington, DC: National Academy Press; 2000. Accessible at http://www.books.nap.edu/books/0309065542/ html/index.html.

Standing Committee on the Scientific Evaluation of Dietary Reference Intakes. *Dietary Reference Intakes for Vitamin A, Vitamin K, Arsenic, Boron, Chromium, Copper, Iodine, Iron, Manganese, Molybdenum, Nickel, Silicon, Vanadium and Zinc.* National Academy of Sciences, Institute of Medicine. Washington, DC: National Academy Press; 2002. Accessible at http://www.bookd.nap.edu/books/0309072794/html/index.html.

Standing Committee on the Scientific Evaluation of Dietary Reference Intakes. *Dietary Reference Intakes for Vitamin C, Vitamin E, Selenium, and Carotenoids.* National Academy of Sciences, Institute of Medicine. Washington, DC: National Academy Press; 2000. Accessible at http://www.books.nap.edu/books/ 0309069351/html/index.html.

Stephens NG, Parsons A, Schofield PM, et al. Randomized controlled trial of vitamin E in patients with coronary disease: Cambridge Heart Antioxidant Study (CHAOS). *Lancet* 1996;347:781-786.

Suarez FL, Savaiano DA, Levitt MD. A comparison of symptoms after the consumption of milk or lactose-hydrolyzed milk by people with self-reported severe lactose intolerance. *N Engl J Med* 1995; 333:1-4.

Suarez FL, Savaiano DA, Levitt MD. Review article: the treatment of lactose intolerance. *Ailment Pharmacol Ther* 1995;9:589-597.

Thomas MG, Thomson JP, Williamson RC. Oral calcium inhibits rectal epithelial proliferation in familial adenomatous polyposis. *Br J Surg* 1993;80:499-501.

Thys-Jacobs S, Starkey P, Bernstein D, Tian J, for the Premenstrual Study Group. Calcium carbonate and the premenstrual syndrome: effects on premenstrual and menstrual symptoms. *Am J Obstet Gynecol* 1998;179:444-452.

Verhoef P, Stampfer MJ, Buring JE, et al. Homocysteine metabolism and risk of myocardial infarction: relation with vitamins B_6, B_{12}, and folate. *Am J Epidemiol* 1996;143:845-859.

Volpe SJ, Taper LJ, Meacham S. The relationship between boron and magnesium status and bone mineral density in the human: a review. *Magnes Res* 1993;6:291-296.

Whiting SJ. Safety of some calcium supplements questioned. *Nutr Rev* 1994;52:95-97.

Willett WC, Stampfer MJ. What vitamins should I be taking, doctor? *N Engl J Med* 2002;345:1819-1824.

Zemel MB, Shi H, Greer B, Dirienzo D, Zemel PC. Regulation of adiposity by dietary calcium. *FASEB J* 2000;14:1132-1138.

Zhang S, Hunter DJ, Hankinson SE, et al. A prospective study of folate intake and the risk of breast cancer. *JAMA* 1999;281:1632-1637.

G.03. OTC hormones

Three over-the-counter (OTC) hormone preparations require special mention: topical progesterone, DHEA, and melatonin. The passing of the US Dietary and Supplement Act allows these products to be marketed in the United States as dietary supplements.

G.03.a. Topical progesterone

Many brands of topical "natural" progesterone can be purchased without a prescription. These products are regulated as dietary supplements. Although lotions and gels are available, by far the most commonly marketed formulation is a cream. The contents and concentration of the various brands of creams vary widely, ranging from no active ingredient to 450 mg progesterone per ounce, whereas custom-compounded prescription progesterone cream usually contains 400 to 450 mg progesterone per ounce. Most of the US sales are of Pro-Gest cream (containing 20 mg progesterone per one-quarter teaspoon or 450 mg/oz). Pro-Gest is available OTC.

Progesterone is the progestogen secreted by the human ovary and, hence, it is called "bioidentical" or "natural" to distinguish it from synthetic progestogens (ie, progestins). However, the term natural progesterone is redundant. By using the term natural, marketers are capitalizing on consumers' perception that natural products are better or safer.

Marketers of OTC topical progesterone creams claim a variety of benefits, including balancing the hyperestrogenic surges of perimenopause, relief of hot flashes, protection against osteoporosis and breast cancer, and even breast enlargement if applied to the breasts. Clinical trial data do not support these claims.

Some practitioners recommend the creams that contain more than 400 mg progesterone per ounce for perimenopausal women to achieve physiologic (not pharmacologic) levels of progesterone during the time of estrogen dominance. A typical regimen includes use of one-quarter teaspoon progesterone cream (450 mg/oz) twice daily on days 8 to 21, then one-quarter to one-half teaspoon twice daily on days 22 to 28, and no therapy on days 1 to 7 (menses). The product can be applied to the palms, inner arms, chest, or inner thighs. Although clinical experience is extensive, scientific evidence of efficacy for menopause-related symptoms is limited.

A 12-month trial of 102 early postmenopausal women who received either Pro-Gest cream (450 mg/oz daily) or placebo found a significant improvement in vasomotor symptoms in the treated group, although no change in bone density was observed. Most clinicians do not recommend OTC progesterone creams for prevention of osteoporosis or any other serious disease.

Practitioners report that women tolerate therapy well and that side effects are minimal. Studies are needed to support this anecdotal safety evidence.

Both anecdotal and limited clinical trial evidence suggest that absorption of transdermal OTC progesterone creams is minimal and varies from woman to woman. In a small (N = 6) study of postmenopausal women measuring hormone absorption of transdermal estradiol and topical progesterone cream (Pro-Gest), progesterone was absorbed as well as the estrogen. However, a randomized, double-blind, placebo-controlled, crossover study of 20 surgically induced menopausal women showed that systemic absorption of progesterone from Pro-Gest was small. The study concluded that this cream should not be substituted for the progestogen in conventional estrogen plus progestogen regimens. No biopsy-confirmed studies exist to document that topical OTC progesterone produces sufficient levels to counteract the effect of estrogen on the endometrium. Both conventional and CAM clinicians agree that women with a uterus who use a topical OTC progesterone and ERT should be treated as if they are using unopposed ERT.

Wild yam creams. Topical creams made from wild yam are marketed as containing progesterone precursors that have the ability to provide the health benefits attributed to progesterone cream. Wild yam creams are available over the counter as nutritional supplements.

Diosgenin, a precursor substance for progesterone, is found in wild yam. *Dioscorea villosa* is one of the 600 species of wild yam that is both abundant and high in diosgenin. However, wild yam progesterone precursors cannot be converted into progesterone within the body.

Some wild yam creams contain progesterone that has been produced in the laboratory from the diosgenin extracted from wild yam and then added to the cream. But some wild yam creams do not contain this synthesized progesterone additive and, thus, do not provide any progesterone at all.

Data do not support any menopause-related health claims of wild yam creams. Diosgenin has been found to have an estrogenic effect on mouse mammary epithelium, although no studies have been conducted in humans. Health risks and side effects are unknown.

G.03.b. DHEA

Dehydroepiandrosterone (DHEA) supplementation appears to be effective in women with adrenal insufficiency. However, many women use DHEA purchased over-the-counter for its marketers' claims of improved immunity, slowed aging, increased energy, improved lipids, weight loss, heightened mood, and increased libido. Most often, DHEA is sold as a single-ingredient supplement, although it is sometimes packaged with herbs or other ingredients.

DHEA, a steroid with androgenic properties, is considered a nonmedicinal dietary supplement and is widely available in US health food stores as a nutritional supplement. DHEA is not a food, and it does not occur naturally in foods consumed by humans. The DHEA products currently marketed are synthesized from wild yam, thereby maintaining its classification as a dietary supplement. Analysis of 16 DHEA-containing dietary supplements revealed only 7 of the 16 products contained DHEA within 90% to 110% of the product specifications stated on the product label.

In women, endogenous DHEA is produced by the adrenal glands (90%) and the ovaries (10%). Almost all DHEA is converted to the sulfated hormone, DHEA-S, which degrades more slowly than does DHEA. In women, DHEA levels peak at age 25, with levels declining steadily after age 30. DHEA becomes almost undetectable by age 70. The fall in secretion of DHEA and DHEA-S by the adrenal gland parallels the decline in formation of androgen and estrogen by steroidogenic enzymes in specific target peripheral tissues. The role of DHEA is not well defined, perhaps acting as an androgen, estrogen, antiglucocorticoid, or all of these. Compared with other hormones, its circulating level is quite high.

In one trial, topical application of DHEA for 2 weeks to postmenopausal women resulted in a significant increase in serum testosterone levels with little change in estradiol and estrone levels. Interestingly, oral administration of DHEA to postmenopausal women was associated with an increase in estradiol and estrone levels in addition to an increase in testosterone levels, likely due to the hepatic first-pass effect.

Very few clinical trials have been conducted regarding DHEA use in humans. Animals exhibit dramatic effects with DHEA supplementation because they have low or nonexistent circulating DHEA levels. The animal data may not translate to humans.

Some results to date indicate DHEA increases physical and psychological well-being and energy, although not all studies have demonstrated a clear relationship between DHEA and psychological variables.

Oral DHEA (50 mg/day) given to 60 symptomatic perimenopausal women for 6 months resulted in little improvement of perimenopausal symptoms or well-being when compared with placebo. Improvement of behavioral symptoms in postmenopausal women is believed to be mediated by neuroendocrine effects of DHEA-S or its active metabolites on pituitary beta-endorphin secretion. DHEA supplementation in early and late postmenopausal women is also associated with an increase in growth hormone and IGF-1 levels.

In 2001, a Cochrane review of four studies measuring cognition (three in normal older women and men and one in perimenopausal women with decreased well-being) found no evidence of an improvement in memory or other aspects of cognitive function following DHEA treatment (typically 25 mg/day for women, 50 mg/day for men). The authors concluded that a neuroprotective effect may be evident in the long term and that ongoing trials may provide clarification.

Administration of DHEA to women results in a slight decrease in HDL cholesterol, but its effect on cardiovascular disease risk is unknown. Long-term studies are needed to elucidate the role of DHEA in altering the risk of CVD in postmenopausal women. Observational studies of DHEA levels in cardiovascular disease in humans are inconsistent. High levels may be associated with lowered cardiovascular risk in men, although they may have the opposite effect.

Increased hip BMD was noted in a small group (N = 14) of women aged 60 to 70 years who used topical 10% DHEA cream, but the results could not be replicated in a 6-month trial of 100 mg oral DHEA.

DHEA appears to have no benefit as an antiobesity drug, although some clinical data support the contention that DHEA supplementation improves lean body mass and glucose tolerance.

The specific effects of DHEA on sexual function are just beginning to be explored. In a double-blind, placebo-controlled, crossover trial among women with naturally occurring adrenal insufficiency, oral DHEA (50 mg daily for 4 months) demonstrated significant increases in sexual function (frequency of thoughts and fantasies, interest, level of mental/physical satisfaction). In a randomized, double-blind, crossover trial of postmenopausal women (N = 16), oral DHEA (single dose of 300 mg) demonstrated significant increases in mental and physical sexual arousal ratings.

Some CAM clinicians recommend a daily oral intake of 50 mg or less of DHEA to postmenopausal women with a loss of vitality and/or low libido. It is believed that, at this level, DHEA is converted to more potent androgens, including testosterone. At pharmacologic levels of 1,600 mg daily, DHEA will be converted to estrone and estradiol.

At doses of 25 to 50 mg/day, DHEA appears to be well tolerated in the older population. At these doses, few adverse effects have been reported, although in some women, androgenic side effects (eg, facial hair growth, acne) can occur. Nausea, vomiting, dermatitis, and jaundice have been noted with chronic use of low-dose DHEA. With higher doses of DHEA, side effects reported by women include jaundice, elevated liver function tests, virilization, adverse effect on lipids and the breast, depressed mood, and, possibly, hepatocarcinogenicity. Clinical trials are needed to support these safety observations. There may be unknown long-term side effects, including increased cancer risks.

DHEA is contraindicated in women of reproductive age, especially if they are at any risk of pregnancy, because of possible masculinization of a female fetus. DHEA is also contraindicated in women who have hormone-responsive tumors. The National Institute on Aging recommends against taking DHEA supplements to reverse the effects of aging.

DHEA is banned in Canada due to lack of safety data. NAMS does not recommend its use because it has not been shown to be effective and safe.

G.03.c. Melatonin

Although melatonin is a hormone, it is regulated as a dietary supplement, not a drug. Melatonin is available OTC in most pharmacies and health food stores. However, the lack of regulation and its availability in small doses with increased vehicle-to-drug ratio increases the likelihood of misformulation and poor release of melatonin.

Melatonin (N-acetyl-5-methoxytryptamine) regulates the central clock and the rest-activity cycles. It is produced in the pineal gland of the brain from its precursor, tryptophan, with the process regulated by the suprachiasmatic nucleus of the hypothalamus.

Endogenous melatonin levels peak in childhood, drop acutely during puberty, and decline steadily thereafter throughout life. Light suppresses melatonin secretion during the day to a virtually nonexistent level. Melatonin levels begin to increase in the evening and peak between midnight and 3 AM, resulting in a direct sedative effect and a drop in body temperature. Approximately 99% of melatonin receptors regulate the general level of arousal; the other 1% regulate the central clock.

Melatonin promotes natural sleep and augments benzodiazepine-induced sleep induction. The active urinary metabolite of melatonin, 6-sulfatoxymelatonin, is significantly lower in subjects with insomnia than those without insomnia, suggesting that melatonin deficiency may be responsible for sleep disturbance in the elderly. Melatonin may also be useful in patients with insomnia requiring benzodiazepines for prolonged periods. In one study, discontinuation of benzodiazepine therapy in patients with insomnia was effectively achieved using 2 mg of a controlled-release melatonin formulation for 6 weeks. Good sleep quality was maintained at 6 months.

Although sleep disturbances are a common complaint during the menopause transition, there are no data demonstrating that melatonin can provide relief for menopause-related sleep disturbances. There is no evidence that melatonin retards aging.

Studies suggest that melatonin has uses other than for sleep. Data support the use of melatonin supplementation to treat jet lag, particularly in those who have crossed several time zones. Two randomized, controlled trials have demonstrated that melatonin allays anxiety in presurgery patients without causing amnesia.

There is some evidence that melatonin when used in conjunction with chemotherapeutic agents may be useful for its oncostatic effects, but this evidence is preliminary. For this indication, melatonin should be used with extreme caution. Melatonin has been shown to retard growth of cancer cell lines. Its oncostatic effects are likely due to the ability of the indole moiety to suppress tumor fatty acid uptake and metabolism. Also, melatonin is known to activate T-helper cells. By virtue of its stimulatory effect on nonspecific immunity and antioxidant properties, it may result in tumor amelioration.

There is little evidence regarding the recommended dose or safety of long-term melatonin therapy. The optimal dose of melatonin is not known. It has been used in doses varying from 0.3 to 10 mg daily, although continued daily use is not recommended. Melatonin is available in two formulations: quick-release and sustained-release. Since melatonin has a short half-life of approximately 30 to 60 minutes, a sustained-release formulation to replicate physiology and maintain sleep appears to be more advantageous.

Certain pharmacologic agents such as nonsteroidal anti-inflammatory drugs, benzodiazepines, and beta adrenergic-receptor blockers can inhibit endogenous melatonin synthesis. Acute and chronic alcohol use, tryptophan deficiency, and caffeine are also associated with decreased melatonin function. Monoamine oxidase (MAO) inhibitors, noradrenergic uptake inhibitors, selective serotonin-reuptake inhibitors, neuroleptics, and psoralens enhance melatonin function.

High doses (>3 mg daily) of melatonin have been associated with adverse effects, such as abdominal cramps, hangover effect, dizziness, fatigue, irritability, and impaired balance. High doses also exacerbate depression; its use is best avoided in women with a history of mental illness. Melatonin should be used with caution in the elderly since it can affect the activity of various neurotransmitters that are altered with advancing age, such as dopamine, serotonin, GABA, and opioid peptides.

In animal studies, melatonin has caused coronary and cerebral artery vasoconstriction, suggesting it be used with caution in women with coronary artery disease. Data regarding its use in postmenopausal diabetic women are conflicting.

Bibliography

Arendt J, Skene DJ, Middleton B, Lockley SW, Deacon S. Efficacy of melatonin treatment in jet lag, shift work, and blindness. *J Biol Rhythms* 1997;12:604-617.

Arlt W, Callies F, Allolio B. DHEA replacement in women with adrenal insufficiency; pharmacokinetics, bioconversion and clinical effects on well-being, sexuality and cognition. *Endocr Res* 2000;26:505-511.

Barnhart KT, Freeman E, Grisso JA, et al. The effect of DHEA supplementation to symptomatic perimenopausal women on serum endocrine profiles, lipid parameters, and health-related quality of life. *J Clin Endocrinol Metab* 1999;84:3896-3902.

Barry NN, McGuire JL, van Vollenhoven RF. Dehydroepiandrosterone in systemic lupus erythematosus: relationship between dosage, serum levels, and clinical response. *J Rheumatol* 1998;25:2352-2356.

Blask DE, Sauer LA, Dauchy RT, et al. Melatonin inhibition of cancer growth in vivo involves suppression of tumor fatty acid metabolism via melatonin receptor-mediated signal transduction events. *Cancer Res* 1999;59:4693-4701.

Brzezinski A. Melatonin in humans. *N Engl J Med* 1997;336:186-195.

Burry KA, Patton PE, Hermsmeyer K. Percutaneous absorption of progesterone in postmenopausal women treated with transdermal estrogen. *Obstet Gynecol* 1999;180:1504-1511.

Cagnacci A, Arangino S, Renzi A, et al. Influence of melatonin administration on glucose tolerance and insulin sensitivity of postmenopausal women. *Clin Endocrinol* 2001;54:339-346.

Callies F, Fassnacht M, van Vlijmen JC, et al. Dehydroepiandrosterone replacement in women with adrenal insufficiency: effects on body composition, serum leptin, bone turnover, and exercise capacity. *J Clin Endocrinol Metab* 2001;86:1968-1972.

Casson PR, Anderson RN, Herrod HG, et al. Oral dehydroepiandrosterone in physiologic doses modulates immune function in postmenopausal women. *Am J Obstet Gynecol* 1993;169:1536-1539.

Clore NJ. Dehydroepiandrosterone and body fat. *Obes Res* 1995; 3(suppl 4):613S-616S.

Cooper A, Spencer C, Whitehead MI, Ross D, Barnard GJ, Collins WP. Systemic absorption of progesterone from Progest cream in postmenopausal women [Letter]. *Lancet* 1998;351:1255-1256.

Diamond P, Cusan L, Gomez JL, et al. Metabolic effects of 12-month percutaneous dehydroepiandrosterone replacement therapy in postmenopausal women. *J Endocrinol* 1996;150(suppl):S43-S50.

Garfinkel D, Loudon M, Nof D, Zisapel N. Improvement of sleep quality in elderly people by controlled-release melatonin. *Lancet* 1995;346:541-544.

Garfinkel D, Zisapel N, Wainstein J, Laudon M. Facilitation of benzodiazepine discontinuation by melatonin: a new clinical approach. *Arch Intern Med* 1999;159:2456-2460.

Hackbert L, Heiman JR. Acute dehydroepiandrosterone (DHEA) effects on sexual arousal in postmenopausal women. *J Womens Health Gend Based Med* 2002;11:155-162.

Hahm H, Kujawa J, Augsburger L. Comparison of melatonin products against USP's nutritional supplements standards and other criteria. *J Am Pharm Assoc* 1999;39:27-31.

Haimov I, Laudon M, Zisapel N, et al. Sleep disorders and melatonin rhythms in elderly people. *BMJ* 1994;309:167.

Hudson T. *Women's Encyclopedia of Natural Medicine: Alternative Therapies and Integrative Medicine.* Los Angeles, CA: Keats Publishing; 1999.

Huppert FA, Van Niekerk JK. Dehydroepiandrosterone (DHEA) supplementation for cognitive function. *Cochrane Database Syst Rev* 2000;2:CD000304.

Katz S, Morales AJ. Dehydroepiandrosterone (DHEA) and DHEA-sulfate (DS) as therapeutic options in menopause. *Semin Reprod Endocrinol* 1998;16:1-70.

Khaw KT. Dehydroepiandrosterone, dehydroepiandrosterone sulfate and cardiovascular disease. *J Endocrinol* 1996;150(suppl): S149-S153.

Labrie F, Bélanger A, Cusan L, Candas B. Physiological changes in dehydroepiandrosterone are not reflected by serum levels of active androgens and estrogens but of their metabolites: intracrinology. *J Clin Endocrinol Metab* 1997;82:2403-2409.

Labrie F, Diamond P, Cusan L, Gomez JL, Bélanger A, Candas B. Effect of 12-month dehydroepiandrosterone replacement therapy on bone, vagina, and endometrium in postmenopausal women. *J Clin Endocrinol Metab* 1997;82:3498-3505.

Labrie F, Luu-The V, Lin SX, et al. Intracrinology: role of the family of 17 beta-hydroxysteroid dehydrogenases in human physiology and disease. *J Mol Endocrinol* 2000;25:1-16.

Lamberg L. Melatonin potentially useful but safety, efficacy remain uncertain. *JAMA* 1996;276:1011-1014.

Leonetti HB, Longo S, Anasti JN. Transdermal progesterone cream for vasomotor symptoms and postmenopausal bone loss. *Obstet Gynecol* 1999;94:225-228.

Morales AJ, Haubrich RH, Hwang JY, et al. The effect of six months treatment with a 100 mg daily dose of dehydroepiandrosterone (DHEA) on circulating sex steroids, body composition, and muscle strength in age-advanced men and women. *Clin Endocrinol* 1998; 49:421-432.

Morales AJ, Nolan JJ, Nelson JC, Yen SS. Effects of replacement dose of dehydroepiandrosterone in men and women of advancing age. *J Clin Endocrinol Metab* 1994;78:1360-1367.

Mortola JF, Yen SS. The effects of oral dehydroepiandrosterone on endocrine-metabolic parameters in postmenopausal women. *J Clin Endocrinol Metab* 1990;71:696-704.

Naguib M, Samarkandi AH. Premedication with melatonin: a double-blind, placebo-controlled comparison with midazolam. *Br J Anaesth* 1999;82:875-880.

Orentreich N, Brind J, Rizer R, Vogelmen JH. Age changes and sex differences in serum dehydroepiandrosterone sulfate concentration throughout adulthood. *J Clin Endocrinol Metab* 1984;59:551-555.

Parasrampuria J, Schwartz K, Petesch R. Quality control of DHEA dietary supplement products [letter]. *JAMA* 1998;280:1565.

Penev PD, Zee PC. Melatonin: a clinical perspective. *Ann Neurol* 1997;42:545-553.

Physicians' Desk Reference for Herbal Medications. 2nd ed. Montvale, NJ: Medical Economics Co; 2000.

Prior JC: Progesterone as a bone-tropic hormone. *Endocr Rev* 1990;11:386-398.

Reiter RJ. Melatonin and human reproduction. *Ann Intern Med* 1998;39:103-108.

Spitzer RL, Terman M, Williams JB, et al. Jet lag: clinical features, validation of a new syndrome-specific scale, and lack of response to melatonin in a randomized, double-blind trial. *Am J Psychiatry* 1999;156:1392-1396.

Stomati M, Rubino S, Spinetti A, et al. Endocrine, neuroendocrine and behavioral effects of oral dehydroepiandrosterone sulfate supplementation in postmenopausal women. *Gynecol Endocrinol* 1999;13:15-25.

van Vollenhoven RF, Park JL, Genovese MC, West JP, McGuire JL. A double-blind, placebo-controlled, clinical trial of dehydroepiandrosterone in severe systemic lupus erythematosus. *Lupus* 1999;8:181-187.

Wolf OT, Neumann O, Hellhammer DH, et al. Effects of a two-week physiological dehydroepiandrosterone substitution on cognitive performance and well-being in healthy elderly men and women. *J Clin Endocrinol Metab* 1997;82:2363-2367.

Yen S, Morales A, Khorram O. Replacement of DHEA in aging men and women: potential remedial effects. *Ann NY Acad Sci* 1995; 774:128-142.

Zhdanova IV, Wurtman RJ, Regan MM, Taylor JA, Shi JP, Leclair OU. Melatonin treatment for age-related insomnia. *J Clin Endocrinol Metab* 2001;86:4727-4730.

Zimmerman RC. Melatonin. In Lobo RA, ed. *Treatment of the Postmenopausal Woman: Basic and Clinical Aspects*. 2nd ed. Philadelphia, PA: Lippincott Williams & Wilkins; 1999:603-609.

G.04. Aspirin

Aspirin continues to show promise in areas other than pain relief. However, its pharmacology is not entirely clear.

The benefit of aspirin use for individuals with heart disease remain unchallenged, and the use of daily low-dose aspirin (81 mg) to prevent recurrence of myocardial infarction (MI) has become common practice. Dozens of studies conducted during the last 30 years have shown that aspirin impairs platelet function, which aids blood flow in those with atherosclerosis.

Meta-analysis of pooled data from five trials examining the effects of aspirin for the primary prevention of cardiovascular events over periods of 4 to 7 years showed that daily or every-other-day aspirin therapy reduced the risk for coronary heart disease by 28%, with no significant effects on mortality and stroke. Most participants were men older than 50 years.

In the Nurses' Health Study, a large trial of healthy women ages 34-59 who were monitored over a 14-year period, those who took aspirin (325 mg, 1-6 times per week) had a lower risk of ischemic stroke, although women who took higher doses (>15 tablets per week) were approximately twice as likely to suffer hemorrhagic strokes. This risk was increased further in older women with hypertension.

Sound evidence from clinical trials shows that aspirin helps in secondary prevention of CHD. The American Heart Association recommends aspirin use for women who have experienced a myocardial infarction (MI), unstable angina, ischemic stroke, or transient ischemic attacks, if not contraindicated.

In 2002, the US Preventive Services Task Force issued a report strongly recommending that aspirin use be considered for primary prevention of coronary events in high-risk adults. The targeted population includes postmenopausal women and those with risk factors such as diabetes, hypercholesterolemia, hypertension, smoking, and a family history of cardiovascular disease. A daily dose of 75 mg is suggested, although the optimal dose is not known. Many experts believe it is too early to recommend that healthy women take aspirin on a regular basis.

The risks of taking aspirin may outweigh the benefits in some individuals. Aspirin is contraindicated for those who are receiving anticoagulant therapy or who have aspirin allergy, tendency for bleeding, recent gastrointestinal bleeding, or clinically active hepatic disease. Even enteric-coated or buffered aspirin may cause damage to the intestinal lining. However, studies have shown that individuals who regularly take aspirin (and other anti-inflammatory drugs) have unusually low rates of digestive tract cancers.

Bibliography

Albers GW, Hart RG, Lutsep HL, Newell DW, Sacco R. Supplement to the guidelines for the management of transient ischemic attacks: a statement from the Ad Hoc Committee on Guidelines for the Management of Transient Ischemic Attacks, Stroke Council, American Heart Association. *Stroke* 1999;30:2502-2511.

Antiplatelet Trialists' Collaboration. Collaborative overview of randomised trials of antiplatelet therapy. I. Prevention of death, myocardial infarction, and stroke by prolonged antiplatelet therapy in various categories of patients. *BMJ* 1994;308:81-106.

Collaborative Group of the Primary Prevention Project (PPP). Low-dose aspirin and vitamin E in people at cardiovascular risk: a randomized trial in general practice. *Lancet* 2001;357:89-95.

Hansson L, Zanchetti A, Carruthers SG, et al. Effects of intensive blood-pressure lowering and low-dose aspirin in patients with hypertension: principal results of the Hypertension Optimal Treatment (HOT) randomised trial. HOT Study Group. *Lancet* 1998;280:1930-1935.

Hayden M, Pignone M, Phillips C, Mulrow C. Aspirin for the primary prevention of cardiovascular events: a summary of the evidence for the US Preventive Services Task Force. *Ann Intern Med* 2002;136:161-172.

Hennekens CH, Dyken ML, Fuster V. Aspirin as a therapeutic agent in cardiovascular disease: a statement for healthcare professionals from the American Heart Association. *Circulation* 1997;96:2751-2753.

Hiroyasu I, Hennekens CH, Stampfer MJ, et al. Prospective study of aspirin use and risk of stroke in women. *Stroke* 1999;30:1764-1771.

Mosca L, Grundy SM, Judelson D, et al. Guide to Preventive Cardiology for Women. AHA/ACC Scientific Statement Consensus Panel Statement. *Circulation* 1999;99:2480-2484.

Roderick PJ, Wilkes HC, Meade TW. The gastrointestinal toxicity of aspirin: an overview of randomized controlled trials. *Br J Clin Pharmacol* 1993;35:219-226.

Stalnikowicz-Darvasi R. Gastrointestinal bleeding during low-dose aspirin administration for prevention of arterial occlusive events. *J Clin Gastroenterol* 1995;21:13-16.

Thrombosis prevention trial: randomised trial of low-intensity oral anticoagulation with warfarin and low-dose aspirin in the primary prevention of ischaemic heart disease in men at increased risk. The Medical Research Council's General Practice Research Framework. *Lancet* 1998;351:233-241.

Wolf PA, Clagett GP, Easton JD, et al. Preventing ischemic stroke in patients with prior stroke and transient ischemic attack: a statement for healthcare professionals from the Stroke Council of the American Heart Association. *Stroke* 1999;30:1991-1994.

G.05. Vaginal lubricants/moisturizers

Nonhormonal vaginal lubricants and moisturizers for the treatment of vaginal dryness are often used by women. Women who are unwilling or unable to use ERT/HRT also choose nonhormonal options, even for more serious atrophic vaginitis. In addition, many women on systemic ERT/HRT experience vaginal dryness during coital activity and prefer to use a nonhormonal vaginal lubricant or moisturizer to prevent dyspareunia rather than increase the ERT/HRT dosage.

Water-based *vaginal lubricants,* such as K-Y Personal Lubricant, Lubrin, Astroglide, and Moist Again, can be purchased over the counter. Vaginal lubricants to coat the vagina before penetration may be suggested to women with atrophic vaginitis but who are otherwise asymptomatic.

In contrast to vaginal lubricants, *vaginal moisturizers,* such as K-Y Long-Lasting Vaginal Moisturizer and Replens, may offer the benefit of longer duration of effect by replenishing and maintaining water content in vaginal epithelium. These products may be preferred by women who have symptoms

of irritation, pressure, and burning that are not limited to episodes of sexual exchange. In addition, moisturizers help maintain an acidic vaginal environment and may be recommended for women with recurrent vaginal infection.

Although women often choose other products for vaginal lubrication, only products designed solely for vaginal use should be used. Ingredients such as alcohol and perfume, which are contained in hand creams, can exacerbate some atrophic symptoms, such as burning and itching. Oil-based products, such as Vaseline petroleum jelly and baby oil, can cause irritation, damage condoms and diaphragms, and, since they tend to cling to vaginal tissue, can also provide a habitat for abnormal vaginal and bladder bacteria. One exception to this rule is vitamin E oil, reported to provide lubrication and relieve itching and irritation without untoward effects.

Vinegar douches or cultures of lactobacilli or yogurt are not effective for moisturizing and are not recommended. Women with vaginal dryness who use antihistamines should be advised that these drugs have a drying effect on all mucous membranes, including the vaginal walls.

Although all postmenopausal women should be counseled on the vaginal changes that occur with both menopause and aging, it is equally as important to counsel perimenopause women about adverse urogenital changes as well. Simple recommendations to alleviate vaginal discomfort are especially important since vaginal atrophy left untreated will predispose women to dyspareunia and vaginal infections. Sexual activity and/or stimulation should be encouraged since fewer atrophic vaginal changes are noted in sexually active women as compared with abstinent women. For severe vaginal atrophy unresponsive to nonhormonal interventions, a short course of vaginal estrogen may be needed to restore vaginal epithelium to the point where sexual exchange is comfortable. The woman may then revert to a nonhormonal method of maintaining vaginal lubrication once vaginal atrophy is ameliorated or reversed.

Bibliography

Bachmann GA, Ebert GA, Burd ID. Vulvovaginal complaints. In: Lobo RA, ed. *Treatment of Postmenopausal Women: Basic and Clinical Aspects.* 2nd ed. Philadelphia, PA: Lippincott Williams & Wilkins; 1999:195-199.

MacLaren A, Woods NF. Midlife women making hormone therapy decisions. *Womens Health Issues* 2001;11:216-230.

Nachtigall LE. Comparative study: Replens versus local estrogen in menopausal women. *Fertil Steril* 1994;61:178-180.

Willhite LA, O'Connell MB. Urogenital atrophy: prevention and treatment. *Pharmacotherapy* 2001;21:464-480.

G.06. Nonhormonal contraception

Despite a decline in fertility during perimenopause, pregnancy is still possible until menopause is reached. Choosing an effective, safe, and appropriate method of birth control is particularly important in midlife, when the benefits and risks can have an impact on health far beyond the reproductive years. Perimenopausal women have an extensive range of excellent nonhormonal contraception options. Not all the options presented here are available over the counter; some require clinician intervention. But all options here are nonhormonal.

Sterilization (tubal ligation and vasectomy) is safe and effective, with a very low failure rate (about 4-8 in 1,000). The primary disadvantages are the surgical procedure and difficulty reversing the process. In addition, sterilization offers no protection from sexually transmitted infections (STIs). Sterilization is a good option for midlife women (or their male partners) if they are in a mutually monogamous, long-term relationship and desire permanent contraception.

Barrier methods include the male condom, female condom, spermicides, diaphragm, and cervical cap. These methods are highly effective if used correctly and consistently during every act of vaginal sex. The condom is the only proven effective protection against both pregnancy and STIs (during vaginal, oral, and anal sex). Barrier methods can be used in combination with other birth control methods. Disadvantages of barrier methods include potential allergic reaction to latex or spermicides, the need to be used during every act of sex, and (with condoms) the potential to break, leak, or spill when removed. The diaphragm and cervical cap are available only from a healthcare provider.

Many women rely on *natural family planning* (NFP; the rhythm method or periodic abstinence) or the *withdrawal method*. These methods have the advantages of no cost, no need for surgery, and no need to take a drug or use a device. Disadvantages include a high failure rate compared with other methods and no protection against sexually transmitted infections. When using NFP, which relies on regular measurements of ovulation-related factors, there is difficulty predicting ovulation during perimenopause because of irregular menstrual periods. Ovulation occurs sporadically during perimenopause, resulting in less reliability with NFP. When using the withdrawal method, which should never be considered reliable birth control, enough sperm to cause pregnancy may seep from the penis prior to ejaculation.

Hormonal contraceptives and intrauterine devices are discussed in Section H.01.

Bibliography

Speroff L, Darney D, eds. *A Clinical Guide for Contraception.* 3rd ed. Philadelphia, PA: Lippincott Williams & Wilkins; 2001.

Many prescription drugs are available to help midlife women with menopause-related complaints and to lower their risk of serious disease in later life. There are also several prescription options for perimenopausal women who require contraception.

H.01. Contraceptives

Despite a decline in fertility during perimenopause, pregnancy is still possible until menopause is reached. Perimenopausal women should be aware that use of oral contraceptives (OCs) or any other hormonal or intrauterine contraceptive method does not reduce the risk of acquiring sexually transmitted infections. Accordingly, at-risk women should protect themselves through use of "safer sex" practices.

Prescription contraceptives are discussed in this section and noncontraceptive use of these prescription products is discussed in Section H.01.e. Transition from hormonal contraception to ERT/HRT is described in Section H.02.e.

H.01.a. Combination (estrogen-progestin) contraceptives

Increasingly more options are available when prescribing a combination (estrogen plus progestin) contraceptive. They include both oral and nonoral contraceptives:

Oral combination contraceptives. Oral products containing combined estrogen plus progestin represent a safe contraceptive option for healthy, nonsmoking, midlife women. Because of the effective contraception as well as important noncontraceptive benefits, combination oral contraceptives (OCs) are increasingly being used by perimenopausal women.

The use of combination OCs by perimenopausal women results in a number of noncontraceptive benefits. These include regulation of irregular uterine bleeding, reduction of vasomotor symptoms, decreased risk for ovarian and endometrial cancer, and maintenance of bone density (with a potential for decreased risk for postmenopausal osteoporotic fractures).

Contraindications to combination OCs include history of thrombophlebitis or thromboembolic disorders; cerebral vascular or coronary artery disease; known or suspected breast, endometrial, or other estrogen-dependent cancer; undiagnosed abnormal uterine bleeding; jaundice during previous pregnancy or OC use; hepatic adenomas or cancer; and known or suspected pregnancy.

FDA labeling for OCs warns that cigarette smoking increases the risk of serious cardiovascular side effects. This risk increases with age and with heavy smoking (15 or more cigarettes per day) and is quite marked in women over 35 years of age. Thus, women over age 35 who smoke should not use OCs.

Obesity, diabetes, hypertension, or classic migraine headaches (with aura) also should be considered contraindications to combination OC use by perimenopausal women. Use of combination OCs increases the risk of venous thromboembolism (VTE). Although the incidence of VTE is very low in reproductive-age women, VTE risk increases with age and body mass index. Use of OCs formulated with desogestrel appears to be associated with a higher VTE risk than with other OCs. As women age, the risk for vascular events associated with diabetes or hypertension mounts. Finally, the risk of stroke appears to be increased in women with classic migraines. Use of combination OCs by women with this history appears to further increase the risk of stroke.

Common side effects of OCs include nausea and breast tenderness, which tend to resolve as OC use continues. Use of combination OCs does not cause weight gain or headaches.

When prescribing combination OCs for perimenopausal women, the 25-μg estrogen formulations represent a prudent choice (although these OCs are not available in Canada). These formulations, when combined with a triphasic regimen of the highly selective progestins desogestrel or norgestimate, achieve the low rates of unscheduled bleeding and spotting characteristic of OCs with higher-dose estrogen. The ultra low-dose OCs formulated with 20 μg of estrogen have been associated with higher rates of breakthrough bleeding and spotting than the 25-μg products.

Nonoral combination contraceptives. Recently approved nonoral combination contraceptives include a monthly injection (Lunelle), a vaginal ring that is worn for 3 out of 4 weeks (NuvaRing), and a 1-week contraceptive transdermal system (Ortho Evra). The injection product combines estradiol cypionate and medroxyprogesterone acetate (MPA), the ring releases ethinyl estradiol and etonogestrel, and the patch delivers ethinyl estradiol and norelgestromin. Etonogestrel and norelgestromin are the biologically active metabolites of desogestrel and norgestimate, respectively, which are both progestins used in commonly prescribed combination OCs. As with combination OCs, use of the monthly injections, the ring, and the patch results in cyclical monthly withdrawal bleeding. Because these methods are longer-acting, patient compliance (and, therefore, contraceptive efficacy) may be higher than with the oral combination products. Side effects and contraindications are similar to those for the combination OCs. (Lunelle and NuvaRing are not available in Canada.)

H.01.b. Progestin-only contraceptives

In contrast with combination contraceptives, progestin-only contraceptives can be used by perimenopausal women in whom contraceptive doses of estrogen are contraindicated (see Table 1).

Table 1. Contraindications for estrogen-containing contraceptives

Cigarette smoking

Hypertension

Migraines

History of coronary artery/cerebrovascular disease

Diabetes mellitus (including women with peripheral vascular disease)

History of venous thromboembolism

The depot form of medroxyprogesterone acetate (DMPA) provides highly effective contraception. The dosage, 150 mg intramuscular injection, given every 3 months, does not need to be adjusted for body weight. Although DMPA contraception is reversible, return of fertility after cessation of therapy may be delayed for 12 to 18 months.

Initially, irregular uterine bleeding or spotting is common with use of DMPA. After four or more injections, at least half of DMPA users will experience amenorrhea. Use of DMPA suppresses ovarian estradiol production, which can reversibly lower bone mineral density. Accordingly, clinicians prescribing DMPA to perimenopausal women may wish to supplement ("add back") with oral or transdermal estrogen, using doses similar to those used in conventional postmenopausal hormone replacement therapy.

Progestin-only oral contraceptives (eg, Nor QD, Micronor) formulated with norethindrone or norgestrel provide effective contraception for perimenopausal women. Because the dose of progestin in these "minipills" is low, maintenance of high contraceptive efficacy may depend on precise daily pill-taking. Women using mini-pills may experience irregular uterine bleeding or spotting or, less commonly, amenorrhea. (Nor QD is not available in Canada.)

The levonorgestrel subdermal contraceptive implant product (Norplant System) consists of six flexible capsules (each containing 36 mg levonorgestrel) that are surgically implanted under the skin of the upper arm. It offers highly effective contraception for at least 5 years. As with minipills, irregular uterine bleeding, spotting, or amenorrhea may occur during use. Problems associated with difficult removals have decreased the popularity of this system. In July 2002, the manufacturer announced plans to discontinue the product. Removal procedures will be reimbursed through December 2002. Newer contraceptive systems with one or two implants are available in other countries.

H.01.c. Emergency contraception

Emergency contraception (EC) may be appropriate in certain cases, including after unprotected sexual intercourse, a condom accident, an IUD partially or totally expelled, and if one or more progestin-only contraceptive pills have been missed. Various oral estrogen plus progestin contraceptives can be used for EC. Most use a dose of 100 to 120 µg ethinyl estradiol plus 0.5 to 0.6 mg levonorgestrel taken within 72 hours after unprotected intercourse and followed by another dose 12 hours later. It must be used within this time, as EC has no effect once a fertilized egg has become implanted. Efficacy is approximately 75%. Side effects include nausea, vomiting, cramping, and headache.

The most-often prescribed products for EC are specifically marketed (and FDA-approved) for this use and are sometimes called the "morning-after pill." In the United States, the first product approved for this use (Preven) contains four pills, each with 0.05 mg ethinyl estradiol and 0.25 mg levonorgestrel, as well as a pregnancy test. A newer product (Plan B) is a progestin-only product. It reportedly reduces the risk of pregnancy by 89% and has fewer side effects than Preven. EC is most effective when taken within 72 hours of unprotected sex.

The only absolute contraindication to emergency contraception is a confirmed pregnancy, because these regimens will not terminate the pregnancy. These products should not be used as a regular method of birth control because they are not as reliable as many ongoing methods of contraception.

H.01.d. Intrauterine devices

Intrauterine devices (IUDs) provide another highly effective and convenient contraceptive option. Throughout the world, the IUD is the most widely used reversible contraceptive, with 85 to 100 million users. In the United States, however, the IUD is used by less than 1% of contraceptive users.

Use of an IUD may represent a particularly desirable contraceptive alternative for midlife women requesting sterilization. Two IUDs are available in North America: the copper IUD (ParaGard T 380A), which is approved for 10 years of contraception, and the levonorgestrel-releasing IUD (Mirena), which provides 5 years of contraception.

The principal side effects associated with use of the copper IUD are increased cramping and menstrual flow. Accordingly, the copper IUD may not be an optimal choice for women who have problems with dysmenorrhea or menorrhagia.

The levonorgestrel-releasing IUD profoundly reduces menstrual blood loss and appears to reduce dysmenorrhea. For this reason, the levonorgestrel-releasing IUD represents an appropriate choice for women with menorrhagia or excessive cramps at baseline. Use of the levonorgestrel IUD is associated with high local endometrial progestin concentrations; thus, it can be combined with systemic estrogen in perimenopausal women. Irregular uterine bleeding and spotting are the most commonly reported side effects. During use, these side effects become considerably less prominent, as women develop either light, cyclical menses; ongoing, unpredictable, light uterine bleeding or spotting; or amenorrhea.

Insertion of IUDs is an office-based procedure, and is different for each of the two types. Although uterine perforation rarely occurs during insertion of modern IUDs, expulsion rates can be relatively high (at least 5%) in the first months following insertion. Clinicians trained in insertion have the lowest rates of IUD expulsions and uterine perforations.

H.01.e. Noncontraceptive use during perimenopause

Oral and other hormonal contraceptives are increasingly being used by perimenopausal women for noncontraceptive purposes. Table 2 lists noncontraceptive benefits of OCs that are applicable to perimenopausal women. The benefits may also apply to the other hormonal contraceptives.

Hormonal contraceptives (including extended use of combined OCs, injectable progestin, and the levonorgestrel-releasing IUD) are often used to reduce the frequency of menses or eliminate menstruation entirely.

OCs with very low hormone doses still provide significantly more hormone than in standard ERT/HRT regimens, which may increase exposure to unnecessary risks with long-term use. Therefore, the lowest effective OC dose should be used, and the woman transitioned to ERT/HRT when appropriate (see Section H.02.e).

Table 2: Noncontraceptive benefits of oral contraceptives

Stabilization of erratic perimenopausal bleeding

Reduction of dysmenorrhea

Reduction of menorrhagia

Reduction of vasomotor symptoms

Stabilization of bone mineral density

Reduction in biopsies for benign breast disease

Reduction in surgery for benign ovarian tumors

Prevention of endometrial and ovarian malignancies

Possible prevention of colorectal cancers

Bibliography

Audet MC, Moreau M, Koltun WD, et al. Evaluation of contraceptive efficacy and cycle control of a transdermal contraceptive patch vs an oral contraceptive: a randomized controlled trial. *JAMA* 2001;285:2347-2354.

Hubacher D, Lara-Ricalde R, Taylor DJ, Guerra-Infante F, Guzman-Rodriguez R. Use of copper intrauterine devices and the risk of tubal infertility among nulligravid women. *N Engl J Med* 2001; 345:561-567.

Kaunitz AM. Injectable long-acting contraceptives. *Clin Obstet Gynecol* 2001;44:73-91.

Kaunitz AM. Oral contraceptive use in perimenopause. *Am J Obstet Gynecol* 2001;185(2 suppl):S32-S37.

Kaunitz AM. The use of hormonal contraception in women with coexisting medical conditions. *ACOG Practice Bulletin* 2000;18:1-13.

Raudaskoski TH, Lahti EI, Kauppila AJ, et al. Transdermal estrogen with a levonorgestrel-releasing intrauterine device for climacteric complaints: clinical and endometrial responses. *Am J Obstet Gynecol* 1995;172:114-119.

Roumen FJ, Apter D, Mulders TM, Dieben TO. Efficacy, tolerability and acceptability of a novel contraceptive vaginal ring releasing etonogestrel and ethinyl oestradiol. *Hum Reprod* 2001;16:469-475.

Trussell J, Rodriguez G, Ellerston C. Updated estimates of the effectiveness of the Yuzpe regimen of emergency contraception. *Contraception* 1999;59:147-151.

H.02. ERT and HRT

Standard estrogen-based pharmacologic therapies for postmenopausal women are divided into two categories:

Estrogen replacement therapy (ERT) is unopposed estrogen, which is usually prescribed for postmenopausal women who have undergone hysterectomy. It may also be prescribed for women with an intact uterus who are intolerant to progestogens, provided that they are fully informed about increased risk for endometrical cancer and are followed with appropriate endometrial surveillance.

Hormone replacement therapy (HRT) is combination estrogen and progestogen (either progesterone or the synthetic form of progesterone, progestin). Although the available data suggest that the benefits of HRT are almost exclusively due to estrogen, progestogen reduces the risk of endometrial adenocarcinoma, which is significantly increased in women with a uterus who use unopposed estrogen.

The term *replacement* is a misnomer, because ERT/HRT provides only a small fraction of the estrogen the ovaries once produced. However, the terms *estrogen replacement therapy* and *hormone replacement therapy* are commonly used to distinguish postmenopausal hormonal therapy from other hormonal therapies (eg, contraceptives, selective estrogen-replacement modulators, thyroid medications). (See box below for more.)

All postmenopausal women should be counseled regarding menopause and ERT/HRT use. This is especially important for women with premature menopause (ie, before age 40), whether natural or induced. In the absence of contraindications, ERT/HRT can be recommended to treat symptoms of the menopausal transition, especially hot flashes and vaginal dryness, and to reduce the risk of osteoporosis.

Few data are available regarding the effects of ERT/HRT in perimenopausal women.

Important Notice

Future materials from NAMS will not use the word "replacement" when describing hormone therapy for menopause. ERT and HRT will be referred to as ET and HT.

H.02.a. Estrogens and ERT

Estrogen is an umbrella term for a variety of chemical compounds that have an affinity for the estrogen receptor.

The natural versus synthetic terminology can be misleading. The term *natural* is sometimes used to refer to the product source (ie, plant or animal) or to the chemical structure (ie, identical to human estrogens). Marketers often call their products natural because consumers believe that if something is natural, it must be better or safer. However, the primary factor in determining usefulness of an estrogen is not its origin, but its chemical structure and biological efficacy.

Estrogens can be divided into the following six main groups:

Human estrogens, such as estrone (E_1), 17β-estradiol (E_2), and estriol. Estradiol is the most biologically active, whereas estrone is 50% to 70% less active and estriol is only 10% as active. Estradiol, the principal estrogen secreted by the ovaries, is metabolized to estrone; both estradiol and estrone can be metabolized to estriol, although exogenous estriol cannot be converted. Of these types of endogenous estrogens, only one exogenous product — micronized 17β–estradiol — is available, in an FDA-approved single-estrogen product (eg, Estrace, Estrace Vaginal Cream, Estring, estrogen-only transdermal products).

Nonhuman estrogens, such as conjugated equine estrogens (Premarin), a mixture of estrogens extracted and purified from pregnant mares' urine. Premarin labeling claims 10 active estrogens, including sodium estrone sulfate (50%) and sodium equilin sulfate (25%), as well as sodium sulfate conjugates, 17β-dihydroequilin, 17β-estradiol, and 17β-dihydroequilin.

Synthetic estrogen mixtures, such as synthetic conjugated estrogens (Cenestin, CES, Congest, PMS Conjugated), and esterified estrogens, which is 75% to 85% sodium estrone sulfate (Estratab, Menest, Neo-Estrone).

Synthetic estrogen analogues with a steroid skeleton, such as ethinyl estradiol (Estinyl) and piperazine estrone sulfate (Ortho-Est, Ogen).

Synthetic estrogen analogues without a steroid skeleton, such as stilbesterol derivatives, which are not used for menopause-related therapy.

Plant-based estrogens without a steroid skeleton, also known as phytoestrogens, which may have weak estrogenic as well as antiestrogenic properties, depending on the target tissue. These are not prescription products.

Estrogen drug products act by regulating the transcription of a number of genes. Estrogens diffuse through cell membranes, distribute themselves through the cell, and bind to and activate the nuclear estrogen receptor, a DNA-binding protein that is found in estrogen-responsive tissues. The activated estrogen receptor binds to specific DNA sequences, or hormone-response elements, which enhance the transcription of adjacent genes and, in turn, lead to the observed effects. In women, estrogen receptors have been identified in tissues of the reproductive tract, breast, pituitary, hypothalamus, liver, and bone.

Clinical pharmacology. Estrogens are largely responsible for the development and maintenance of the female reproductive system and secondary sex characteristics. By a direct action, they cause growth and development of the uterus, fallopian tubes, and vagina. With other hormones, such as pituitary hormones and progesterone, they cause enlargement of the breasts through promotion of ductal growth, stromal development, and the accretion of fat. Estrogens are intricately involved with other hormones, especially progesterone, in the processes of the ovulatory menstrual cycle and pregnancy, and affect the release of pituitary gonadotropins. They also contribute to the shaping of the skeleton, maintenance of tone and elasticity of urogenital structures, changes in the epiphyses of the long bones that allow for the pubertal growth spurt and its termination, and pigmentation of the nipples and genitals.

Estrogens occur naturally in several forms. The primary source of estrogen in normally cycling adult women is the ovarian follicle, which secretes 70 to 500 µg of estradiol daily, depending on the phase of the menstrual cycle. This is converted primarily to estrone, which circulates in roughly equal proportion to estradiol, and to small amounts of estriol. After menopause, most endogenous estrogen is produced by conversion to androstenedione (secreted by the adrenal cortex) to estrone by peripheral tissues. After menopause, estrone and the sulfate conjugated form, estrone sulfate, are the most abundant circulating estrogens. Although circulating estrogens exist in a dynamic equilibrium of metabolic interconversions, estradiol is the principal intracellular human estrogen and is substantially more potent than estrone or estriol at the receptor.

Circulating estrogens modulate the pituitary secretion of the gonadotropins, luteinizing hormone (LH) and follicle-stimulating hormone (FSH) through a negative feedback mechanism and estrogen replacement therapy acts to reduce the elevated levels of these hormones in postmenopausal women.

Pharmacokinetics. Estrogens used in oral estrogen replacement therapy are well-absorbed from the gastrointestinal tract after release from the drug formulation. Maximum plasma concentrations are attained within 4 to 10 hours after oral administration. Estrogens are also well-absorbed through the skin and mucous membranes; when applied for a local action, absorption is usually sufficient to cause systemic effects. Systemic availability of estradiol after transdermal administration is about 20 times higher than after oral administration. The rate of absorption of parenteral administration is slowed with a prolonged duration of action over several weeks.

Although naturally occurring estrogens circulate in the blood largely bound to sex hormone-binding globulin (SHBG) and albumin, only unbound estrogens enter target tissue cells. The half-life of the different estrogens in CEE ranges from 10 to 25 hours; with estradiol, half-life is approximately 16 hours (oral) and 4 to 8 hours (transdermal). After removing transdermal patches, serum estradiol levels decline in about 12 to 24 hours to preapplication levels.

The skin metabolizes transdermal estrogen only to a small extent. In contrast, orally administered, naturally occurring estrogens and their esters are rapidly metabolized in the liver (ie, first-pass effect). A significant portion of the circulating estrogens exists as sulfate conjugates, especially estrone sulfate, which serves as a circulating reservoir for the formation of more active estrogens. This results in limited oral potency. In contrast, synthetic estrogens are degraded very slowly in the liver and other tissues, which results in their high intrinsic potency. Estrogen drug products administered by nonoral routes are not subject to first-pass metabolism, but also undergo significant hepatic uptake, metabolism, and enterohepatic recycling. Transdermal administration produces therapeutic plasma levels of estradiol with lower circulating levels of estrone and estrone conjugates and requires smaller total doses than does oral therapy.

Marketed estrogens

Estrogens are available in many prescription preparations, both as single agents and in combination with progestogens. The following are the most common types of estrogen products used in prescription preparations.

Conjugated equine estrogens. The most widely used estrogen product in the world is conjugated equine estrogens (CEE, marketed as Premarin; the official generic name has recently been changed to conjugated estrogens). CEE is also available in a vaginal cream formulation and used in HRT products.

CEE is a mixture of 50% estrone and 25% equilin sulfate along with eight other "active" estrogens and other components derived from the urine of pregnant mares. Most clinical studies have used CEE. As a result, more is known about its efficacy and safety than any other estrogen product. Premarin is FDA-approved for the treatment of moderate to severe vasomotor symptoms, vaginal atrophy, and the prevention of osteoporosis. Although Premarin has been on the US market for over 60 years, no generic equivalent has been FDA approved because of its unique composition. In Canada, other conjugated estrogens have been approved as generic substitutes for Premarin. Concern has been raised that these are not pharmacologically identical to Premarin and therefore may not provide the same therapeutic benefits. The standard CEE oral dose is 0.625 mg daily. Recent studies have shown that many women receive substantial benefit from lower doses (0.45 mg or 0.3 mg/day), although some women require higher doses for symptom relief and osteoporosis prevention.

Synthetic conjugated estrogens. Currently, the only synthetic conjugated estrogens product in the United States is Cenestin. This oral tablet contains 9 of the 10 CEE "active" components in a slow-release formulation approved by the FDA for the treatment of moderate to severe vasomotor symptoms. There are no long-term data on this product.

Estradiol. Initially, 17β-estradiol could only be administered by injection because it was not absorbed from the gastrointestinal tract. An oral product (Estrace) became available when micronization was developed; various generics are also available. Subsequently, transdermal delivery systems (reservoir, then matrix, each with different adhesives) were developed, followed by the vaginal ring (Estring) and, in Canada, topical gel (Estragel). All of the transdermal products and the vaginal ring use estradiol. It is also used in oral and transdermal HRT products. Estradiol is the most widely used estrogen in Europe.

Esterified estrogens. Esterified estrogens (Estratab, Menest, Neo-Estrone) are plant-derived products containing esterified estrogens (principally estrone).

Estropipate (piperazine estrone sulfate). This is a form of estrone sulfate that has been solubilized and stabilized by piperazine. It is marketed as Ogen and Ortho-Est, as well as in generic formulations.

Ethinyl estradiol. This synthetic steroid is widely used in combination contraceptives but is also available alone as Estinyl and is used in HRT products.

Estradiol valerate. This product is widely used in Europe but is not available in the United States. It is available as an injectable estrogen (Delestrogen) in Canada.

Estradiol hemihydrate. This product is available in tablet form for use locally in the vagina (Vagifem).

Measuring estrogen potency presents challenge. Estrogens vary in their dose equivalency and their effects on various target tissues. Oral micronized estradiol 1.0 mg is equivalent to CEE 0.625 mg with respect to effects on liver function, whereas 0.5 mg oral micronized estradiol produces changes in bone density equivalent to CEE 0.625 mg. (See Table 3 for an approximation of equivalency.) Very few head-to-head trials have compared different estrogens. Clinicians tend to view estrogen products as equivalent on a dose-for-dose basis, although data do not support this assumption; their metabolic pathways and side effects can vary in general and from woman to woman. Estrogen therapy should be tailored to the individual.

Table 3. Approximate equivalent estrogen doses for menopausal use

conjugated equine estrogens	0.625 mg
synthetic conjugated estrogens	0.625 mg
esterified estrogens	0.625 mg
piperazine estrone sulfate (0.75 mg)	0.625 mg
ethinyl estradiol	0.005-0.015 mg
17β-estradiol (oral)	1.0 mg
17β-estradiol (transdermal patch)	50 μg
17β-estradiol (transdermal gel)	1.5 mg/2 metered pumps

Route of administration. For menopause-related therapy, estrogen can be administered orally, transdermally, or locally in the vagina. Intramuscular preparations are rarely used. A woman's preference should be a primary factor in determining the estrogen delivery route, with the primary goal being enhancing continuance of therapy. In some women, medical factors may determine the route (eg, vaginal administration to treat vaginal atrophy or transdermal administration for women with hypertriglyceridemia).

Oral products. With oral estrogen products, estrone will be the predominant estrogen in the circulation owing to the first-pass uptake and metabolism in the liver. This hepatic effect is associated with the production of HDL cholesterol.

Table 4. Oral ERT products for postmenopausal use in the United States and Canada

Composition	Product name	Available dose forms (mg)
Conjugated equine estrogens	Premarin	0.3, 0.9, 0.625, 1.25, 2.5
Synthetic conjugated estrogens	Cenestin*	0.625, 0.9
	Congest**	0.3, 0.625, 0.9, 1.25, 2.5
	CES**	0.3, 0.625, 0.9, 1.25
	PMS-conjugated**	0.3, 0.625, 0.9, 1.25
Esterified estrogens	Estratab*	0.3, 0.625, 2.5
	Menest*	0.3, 0.625, 1.25, 2.5
	Neo-Estrone**	0.3, 0.625, 1.25
Micronized 17β-estradiol	Estrace	0.5, 1.0, 2.0
	Various generics*	0.5, 1.0, 2.0
Estropipate (piperazine estrone sulfate)	Ortho-Est*	0.625, 1.25
	Ogen	0.625, 1.25, 2.5
	Various generics*	0.625, 1.25
Ethinyl estradiol	Estinyl*	0.02, 0.05

* Available only in the United States.
** Available only in Canada.
Products not marked are available in the United States and Canada.

Local estrogen products refer to products formulated specifically for use in the vagina: vaginal creams, a vaginal ring, and a vaginal tablet. Vaginal creams have been available in the United States for decades; the tablet and ring were more recently marketed. Small amounts of estrogen administered locally are effective for treating atrophic vaginitis. Vaginal estrogens are not used for systemic effects (eg, hot flashes, osteoporosis), although systemic absorption of vaginal estrogen cream has been documented, and women may notice breast tenderness when initiating therapy.

A relatively new method of vaginal ERT administration is a ring containing 2 mg of estradiol (marketed as Estring). The ring is inserted into the vagina similar to a diaphragm and changed every 3 months. A small estrogen surge is measurable within 24 to 48 hours of insertion, but estrogen levels subsequently fall to within the menopausal range.

Table 5. Transdermal ERT products for postmenopausal use in the United States and Canada

Composition	Product name	Release rate (mg/day)	Dosing
17β-estradiol matrix patch	Alora*	0.05, 0.075, 0.1	twice weekly
	Climara	0.025, 0.05, 0.075, 0.1	once weekly
	Esclim*	0.025, 0.0375, 0.05, 0.075, 0.1	twice weekly
	Oesclim**	0.025, 0.05	twice weekly
	Vivelle	0.0375, 0.05, 0.075, 0.1	twice weekly
	Vivelle-Dot*	0.025, 0.0375, 0.05, 0.075, 0.1	twice weekly
	Estradot**	0.0375, 0.050, 0.075, 0.1	twice weekly
17β-estradiol reservoir patch	Estraderm	0.025, 0.05, 0.1	twice weekly (patch cannot be cut)
17β-estradiol transdermal gel	Estrogel**	1.5 mg per 2 metered pumps	daily application

* Available only in the United States.
** Available only in Canada.
Products not marked are available in the United States and Canada.

However, oral estrogen is also associated with about a 25% increase in triglycerides. Several oral forms of estrogen are available (see Table 4).

Transdermal or topical estrogens can be used in lower doses because they are not dependent on gastrointestinal absorption or subjected to first-pass hepatic metabolism. There is variation in absorption among topical estrogens, depending on the carrier vehicle and how the patches are applied. In contrast to oral estrogen, high-density lipoprotein and triglyceride levels do not increase with transdermal estrogen.

Transdermal products have the advantage of theoretically delivering a more consistent blood level of estrogen, which may result in fewer headaches. Because of less liver exposure, it has been speculated that transdermal estrogen might have less effect on gallbladder disease and coagulation factors, but this has not been proven.

Estraderm was the first transdermal patch approved for use in the United States. Other patches are now available, each with different technology. A transdermal gel is available in Canada but not in the United States. Transdermal administration is less popular than oral ERT in North America. Transdermal products are listed in Table 5.

The vaginal tablet (Vagifem) is a 6-mm tablet containing 25 µg of estradiol hemihydrate. Only a small amount of estrogen is systemically absorbed, but more than with the vaginal ring. In a head-to-head study with estrogen cream, women preferred the tablet because it was less messy.

Vaginal ERT products are listed in Table 6. The initial daily dose is usually tapered to once or twice weekly, as is required to provide symptomatic relief.

Table 6. Vaginal ERT products used for atrophic vaginitis in the United States and Canada

Composition	Product name	Dosage
Vaginal creams		
17β-estradiol	Estrace Vaginal Cream*	2-4 g/d for 2-4 wk then 1 g/d 1-3/wk
conjugated equine estrogens	Premarin Vaginal Cream	0.5-2 g/d for 3 wk then 1 wk off
estrone	Neo-Estrone Vaginal Cream**	1.0 mg/g
	Oestrilin**	1.0 mg/g
Vaginal ring		
17β-estradiol	Estring	Device releases 7.5 µg/d for 90 days
Vaginal tablet		
estradiol hemihydrate	Vagifem	25 µg/d for 2 wk then 25 µg 2/wk

* Available only in the United States.
** Available only in Canada.
Products not marked are available in the United States and Canada.

H.02.b. Progestogens and HRT

For women with a uterus, progestogen is usually added to ERT (ie, HRT) to reduce the risk of endometrial hyperplasia and cancer associated with ERT. Unopposed oral ERT used for 1 or 2 years has a relative risk for endometrial cancer of approximately 2.4, which increases to 8.0 after 10 years.

The clinical goal of HRT, therefore, is to provide the beneficial effect of estrogen while protecting the uterus and to minimize side effects. Because the side effects of progestogens, especially uterine bleeding, have an adverse effect on continuance, many dosing patterns have been tested.

In one study of women who used HRT, 30% stopped taking the progestogen at some point and continued taking ERT. A more recent study in a managed care organization documented use of estrogen without progestogen in a substantial number of cases.

The term *progestogen* refers to a wide range of hormones with the properties of the naturally occurring steroid progesterone. Progestogens include both *progesterone* and the synthetic progestational compounds referred to as *progestins*.

Progesterone is the compound produced by the ovary after ovulation and by the placenta during pregnancy. Exogenous progesterone is a compound identical to endogenous progesterone. It can be synthesized in the laboratory for therapeutic use, and it is available in the United States as progesterone USP (ie, meets specifications of the *US Pharmacopeia*). The bioavailability of oral progesterone has been enhanced with micronization.

Progestins are synthetic products that have progesterone-like activity but are not identical to progesterone produced in the human body. Progestins can be classified as those that more closely resemble either progesterone or testosterone in chemical structure. Progestins obtained from a plant-derived precursor (eg, diosgenin, which is found in plants such as the wild yam or soybean) should not be referred to as natural progestogens because they undergo multiple chemical reactions during synthesis.

The pharmacokinetics of the progestogens used in menopause are poorly characterized. Many were investigated at high doses used in contraceptives or to oppose higher estrogen doses than those currently prescribed with modern HRT. At adequate doses, all progestogens will convert an estrogen-primed endometrium into secretory endometrium, reducing the endometrial cancer risk to that found in never users.

Progestogens come in many forms, including oral, transdermal, and injectable preparations (rarely used), as well as in combination with estrogen. Use of the vaginal gel or levonorgestrel IUD results in some systemic absorption. Table 7 lists the progestogens available to oppose the stimulating effect of estrogen on the endometrium.

Table 7. Progestogens used for HRT in the United States and Canada

Composition	Product name	Available dosages
Progestins: Oral tablets		
A. Structurally related to progesterone		
medroxyprogesterone acetate (MPA)	Amen,* Provera Alti-MPA,** Curretab,* Cycrin,* Gen-Medroxy,** Novo-Medrone, ** various generics	10.0 mg 2.5, 5.0, 10.0 mg
B. Structurally related to testosterone (19-nortestosterone)		
norethindrone (norethisterone)	Micronor, Nor-QD*	0.35 mg
norethindrone acetate	Aygestin,* Norlutate, generic	5.0 mg
norgestrel	Ovrette*	0.075 mg
levonorgestrel IUD	Mirena	20 µg/day approximate release rate 52 mg/IUD; 5-yr use
Progesterone: Oral capsule		
micronized progesterone USP (in peanut oil)	Prometrium	100, 200 mg
Progesterone: Oral liquid	Cytex**	50/mL
Progesterone: Vaginal gel	Crinone	4% or 8% gel (45 or 90 mg/dose)

* Available only in the United States.
** Available only in Canada.
Products not marked are available in the United States and Canada.

All progestogens affect metabolism to some degree. High doses of oral progestogens affect insulin sensitivity and elevate low-density lipoprotein (LDL) cholesterol, while standard HRT progestin doses lower high-density lipoprotein (HDL) cholesterol. Norethindrone acetate lowers triglycerides. Procoagulant changes are not different with added progestogen, and there are no apparent adverse effects of added progestogens on coagulation risk factors, although this is often discussed. More research is needed to determine the overall effects of progestogens.

The FDA approval of progestogen products to oppose postmenopausal ERT is relatively recent, although progestogens have been used in this way for decades. The most commonly used progestogen formulation for endometrial protection among US women is the oral progestin medroxyprogesterone acetate (MPA). It is also the most widely studied progestogen for postmenopausal use.

Currently, only transdermal progestogen is the progestin norethindrone (NET), which is marketed combined with estradiol (CombiPatch, Estalis, Estalis sequi, Estracomb). Low doses of transdermal progestogens theoretically have metabolic advantages over higher doses of oral therapy because they avoid the first-pass effects; however, clinical data are limited.

Since vaginal administration at typical doses avoids systemic effects, vaginal progestogen is an attractive option. A vaginal bioadhesive gel containing micronized progesterone (Crinone) provides sustained and controlled delivery of progesterone to the vaginal tissue. In a trial using cyclic administration of the gel, no hyperplasia was observed after 3 months. However, experts consider the trial duration of 3 months to be inadequate.

It is important to note that transdermal progesterone cream or gel preparations obtained either over-the-counter or custom-compounded by prescription may not exert sufficient activity to protect the endometrium from unopposed estrogen. These products should not be used for this purpose until optimum therapeutic doses and serum levels of topical progesterone are established.

The use of a progestogen-releasing IUD is appealing because it delivers the progestogen in the highest concentration directly to the endometrium where protection is needed. The only progestogen-containing IUD available in the United States, Mirena, is not FDA-approved for this use, although there are small studies suggesting it is effective. There is some systemic absorption of levonorgestrel with Mirena. Its relatively low dose (20 µg/day) and 5-year lifespan makes it an attractive alternative for perimenopausal women. The progesterone IUD, Progestasert, is no longer marketed.

Prior to the late 1990s, US women seeking progesterone products had to rely on custom-compounded formulations. Prometrium, an oral capsule containing micronized progesterone, was the first FDA-approved option for use in HRT. Anecdotal data suggest that women who experience unpleasant side effects with a synthetic progestin, especially mood changes, sometimes respond more favorably to progesterone. However, this product should never be used by a woman allergic to peanuts, as the active ingredient is suspended in peanut oil. In addition, a small percentage of women may experience extreme dizziness and/or drowsiness during initial therapy, so women should use caution when driving or operating machinery. Bedtime dosing is advised.

Micronized progesterone formulations (eg, cream, lotion, gel, oral capsule, suppositories) are also available by prescription through custom-compounding pharmacies. Most third-party payors do not cover the cost of these experimental therapies.

HRT regimens. There are many HRT regimens from which to choose, and there is no consensus on the preferred regimen. Regimens may be classified into cyclic, cyclic-combined, continuous-cyclic, continuous long-cycle, continuous-combined, and intermittent-combined (see Table 8).

Table 8. Terminology defining types of HRT regimens

Regimen	Estrogen	Progestogen
Cyclic	Days 1-25	Last 10-14 days of ERT cycle
Cyclic-combined	Days 1-25	Days 1-25
Continuous-cyclic (sequential)	Daily	10-14 days every month
Continuous long-cycle	Daily	14 days every 3-6 months
Continuous-combined	Daily	Daily
Intermittent-combined (pulsed-progestogen; continuous-pulsed)	Daily	Repeated cycles of 3 days on, 3 days off

Cyclic HRT. Estrogen is taken from day 1 to day 25 of the calendar month with progestogen added the last 10 to14 days. This allows for a hormone-free interval of 3 to 6 days and is designed to mimic the normal premenopausal ovulatory cycle. Progestogen therapy should be used for 10 days or more.

With this regimen and standard HRT dosing, about 80% of women have withdrawal uterine bleeding after the progestogen cycle. This bleeding usually starts 1 to 2 days after the last progestogen dose and continues a few days during the therapy-free interval. Estrogen should be resumed at the beginning of the next month irrespective of bleeding.

Some women will experience vasomotor symptoms during the therapy-free interval, due to the relatively short half-life of estrogens (eg, the half-life of oral estradiol has been reported to be 15-20 hours).

This is the oldest of the regularly used HRT regimens and is decreasing in popularity in North America, primarily because newer regimens have lower uterine bleeding rates.

Cyclic-combined HRT. Estrogen is combined with a progestogen on days 1 to 25, followed by a hormone-free interval of approximately 5 days. This regimen provides a low rate of uterine bleeding and a high rate of tolerability in studies using oral micronized progesterone. In one trial, endometrial biopsies performed before and after 4 months of cyclic-combined HRT (2 mg/day 17β-estradiol plus 50, 100, or 200 mg/day oral micronized progesterone) showed an atrophic endometrium in all women receiving 200 mg/day oral micronized progesterone and in most women receiving 100 mg/day. Uterine bleeding occurred in the first few cycles, but decreased with time. However, the trial duration of 4 months is considered inadequate for evaluating the regimen's effect on endometrial hyperplasia.

Continuous-cyclic HRT. This regimen is sometimes referred to as *sequential HRT*. Estrogen is used daily with progestogen added cyclically for 10 to 14 days during each month. The combination pill Premphase provides a sequential regimen of estrogen for 14 days followed by estrogen and progestin for 14 days, similar to oral contraceptives. In a typical continuous-cyclic regimen, progestogen is started on the 1st or 15th of the month. Starting the first day of the month makes it easier for some women to track their uterine bleeding, as the cycle day corresponds with the day of the month.

Uterine bleeding occurs in about 80% of women when a progestogen is withdrawn, although it sometimes starts 1 or 2 days earlier, depending on the dose and type of progestogen used. The main advantage of the continuous-cyclic regimen compared with cyclic HRT is the absence of an estrogen-free period during which vasomotor symptoms may occur.

Continuous long-cycle HRT. To lessen the incidence of uterine bleeding, a modified continuous-cyclic HRT regimen of daily estrogen with cyclic progestogen (eg, 10 mg/day MPA for 14 days during the month) added every 3 to 6 months has been evaluated. Although this regimen reduces the number of withdrawal bleeding episodes, it has resulted in heavier and longer periods.

The effect on endometrial protection is undetermined. Two studies did not find evidence of endometrial hyperplasia after 1 year in women using estrogen at standard (0.625 mg/day CEE) or one-half standard (0.3 mg/day CEE) doses with MPA administered either quarterly or every 6 months. However, the Scandinavian Long Cycle Study, which used 2 mg/day of 17β-estradiol (twice the standard dose) with a progestin administered quarterly, was stopped after 3 of 5 scheduled years because of an increased incidence of hyperplasia compared with a monthly progestogen regimen. Until more data are available, the continuous long-cycle regimen is not recommended as standard therapy.

Continuous-combined HRT. These regimens were developed to address uterine withdrawal bleeding, which is annoying to women and decreases continuance. In this regimen, a woman uses estrogen and progestogen every day. Within several months, the endometrium can become atrophic and amenorrhea results.

Currently marketed continuous-combined HRT preparations do not have significant rates of endometrial cancer, based on short-term studies usually no longer than 1 year. The continuous-combined regimen is the predominant regimen used in North America.

Various HRT doses in continuous-combined fixed-dose regimens have demonstrated a low incidence of endometrial hyperplasia. The use of combined oral CEE plus MPA (CEE 0.625/MPA 2.5 mg/day; CEE 0.45/MPA 2.5 mg/day; CEE 0.45/MPA 1.5 mg/day; CEE 0.3/MPA 1.5 mg/day) produced hyperplasia rates equal to those found in the placebo arms of clinical trials (<1%). Use of oral continuous-combined regimens of 17β-estradiol (1 mg/day) with NETA (0.1, 0.25, or 0.5 mg/day), as well as oral ethinyl estradiol (1.0, 2.5, 5.0, or 10 μg/day) combined with NETA (0.2, 0.5, 1.0, or 1.0 mg/day,

respectively), also resulted in hyperplasia rates less than 1%. Use of transdermal 17β-estradiol (50 μg/day) combined with NETA (0.14 or 0.25 mg/day) did not result in any measurable hyperplasia after 1 year of treatment. A continuous-combined transdermal patch delivering 17β-estradiol (25 μg/day) and NETA (0.125 mg/day) provided endometrial protection and maintained a high rate of amenorrhea in a 2-year clinical trial.

Intermittent-combined HRT. This regimen (also called *pulsed-progestogen* or *continuous-pulsed HRT*) provides a daily dose of estrogen while the progestogen dose is intermittently administered in cycles of 3 days on and 3 days off, which is repeated without interruption. This regimen is designed to lower the incidence of uterine bleeding while avoiding the down-regulation of progesterone receptors that may result with continuous progestogen, a mechanism that may not fully protect the endometrium. By interrupting the progestogen for 3 of every 6 or 7 days, up-regulation of progesterone receptors occurs intermittently.

In clinical trials, the use of pulsed regimens has resulted in amenorrhea rates of 80% after 1 year with favorable endometrial hyperplasia safety profiles. However, almost all prospective studies of this regimen were only 1 year in length. Longer-term surveillance of endometrial effects will be needed to more fully ascertain efficacy and safety.

Comparing regimens: endometrial hyperplasia. A 1999 Cochrane review reports that the addition of oral progestin to ERT, administered either as continuous-cyclic or continuous-combined, is associated with reduced rates of hyperplasia. Cyclic progesterone added to ERT also has been shown to inhibit the development of endometrial hyperplasia. In the Postmenopausal Estrogen/Progestin Interventions Trial (PEPI), combining CEE (0.625 mg/day) with progesterone (200 mg/day for 12 days/mo) for 3 years did not result in an increase in endometrial hyperplasia compared with placebo.

It has been suggested that continuous-combined HRT may not be as protective as continuous-cyclic HRT, citing the possibility that some buildup of the endometrium may not be shed, and that continuous progestogen may completely down-regulate progesterone receptors, thereby reducing endometrial protection. However, epidemiologic studies of continuous-combined HRT indicate no increased risk and may even suggest added protection over continuous-cyclic HRT against endometrial cancer. A 9-month study of postmenopausal women using cyclic progestin for 10 to 13 days a month found an incidence of complex endometrial hyperplasia and atypical hyperplasia of 5.3% and 0.7%, respectively.

Comparing regimens: uterine bleeding. Many postmenopausal women dislike having episodes of uterine bleeding and this progestogen-related side effect decreases HRT continuance. Various regimens have been designed to lessen or eliminate bleeding.

Retrospective trials have suggested that regular uterine bleeding occurring after day 11 of a cyclic 12-day progestogen course reflects a normal secretory pattern of the endometrial tissue. However, prospective trials have not confirmed these findings, and no correlation has been established between day of bleeding onset and histological findings. Nevertheless, most studies with cyclic administration of progestogen have shown a high percentage of regular withdrawal uterine bleeding in women with a normal secretory endometrium. Bleeding pattern is a less reliable indicator of endometrial safety when continuous-combined regimens are used.

Breakthrough uterine bleeding (not called *withdrawal* uterine bleeding because it does not result from progestogen withdrawal) is the unpredictable and irregular bleeding associated with regimens using continuous progestogen. It has been observed in 40% of women using a continuous-combined regimen during the first 3 to 6 months. The probability of achieving amenorrhea is greater if HRT is started 12 months or more after menopause; women who are recently postmenopausal exhibit more breakthrough bleeding. Most of the women (75%-89%) who continued therapy became amenorrheic within 12 months. However, bleeding may persist intermittently for months or years. Persistent breakthrough bleeding with continuous-combined HRT may necessitate switching to another regimen.

A study comparing two continuous-combined regimens — CEE 0.625 mg/day plus MPA 2.5 mg/day and 17β-estradiol 1 mg/day plus NETA 0.5 mg/day — found that within 3 months, 71.4% of the estradiol-NETA users reached amenorrhea compared with 40.0% of the CEE-MPA users, but after 6 months, the differences were not statistically significant. This study confirmed other findings that recently postmenopausal women (within 1-2 years of last menses) experienced more bleeding than women more than 3 years postmenopausal.

Table 9. Combination estrogen-progestogen products for postmenopausal use in the United States and Canada

Composition	Product name	Available dosages
Oral continuous-cyclic regimen		
conjugated equine estrogens (E) + medroxyprogesterone acetate (P) (E alone for days 1-14, followed by E+P on days 15-28)	Premphase* Premplus**	0.625 mg (E) + 5.0 mg (P) two tablets: E; E + P
Oral continuous-combined regimen		
conjugated equine estrogens (E) + medroxyprogesterone acetate (P)	Prempro* Premplus**	0.625 mg (E) + 2.5 or 5.0 mg (P)
ethinyl estradiol (E) + norethindrone acetate (P)	Femhrt	5 μg (E) + 1 mg (P)
17β-estradiol (E) + norethindrone acetate (P)	Activella*	1 mg (E) + 0.5 mg (P)
Oral intermittent-combined regimen		
17β-estradiol (E) + norgestimate (P) (E alone for 3 days, followed by E+P for 3 days; repeated continuously)	Ortho-Prefest*	1 mg (E) + 0.09 mg (P) two tablets: E; E + P
Transdermal continuous-combined regimen		
17β-estradiol (E) + norethindrone acetate (P)	CombiPatch* Estalis** Estalis sequi**	0.05 mg (E) + 140 μg (P)
	CombiPatch* Estalis**	0.05 mg (E) + 250 μg (P)
	Estalis sequi** Estracomb**	

* Available only in the United States.
** Available only in Canada.
Products not marked are available in the United States and Canada.

The 19-nortestosterone derivatives (eg, NET, NETA, levonorgestrel, norgestimate) tend to produce less breakthrough uterine bleeding during the first few months of use because of atrophy caused by increased progestational activities. Conversely, micronized oral progesterone when given sequentially may lead to less uterine bleeding than other progestogens. In this setting, the endometrium is weakly proliferative and does not exhibit a strong progestational effect.

Among women using HRT beyond 2 years, those using a continuous-combined regimen have a lower rate of breakthrough uterine bleeding and fewer endometrial biopsies than those using the cyclic regimen. These findings confirm other studies that show decreased breakthrough uterine bleeding over time in women using the continuous-combined regimen. Nevertheless, continuance rates at 3 years are slightly higher in cyclic HRT users than in continuous-combined HRT users.

Intrauterine-administered progestogen is an option to avoid systemic side effects, although the marketed levonorgestrel IUD (Mirena) was developed for contraception, not HRT use. This IUD, which releases levonorgestrel at a rate of 20 μg/day, appears to be effective in postmenopausal women in opposing ERT's proliferative effects on the endometrium. Similar effects had been observed with the progesterone IUD, now withdrawn from the market. A lower-dose levonorgestrel-containing IUD (10 μg/day) also appears to protect the endometrium and produces minimal uterine bleeding. However, more experience and longer duration of use are required before conclusions regarding its clinical endometrial response profile can be reached.

Marketed HRT combination products. Several combination estrogen/progestogen products are available (see Table 9). Although these are convenient and many women prefer to take one pill or use one patch, they do reduce dosing flexibility.

H.02.c. Custom-compounded formulations

Custom compounding allows individualized dosing and combinations of therapy, depending on a woman's preference or tolerance. It also allows for different modes of administration of hormones, including subdermal implants, sublingual tablets, rectal suppositories, and nasal sprays. Products can be prepared without the binders, fillers, preservatives, or adhesives found in patented products. However, because these formulations are not FDA-approved, they often have not been as thoroughly tested as patented products. Their safety, reliability, and efficacy may be

uncertain. These products should be used with caution and only with informed patient consent. More research is needed to determine the risk-benefit ratio of using compounded hormones.

Compounded ERT/HRT formulations are used by many practitioners of complementary and alternative medicine. Traditional clinicians also utilize compounding pharmacies for women who need hormonal therapy not available in marketed products. Women also request compounded formulations, sometimes when they are misled by health claims that are not government regulated. Often, women are attracted to hormones marketed as "natural," which they perceive as better or safer than other formulations.

Transdermal creams and pills of many varieties are compounded. Some of the most widely used custom estrogen products contain estriol, a weak estrogen having 5% to 10% the effect of estradiol. Limited data show that oral estriol helps to relieve hot flashes. Estriol alone or in an oral "tri-estrogen" mixture of three estrogens (usually 80% estriol, 10% estrone, and 10% estradiol, and sometimes called Tri-Est) is often promoted as providing the benefits of FDA-approved estrogen formulations without increasing the risk of breast or endometrial cancer. Although estriol is a weak estrogen, it can still have a stimulatory effect on the breast and endometrium. Most data supporting estriol or any compounded formulation as safer than the standard products are anecdotal. Until more is known, women with an intact uterus using custom-compounded estrogen should also use a progestogen to counter estrogen's stimulatory effect on the endometrium.

Before the micronized progesterone product Prometrium was marketed in the United States, oral micronized progesterone (USP) was a frequently prescribed compound. Custom products are still used and may be especially appropriate for women with peanut allergies, since Prometrium contains progesterone suspended in peanut oil. A 200-mg dose of micronized progesterone USP is equivalent to about 5 mg MPA. The available strengths of Prometrium preclude continuous-combined HRT; custom products can provide lower strengths for daily dosing.

Custom topical preparations of progesterone are also available, although the strength typically used is available in over-the-counter products (eg, Pro-Gest cream). Topical progesterone products do not achieve adequate serum levels to counter the stimulatory effect of estrogen on the uterus.

H.02.d. ERT/HRT safety issues

The contraindications to ERT/HRT, as established by the FDA, include known or suspected pregnancy or breast cancer, estrogen-dependent neoplasia, undiagnosed abnormal uterine bleeding, and an active thromboembolic disorder. As with all therapies, the contraindications may not be absolute, provided that the potential benefits outweigh the potential risks and the woman makes an informed decision. Some of the relevant safety issues when considering HRT are presented in Table 10.

Estrogen may affect liver function. The variety and intensity of these hepatic effects depend on both the type of preparation (oral or transdermal) and the dose. Oral estrogen formulations cause an increase in plasma renin substrate, triglycerides, sex hormone binding and cortisol-binding globulins, ceruloplasmin, and the estrone-to-estradiol ratio as well as a decrease in antithrombin III activity. Most transdermal, vaginal, intramuscular, and subcutaneous estrogen preparations do not significantly affect these hepatic parameters.

Both oral and nonoral administration of ERT increase the risk of gallbladder disease. In the HERS study, the risk of gallbladder disease was 38% higher in the oral estrogen recipients than in placebo recipients. (For more, see Section P.07.)

Unopposed ERT, when used for more than 3 years, is associated with a 5-fold increased risk of endometrial cancer; if used for 10 years, the risk increases 10-fold. Adding progestogen therapy to ERT reduces that risk to the level found in women not taking hormones. (For more, see Section N.01.)

Breast cancer (history of or having a high-risk profile) is generally considered a contraindication to ERT/HRT use. In special situations, a clinician in consultation with a woman's oncologist may decide with the woman that the benefits outweigh the risks. This decision must be made with full awareness that therapy might promote more rapid tumor growth or recurrence. (For more, see Section N. 02.)

The role of ERT/HRT in primary and secondary cardiovascular disease prevention is discussed in Section L.

Table 10. Potential contraindications for ERT/HRT

Breast cancer	Therapy generally contraindicated unless decision to treat follows an informed discussion.
Endometrial cancer within 5 years	For higher grades/stages, therapy generally contraindicated unless decision to treat follows an informed decision. For grade I, stage I, cautious use of therapy after hysterectomy.
Unexplained uterine bleeding	Therapy contraindicated.
Active liver disease	Therapy contraindicated.
Chronic severe hepatic dysfunction (ALT more than twice normal)	Therapy contraindicated.
Recent vascular thrombosis	Therapy contraindicated.
Familial mixed hyperlipidemia or hypertriglyceridemia (TG > 300 mg/dL)	Oral ERT may increase triglycerides. Consider nonoral formulations and monitor triglycerides.
History of coronary artery disease or myocardial infarction	Initiating ERT/HRT may increase CVD risk.
History of thromboembolic event	Consider workup for coagulability disorder. Relative contraindication.
History of endometriosis	ERT/HRT may exacerbate endometriosis.
History of leiomyomas	Effect of ERT/HRT is variable. May make fibroids grow occasionally; if fibroids have submucosal component, bleeding can be a concern.
History of gallbladder disease and no cholecystectomy	Relative contraindication. Counsel regarding the increased risk for surgical intervention.
Seizure disorders	Cautious use of therapy.
Migraine headaches	Cautious use of therapy.
Cigarette smoking	Not a contraindication, although smokers are urged to stop on general health principles.

Side effects. A number of side effects are associated with ERT/HRT (see Table 11), and these often lead to premature discontinuance of therapy.

Table 11. Potential side effects of ERT/HRT

- Uterine bleeding (starting or returning)
- Breast tenderness (sometimes enlargement)
- Nausea
- Abdominal bloating
- Fluid retention in extremities
- Changes in the shape of the cornea (sometimes leading to contact lens intolerance)
- Headache (sometimes migraine)
- Dizziness
- Mood changes with HRT, particularly with progestin

Scientific evidence has absolved ERT/HRT from culpability in weight gain. The Rancho Bernardo prospective cohort found no significant differences in weight between hormone users and nonusers after 15 years of follow-up. These results persisted even after adjustments for a number of confounding factors including age, initial body mass index, smoking, and exercise. The results generally concur with those from the Postmenopausal Estrogen/Progestin Intervention trial (PEPI). A longitudinal study of perimenopausal weight gain in the Massachusetts Women's Health Study also reported similar results.

In some women, ERT causes fluid retention in the hands and feet and/or abdominal bloating with gaseous distention. A few women experience gastrointestinal irritation and nausea from oral HRT administration.

The most common side effect of transdermal ERT is skin irritation at the patch application site. This can sometimes be alleviated by rotating the patch, putting it on the buttock, and being sure the site is very clean. Using over-the-counter hydrocortisone cream can help as well as switching to a different ERT patch.

Women using HRT often experience uterine bleeding. Some women regard this HRT-induced bleeding as an unacceptable nuisance, although the bleeding often diminishes or stops over time. Manipulating dosages and evaluating for other gynecologic disease is indicated. In studies using low-dose hormone replacement (0.3 mg of CEE or the equivalent), bleeding is a less common side effect.

Although the vaginal estrogen ring is generally well tolerated, headache, abdominal pain, and vaginal pain or irritation have been reported. If the ring falls out, it can be rinsed off and reinserted. The ring does not usually interfere with sexual intercourse, although it can be removed if it is uncomfortable for either partner.

Estrogen vaginal creams are considered messy by some women. There are anecdotal reports of estrogen absorption by the male partner during sexual intercourse leading to gynecomastia.

A number of strategies exist for dealing with ERT/HRT side effects (see Table 12). Although there is limited scientific evidence to support these tips, clinical experience has determined they are helpful in some women.

Table 12. Dealing with ERT/HRT side effects

Side effect	Strategy
Fluid retention	Restrict salt intake, maintain adequate water intake, exercise, try a herbal diuretic or mild prescription diuretic.
Bloating	Switch to low-dose transdermal estrogen, lower the progestogen dose to a level that still protects the uterus, switch to another progestin or to micronized progesterone.
Breast tenderness	Lower the estrogen dose, switch to another estrogen, restrict salt intake, switch to progesterone or to another progestin, cut down on caffeine and chocolate.
Headaches	Switch to transdermal estrogen, lower the dose of estrogen and/or progestogen, switch to a continuous-combined regimen, switch to progesterone or a 19-norpregnane derivative, ensure adequate water intake, restrict salt, caffeine, and alcohol intake.
Mood changes	Lower the progestogen dose, switch progestogens, change to a continuous-combined HRT regimen, ensure adequate water intake, restrict intakes of salt, caffeine, and alcohol.
Nausea	Take oral estrogen tablets with meals, switch to another oral estrogen, switch to transdermal estrogen, lower the estrogen or progestogen dose.

An extremely important principle to consider when prescribing HRT, and especially when managing side effects, is that each woman is an individual with her own psychology and physiology. A trial of more than one or two products or regimens may be required to find the most appropriate one.

H.02.e. Transition from hormonal contraception to HRT

Transitioning a woman's therapy from hormonal contraception to postmenopausal estrogen-progestogen therapy (HRT) should be done as soon as is appropriate. Even oral contraceptives (OCs) with very low hormone doses provide significantly higher hormone levels than in standard HRT. Clinicians should consider the woman's need for contraception when making this transition. Perimenopausal women can ovulate sporadically and are potentially fertile

Timing of the switch is often difficult, because cessation of menses — the hallmark of menopause — is not observed while using OCs and some other forms of hormonal contraception. Some clinicians choose age 51, the median age of natural menopause in Western women, to make the switch to HRT. Other clinicians choose age 53 in an effort to provide contraception for those women who reach menopause later than the median age.

Another approach is to base the switch on serum levels of follicle-stimulating hormone (FSH). If the woman's FSH level is consistently above 30 mIU/mL, she has reached menopause and the transition can be safely made. However, use of hormones must cease 2 weeks prior to the FSH measurement, as hormone therapy renders the test invalid. A nonhormonal method of contraception should be used during this time by women who are sexually active.

As an alternative, perimenopausal women may be switched at any time, with counseling to use another form of contraception. If menstrual periods resume, switching back to a contraceptive is an option. If a perimenopausal woman has no further need for contraception, the switch from a contraceptive to lower-dose HRT can occur at any time.

Counseling regarding the potential progestogen-related uterine bleeding with HRT is particularly important when transitioning from hormonal contraceptives to HRT. Some women may misconstrue this bleeding as a menstrual period, misleading them into believing that they are still fertile.

Bibliography

Archer DF, Furst K, Tipping D, Dain MP, Vandepol C. A randomized comparison of continuous combined transdermal delivery of estradiol-norethindrone acetate and estradiol alone for menopause. CombiPatch Study Group. *Obstet Gynecol* 1999;94:498-503.

Archer DF, Pickar JH, Bottiglioni F, for the Menopause Study Group. Bleeding patterns in postmenopausal women taking continuous combined or sequential regimens of conjugated estrogens with medroxyprogesterone acetate. *Obstet Gynecol* 1994;83:686-692.

Badimon L, Bayes-Genis A. Effects of progestogens on thrombosis and atherosclerosis. *Hum Reprod Update* 1999;5:191-199.

Barrett-Connor E. Postmenopausal estrogen therapy and selected (less-often-considered) disease outcomes. *Menopause* 1999;6:14-20.

Barrett-Connor E, Slone S, Greendale G, et al. The Postmenopausal Estrogen/Progestin Interventions Study: primary outcomes in adherent women. *Maturitas* 1997;27:261-274.

Bélisle S, Derzko C. Hormone replacement therapy and cancer: Canadian consensus on menopause and osteoporosis. *J SOGC* 2001;23:1198-1203.

Berman RS, Epstein RS, Lydick E. Risk factors associated with women's compliance with estrogen replacement therapy. *J Womens Health* 1997;6:219-226.

Bjarnason K, Cerin A, Lindgren R, Weber T. Adverse endometrial effects during long cycle hormone replacement therapy. Scandinavian Long Cycle Study Group. *Maturitas* 1999;32:161-170.

Bolaji II, Mortimer G, Grimes H, Tallon DF, O'Dwyer E, Fottrell PF. Clinical evaluation of near-continuous oral micronized progesterone therapy in estrogenized postmenopausal women. *Gynecol Endocrinol* 1996;10:41-47.

Brynhildsen J, Hammar M. Low dose transdermal estradiol/ norethisterone acetate treatment over 2 years does not cause endometrial proliferation in postmenopausal women. *Menopause* 2002;9:137-144.

Buck A, Shen L, Kelly S, et al. Steady-state bio availability of estradiol from two matrix transdermal delivery systems, Alora and Climara. *Menopause* 1998;5:107-112.

Casper RF, Chapdelaine A. Estrogen and interrupted progestin: a new concept for menopausal hormone replacement therapy. *Am J Obstet Gynecol* 1993;168:1188-1196.

Chetkowski RJ, Meldrum DR, Steingold KA, et al. Biologic effects of transdermal estradiol. *N Engl J Med* 1986;314:1615-1620.

Chen C-L, Weiss NS, Newcomb P, Barlow W, White E. Hormone replacement therapy in relation to breast cancer. *JAMA* 2002; 287:734-741.

Corson SL, Richart RM, Caubel P, et al. Effect of a unique constant-estrogen, pulsed-progestin hormone replacement therapy containing 17β-estradiol and norgestimate on endometrial histology. *Int J Fertil* 1999;44:279-285.

Crawford SL, Casey VA, Avis NE, McKinlay SM. A longitudinal study of weight and the menopause transition: results from the Massachusetts Women's Health Study. *Menopause* 2000;7:96-104.

Daly E, Vessey MP, Hawkins MM, Carson JL, Gough P, Marsh S. Risk of venous thromboembolism in users of hormone replacement therapy. *Lancet* 1996;348:977-980.

Darj E, Nilsson S, Axelsson O, Hellberg D. Clinical and endometrial effects of oestradiol and progesterone in post-menopausal women. *Maturitas* 1991;13:109-115.

de Lignieres B. Endometrial hyperplasia: risks, recognition and the search for a safe hormone replacement regimen. *J Reprod Med* 1999;44:191-196.

de Ziegler D, Ferriani R, Moraes LA, Bulletti C. Vaginal progesterone in menopause: Crinone 4% in cyclical and constant combined regimens. *Hum Reprod* 2000;15(suppl 1):149-158.

Dupont A, Dupont P, Cusan L, et al. Comparative endocrinological and clinical effects of percutaneous estradiol and oral conjugated estrogen as replacement therapy in menopausal women. *Maturitas* 1991;13:297-311.

Englund DE, Johansson ED. Plasma levels of oestrone, oestradiol and gonadotropins in postmenopausal women after oral and vaginal administration of conjugated equine oestrogens. *Br J Obstet Gynaecol* 1978;85:957-964.

Eriksen BC. A randomized, open, parallel-group study on the preventive effect of an estradiol-releasing vaginal ring (Estring) on recurrent urinary tract infections in postmenopausal women. *Am J Obstet Gynecol* 1999;180:1072-1079.

Ettinger B, Li D-K, Klein R. Continuation of postmenopausal hormone replacement therapy: comparison of cyclic versus continuous combined schedule. *Menopause* 1996;3:185-189.

Ettinger B, Li D-K, Klein R. Unexpected vaginal bleeding and associated gynecologic care in postmenopausal women using hormone therapy: comparison of cyclic versus continuous combined schedules. *Fertil Steril* 1998;69:865-869.

Ettinger B, Pressman A, Van Gessel A. Low-dosage esterified estrogen opposed by progestin at 6-month intervals. *Obstet Gynecol* 2001;98:205-211.

Ettinger B, Selby J, Citron JT, et al. Cyclic hormone replacement therapy using quarterly progestin. *Obstet Gynecol* 1994;83:693-700.

Fanchin R, De Ziegler D, Bergeron C, Righini C, Torrisi C, Frydman R. Transvaginal administration of progesterone. *Obstet Gynecol* 1997;90:396-401.

Ferreira E, Brown TER. Pharmacotherapy: Canadian consensus on menopause and osteoporosis. *J SOGC* 2001; 23:1115-1114.

Fitzpatrick LA, Good A. Micronized progesterone: clinical indications and comparison with current treatments. *Fertil Steril* 1999;72:389-397.

Gambrell RD Jr. Strategies to reduce the incidence of endometrial cancer in postmenopausal women. *Am J Obstet Gynecol* 1997; 177:1196-204.

Gillet JY, Andre G, Faguer B. Induction of amenorrhea during hormone replacement therapy: optimal micronized progesterone dose: a multicenter study. *Maturitas* 1994;19:103-115.

Grady D, Rubin SM, Petitti DB, et al. Hormone therapy to prevent disease and prolong life in postmenopausal women. *Ann Intern Med* 1992;117:1016-1037.

Grodstein F, Stampfer MJ. The epidemiology of coronary heart disease and estrogen replacement in postmenopausal women. *Prog Cardiovasc Dis* 1995;38:199-210.

Grodstein F, Stampfer MJ, Colditz GA, et al. Postmenopausal hormone therapy and mortality. *N Engl J Med* 1997;336:1769-1775.

Grodstein F, Stampfer MJ, Goldhaber SZ, et al. Prospective study of exogenous hormones and risk of pulmonary embolism in women. *Lancet* 1996;348:983-987.

Grodstein F, Stampfer MJ, Mason JE, et al. Postmenopausal estrogen and progestin use and the risk of cardiovascular disease. *N Engl J Med* 1996;335:453-461.

Guetta V, Cannon RO III. Cardiovascular effects of estrogen and lipid-lowering therapies in postmenopausal women. *Circulation* 1996; 93:1928-1937.

Gutthann SP, Rodriguez LAG, Castellsague J, et al. Hormone replacement therapy and risk of venous thromboembolism: population based case-control study. *BMJ* 1997;314:796-800.

Haas S, Walsh B, Evans S, Krache M, Ravnikar V, Schiff I. The effect of transdermal estradiol on hormone and metabolic dynamics over a six-week period. *Obstet Gynecol* 1988;71:671-676.

Hemminki E, Malin M, Topo P. Selection to postmenopausal therapy by women's characteristics. *J Clin Epidemiol* 1993;46:211-219.

Hill DA, Weiss NA, Beresford SAA, et al. Continuous combined hormone replacement therapy and risk of endometrial cancer. *Am J Obstet Gynecol* 2000;183:1456-1461.

Holmgren PA, Lindskog M, von Schoultz B. Vaginal rings for continuous low-dose release of oestradiol in the treatment of urogenital atrophy. *Maturitas* 1989;11:55-63.

Hudson T. *Women's Encyclopedia of Natural Medicine: Alternative Therapies and Integrative Medicine.* Los Angeles, CA: Keats Publishing; 1999.

Hulley S, Grady D, Bush T, et al. Randomized trial of estrogen plus estrogen for secondary prevention of coronary heart disease in postmenopausal women: Heart and Estrogen/progestin Replacement Study (HERS) Group. *JAMA* 1998;280:605-613.

Jick H, Darvy LE, Myers MW, et al. Risk of hospital admission for idiopathic venous thromboembolism among users of postmenopausal estrogens. *Lancet* 1996;348:981-983.

Johnson JV, Davidson M, Archer D, Bachmann G. Postmenopausal uterine bleeding profiles with two forms of combined continuous hormone replacement therapy. *Menopause* 2002;9:16-22.

Jondet M, Maroni M, Yaneva H, Brin S, Peltier-Pujol F, Pelissier C. Comparative endometrial histology in postmenopausal women with sequential hormone replacement therapy of estradiol and, either chlormadinone acetate or micronized progesterone. *Maturitas* 2002;41:115-121.

Kim S, Korhonen M, Wilborn W, et al. Antiproliferative effects of low-dose micronized progesterone. *Fertil Steril* 1996;65:323-331.

Kritz-Silverstein D, Barrett-Connor E. Long-term postmenopausal hormone use, obesity, and fat distribution in older women. *JAMA* 1996;275:987-988.

Kurman RJ, Felix JC, Archer DF, Nanavati N, Arce J, Moyer DL. Norethindrone acetate and estradiol-induced endometrial hyperplasia. *Obstet Gynecol* 2000;96:373-379.

Lethaby A, Farquhar C, Sarkis A, Roberts H, Jepson R, Barlow D. Hormone replacement therapy in postmenopausal women: endometrial hyperplasia and irregular bleeding. *Cochrane Database Syst Rev* 2000;2:CD00042.

Levine H, Watson N. Comparison of the pharmacokinetics of Crinone 8% administered vaginally versus Prometrium administered orally in postmenopausal women. *Fertil Steril* 2000;73:516-521.

Ley CJ, Lees B, Stevenson JC. Sex- and menopause-associated changes in body-fat distribution. *Am J Clin Nutr* 1992;55:950-954.

Lobo RA. Clinical aspects of hormone replacement. In Lobo RA, ed. *Treatment of the Postmenopausal Woman: Basic and Clinical Aspects.* 2nd ed. Philadelphia, PA: Lippincott Williams and Wilkins; 1999:125-139.

Lobo RA, Zacur HZ, Caubel P, et al. A novel intermittent regimen of norgestimate to preserve the beneficial effects of 17β-estradiol on lipid and lipoprotein profiles. *Am J Obstet Gynecol* 2000;182:41-49.

Melamed M, Castano E, Notides A, Sasson S. Molecular and kinetic basis for the mixed agonist/antagonist activity of estriol. *Mol Endocrinol* 1997;11:1868-1878.

Miles RA, Press MF, Paulson RJ, Dahmoush L, Lobo RA, Sauer MV. Pharmacokinetics and endometrial tissue levels of progesterone after administration by intramuscular and vaginal routes: a comparative study. *Fertil Steril* 1994;62:485-490.

Nachtigall LE. Clinical trial of the estradiol vaginal ring in the US. *Maturitas* 1995;22(suppl):S43-S47.

Nilsson K, Heimer G. Low-dose 17 beta-oestradiol during maintenance therapy: a pharmacokinetic and pharmacodynamic study. *Maturitas* 1995;21:33-38.

The North American Menopause Society. Clinical challenges of perimenopause: consensus opinion of The North American Menopause Society. *Menopause* 2000;7:5-13.

The North American Menopause Society. Role of progestogens in hormone replacement therapy for postmenopausal women: position statement of The North American Menopause Society. *Menopause.* In progress.

Notelovitz M, Funk S, Nanavati N, Mazzeo M. Estradiol absorption from vaginal tablets in postmenopausal women. *Obstet Gynecol* 2002;99:556-562.

Pelissier C, Maroni M, Yaneva H, Brin S, Peltier-Pujol F, Jondet M. Chlormadinone acetate versus micronized progesterone in the sequential combined hormone replacement therapy of the menopause. *Maturitas* 2001;40:85-94.

Phillips A, Demarest K, Hahn DW, et al. Progestational and androgenic receptor binding affinities and in vivo activities of norgestimate and other progestins. *Contraception* 1990;41:399-410.

Pickar JH, Yeh I, Wheeler JE, Cunnane MF, Speroff L. Endometrial effects of lower doses of conjugated equine estrogens and medroxyprogesterone acetate. *Fertil Steril* 2001;76:25-31.

Raudaskoski T, Tapanainen J, Tomás E, et al. Intrauterine 10µg and 20µg levonorgestrel systems in postmenopausal women receiving oral oestrogen replacement therapy: clinical, endometrial and metabolic response. *Br J Obstet Gynaecol* 2002;109:136-144.

Raz R, Stamm W. A controlled trial of intravaginal estriol in postmenopausal women with recurrent urinary tract infections. *N Engl J Med* 1993;329:753-756.

Reubinoff BE, Wurtman J, Rojansky N, et al. Effects of hormone replacement therapy on weight, body composition, fat distribution, and food intake in early postmenopausal women: a prospective study. *Fertil Steril* 1995;64:963-968.

Robson M, Gilewski T, Haas B, et al. BRCA-associated breast cancer in young women. *J Clin Oncol* 1998;16:1642-9.

Ross AH, Boyd ME, Colgan TJ, Ferenczy A, Fugere P, Lorrain J. Comparison of transdermal and oral sequential progestogen in combination with transdermal estradiol: effects on bleeding patterns and endometrial histology. *Obstet Gynecol* 1993;82:773-779.

Ross D, Cooper AJ, Pryse-Davies J, Bergeron C, Collins WP, Whitehead MI. Randomized, double-blind, dose-ranging study of the endometrial effects of a vaginal progesterone gel in estrogen-treated postmenopausal women. *Am J Obstet Gynecol* 1997;177: 937-941.

Schairer C, Byrne GM, Rosenberg PS, et al. Estrogen replacement therapy and breast cancer survival in a large screening study. *J Nat Cancer Inst* 1999;91:264-70.

Schiff I, Tulchinsky D, Cramer D, Ryan KJ. Oral medroxyprogesterone in the treatment of postmenopausal symptoms. *JAMA* 1980;244: 1443-1445.

Schoonen WG, Joosten JW, Kloosterboer HJ. Effects of two classes of progestagens, pregnant and 19-nortestosterone derivatives, on cell growth of human breast tumor cells: I. MCF-7 cell lines. *J Steroid Biochem Mol Biol* 1995;55:423-437.

Sellers TA, Mink PJ, Cerhan JR, et al. The role of hormone replacement therapy in the risk for breast cancer and total mortality in women with a family history of breast cancer. *Ann Intern Med* 1997;127:973-80.

Shau W-Y, Hsieh C-C, Hsieh T-T, Hung T-H, Huang K-E. Factors associated with endometrial bleeding in continuous hormone replacement therapy. *Menopause* 2002;9:188-194.

Shoupe D, Meme D, Mezrow G, Lobo RA. Prevention of endometrial hyperplasia in postmenopausal women with intrauterine progesterone. *N Engl J Med* 1991;325:1811-1812.

Speroff L, Rowan J, Symons J, Genant H, Wilborn W, for the CHART Study Group. The comparative effect on bone density, endometrium, and lipids of continuous hormones as replacement therapy (CHART Study): a randomized controlled trial. *JAMA* 1996;276:1397-1403.

Sturdee DW, Ulrich LG, Barlow DH, et al. The endometrial response to sequential and continuous combined oestrogen-progestogen replacement therapy. *Br J Obstet Gynecol* 2000;107:1392-1400.

Suhonen SP, Allonen HO, Lahteenmaki P. Sustained-release estradiol implants and a levonorgestrel-releasing intrauterine device in hormone replacement therapy. *Am J Obstet Gynecol* 1995;172:562-567.

Suhonen SP, Holmström T, Allonen HO, Lähteenmäki P. Intrauterine and subdermal progestin administration in postmenopausal hormone replacement therapy. *Fertil Steril* 1995;63:336-342.

United States Pharmacopeia — National Formulary. Washington, DC: US Pharmacopeia; 2001.

Varila E, Wahlström T, Rauramo I. A 5-year follow-up study on the use of levonorgestrel intrauterine system in women receiving hormone replacement therapy. *Fertil Steril* 2001;76:969-973.

Van Haaften M, Donker G, Sie-Go D, et al. Biochemical and histological effects of vaginal estriol and estradiol applications on the endometrium, myometrium and vagina of postmenopausal women. *Gynecol Endocrinol* 1997;11:175-185.

Vasilakis C, Jick H, del Mar Melero-Montes M. Risk of idiopathic venous thromboembolism in users of progestagens alone. *Lancet* 1999;354:1610-1611.

Vooijs G, Geurts T. Review of the endometrial safety during intravaginal treatment with estriol. *Eur J Obstet Gynecol Reprod Biol* 1995;62:101-106.

Wagner TM, Moslinger RA, Muhr D, et al. BRCA1-related breast cancer in Austrian breast and ovarian cancer families: specific BRCA1 mutations and pathological characteristics. *Int J Cancer* 1998;77:354-360.

Walsh BW, Paul S, Wild RA, et al. The effects of hormone replacement therapy and raloxifene on C-reactive protein and homocysteine in healthy postmenopausal women: a randomized, controlled trial. *J Clin Endocrinol Metab* 2000;85:214-218.

Weiderpass E, Adami H-O, Baron JA, et al. Risk of endometrial cancer following estrogen replacement with and without progestins. *J Natl Cancer Inst* 1999;91:1131-1137.

White VE, Bennett L, Raffin S, Emmett K, Coleman MJ. Use of unopposed estrogen in women with uteri: prevalence, clinical implications, and economic consequences. *Menopause* 2000; 7:123-128.

The Writing Group for the PEPI Trial. Effects of estrogen or estrogen/progestin regimens on heart disease risk factors in postmenopausal women. *JAMA* 1995;273:199-208.

The Writing Group for the PEPI Trial. Effects of hormone replacement therapy on endometrial histology in postmenopausal women. *JAMA* 1996;275:370-375.

The Writing Group for the PEPI Trial. Effects of hormone therapy on bone mineral density: results from the postmenopausal estrogen/progestin interventions trial. *JAMA* 1996;276:1389-1396.

H.03. Androgen

Androgens are defined as hormones that promote the development and maintenance of male secondary sex characteristics and structures, but these hormones are important for women as well. In women, androgens are responsible for the development of reproductive function and hormonal homeostasis, and they also represent the immediate precursors for estrogen biosynthesis. They affect sexual desire, muscle mass and strength, bone density, distribution of adipose tissue, energy, and psychological well-being, including mood.

The major androgens in women (and men) are testosterone, androstenedione, dehydroepiandrosterone (DHEA), and the peripheral metabolite dihydrotestosterone. Androgens are synthesized primarily in the ovary and adrenal glands, although significant peripheral conversion occurs. Most circulating testosterone is tightly bound to the sex hormone-binding globulin (SHBG), and it is only the free, or unbound, fraction that is bioactive. Serum testosterone concentrations in women are approximately 10% those of males.

Although production of both ovarian and adrenal androgen decreases with age, there is not an abrupt decline in these hormones with menopause, as occurs with ovarian estradiol production. Surgical menopause is an exception, as testosterone levels decrease by approximately 50% following a bilateral oophorectomy. A number of factors cause androgen deficiency, including hypopituitarism, oophorectomy, adrenal insufficiency, corticosteroid use, and the use of drugs (eg, oral ERT/HRT) that increase SHBG concentrations, resulting in decreased bioavailable testosterone.

The recent Princeton consensus statement, developed by a multidisciplinary panel from around the world, concludes that the role of androgens in women's health has been generally neglected and is not well understood. The term *female androgen insufficiency* was proposed to describe a condition that meets three specific criteria: (1) dysphoric mood (ie, diminished sense of well-being), (2) persistent, unexplained fatigue, and (3) changes in sexual function (eg, decreased libido, sexual receptivity, pleasure). Fatigue is the most common symptom. Androgen insufficiency in women is not a specific consequence of spontaneous menopause. However, it can occur secondary to the age-related decline in adrenal and ovarian androgen production.

Symptoms alone are not sufficient for the diagnosis of androgen insufficiency, as this symptom complex is associated with other common disorders, including depression. Moreover, a diagnosis of androgen insufficiency should be made only if the woman has adequate levels of estrogen, as many of the symptoms are also linked to estrogen effects. Finally, although the panelists recognized the lack of a sensitive assay or absolute threshold for androgen insufficiency in women, they recommended that free testosterone (T) values must be at or below the lowest quartile of the normal range for reproductive age women (20-40 years). Low androgen levels alone do not provide a sufficient basis for establishing the diagnosis. (For more about androgen assays, see Section E.02.)

Further recommendations include addressing certain symptoms before considering a trial of androgen therapy, such as (1) major life stress or relationship conflicts, (2) hypo- or hyperthyroidism, (3) major metabolic or nutritional disorders (eg, low levels of iron or vitamin D) or other potential causes of chronic fatigue (eg, chronic fatigue syndrome, Lyme disease), and (4) psychiatric disorders (eg, depression). However, any of these conditions could exist concomitantly with androgen insufficiency.

Potential types of etiologic conditions leading to androgen insufficiency include (1) ovarian (eg, induced menopause), (2) adrenal, (3) hypothalamic-pituitary, (4) drug-related (eg, corticosteroids, oral contraceptives, oral estrogen therapy), and (5) idiopathic.

Pharmacokinetics. Oral testosterone is metabolized by the gut and 44% is cleared by the liver in the first pass. Oral doses as high as 400 mg/day are needed to achieve clinically effective blood levels for full replacement therapy. The synthetic androgens (methyltestosterone and fluoxymestrone) are less extensively metabolized by the liver and have longer half-lives. They are more suitable than testosterone for oral administration.

Testosterone in plasma is 98% bound to a specific testosterone-estradiol-binding globulin, and about 2% is free. Generally, the amount of this sex hormone-binding globulin in the plasma will determine the distribution of testosterone between free and bound forms, and the free testosterone concentration will determine its half-life.

About 90% of a dose of testosterone is secreted in the urine as glucuronic acid conjugates of testosterone and its metabolites; about 6% of a dose is excreted in the feces, mostly in unconjugated form. Inactivation of testosterone occurs primarily in the liver. Testosterone is metabolized to various 17-keto steroids through two different pathways. There are considerable variations of the half-life of testosterone reported in the literature, ranging from 10 to 100 minutes.

In many tissues, the activity of testosterone appears to depend on reduction to dihydrotestosterone, which binds to cytosol receptor proteins. The steroid-receptor complex is transported to the nucleus where it initiates transcription events and cellular changes related to androgen action.

Effects of androgen therapy in postmenopausal women. No large studies in postmenopausal women have found a consistent association of specific clinical signs and symptoms with low androgen levels that improve with androgen replacement. There is a need for large randomized, controlled trials assessing the efficacy and safety of androgen therapies for women.

Androgen therapy is receiving increasing attention for treating postmenopausal women with sexual dysfunction. In women with surgically induced menopause, high doses of intramuscular testosterone have resulted in significantly higher scores of sexual desire, fantasy, and arousal than treatment with either ERT alone or placebo. In one study, postmenopausal women randomized to treatment with esterified estrogens plus methyltestosterone reported significantly improved sexual sensation and desire compared with estrogen alone. In a single-blind study of testosterone implants, postmenopausal women randomized to combination estradiol and testosterone therapy had significantly greater scores for sexual activity, satisfaction, pleasure, and orgasm compared with women receiving estradiol alone. In a recent double-blind, randomized, placebo-controlled, crossover trial, testosterone replacement administered by a transdermal patch significantly increased the frequency of sexual activity, pleasure, and positive well-being in estrogen-treated surgically menopausal women with sexual dysfunction. Oral administration of the adrenal androgen DHEA also has been shown to improve sexual interest and satisfaction in women with adrenal insufficiency (from dexamethasone administration), but not in those experiencing natural menopause.

Androgens also may play a role in the maintenance of bone mineral density (BMD) and body composition in women. In a 9-week randomized study of the effects of ERT compared with combined ERT-methyltestosterone therapy on bone markers, both treatments reduced urinary markers of bone resorption, but only combination estradiol-methyltestosterone therapy resulted in an increase in serum markers of bone formation. In a 2-year study, BMD increased more in women randomized to estradiol-methyltestosterone than in those receiving ERT alone. In a study of physiological testosterone and estradiol replacement administered by implants, women randomized to combined estradiol and testosterone had significantly greater BMD increases than those who received estradiol alone. In addition, women who received both estradiol and testosterone implants experienced an increase in fat-free mass and a reduced ratio of fat mass to fat-free mass.

There are two important caveats when considering androgen therapy:

1. Androgen must always be administered in combination with estrogen;

2. Because androgen does not protect the endometrium against estrogen-induced hyperplasia, a progestogen should be added to the estrogen-androgen regimen in all women with an intact uterus.

Marketed androgen preparations for women. Currently, there are no FDA-approved androgen therapies for sexual dysfunction in women. The only androgen-containing product with FDA approval for women is a combination of esterified estrogens and methyltestosterone, marketed as Estratest (1.25 mg esterified estrogens and 2.5 mg methyltestosterone) and Estratest HS (0.625 mg esterified estrogens and 1.25 mg methyltestosterone). These oral tablets are indicated for the treatment of moderate to severe vasomotor symptoms unresponsive to estrogen.

In Canada, two oral testosterone products are used in women: methyltestosterone (Metandren), typically administered using one-quarter or one-eighth of a 10-mg tablet, and testosterone undecanoate (Andriol), typically used at 40-mg/day. However, the optimal dosing for women has yet to be determined. An intramuscular product, containing a combination of estradiol dienanthate, estradiol benzoate, and testosterone enanthate (Climacteron), administered 0.5 to 1.0 mL intramuscularly every 4 to 6 weeks, is also available.

Custom-compounded preparations of nonmethylated micronized testosterone USP are available, although no definitive studies have determined absorption and utilization rates. Topical 2% testosterone USP (cream, ointment) may be applied directly to the vagina and clitoral area (or any skin surface) several times weekly. Testosterone can be well absorbed through the skin and supraphysiologic levels will be obtained if large amounts are applied. Extensive anecdotal evidence supports this mode of administration for improving libido; however, no controlled studies have confirmed the safety or efficacy of topical testosterone for sexual dysfunction in women.

Testosterone administered by intramuscular injection or custom-prepared implants often results in supraphysiologic levels with the highest levels occurring near the time of administration and, thus, are not recommended. In Canada, the accepted IM dosing is a combination of 0.5 mL estradiol dienanthate, estradiol benzoate, and testosterone enanthate (Climacteron) plus 0.5 mL estradiol valerate (Delestrogen).

In the United States, DHEA is available as a dietary supplement and may be purchased without a prescription. It is not available in Canada. Although the typical replacement dose for women with low androgen levels is 50 mg daily, there is no regulation of available products and, therefore, great variability is found in the actual amount of hormone present. Thus, DHEA is not recommended. (For more, see Section G.03.b.)

Products available for men, including skin patches (Androderm, Testoderm) and gels (Androgel), are inappropriately dosed for women and should be used only for men.

Several androgen products are under investigation for use in postmenopausal women, particularly for sexual dysfunction.

Potential risks and side effects. Due to the lack of scientific evidence, the potential risks of androgen therapy for women are relatively unknown. When recommending such therapy, clinicians should fully inform women and monitor for adverse reactions. Based on current clinical trial data, potential side effects include acne, weight gain, excess facial and body hair, permanent lowering of the voice, clitoral enlargement, changes in emotion (eg, increased anger), and adverse changes in lipids. However, these effects are infrequent if androgen levels are maintained within normal physiologic ranges. Estrogenic side effects are also possible, since androgens are converted to estrogens.

Symptoms should be re-evaluated after an initial trial of 2 to 3 months of androgen therapy. Monitoring of liver function tests and lipids is advisable after 3 to 6 months and periodically thereafter in long-term users. If abnormal lipids are found, androgen therapy should be discontinued. If lipid tests do not return to normal, investigation into another cause is appropriate.

Bibliography

Arlt W, Justl HG, Callies F, et al. Oral dehydroepiandrosterone for adrenal androgen replacement: pharmacokinetics and peripheral conversion to androgens and estrogens in young healthy females after dexamethasone suppression. *J Clin Endocrinol Metab* 1998;83:1928-1934.

Bachmann G, Bancroft J, Braunstein G, et al. Female androgen insufficiency: the Princeton consensus statement on definition, classification, and assessment. *Fertil Steril* 2002;77:660-665.

Barrett-Connor E, Young R, Notelovitz M, et al. A two-year, double-blind comparison of estrogen-androgen and conjugated estrogens in surgically menopausal women: effects on bone mineral density, symptoms and lipid profiles. *J Reprod Med* 1999;44:1012-1020.

Buckler HM, Robertson WR, Wu FC. Which androgen replacement therapy for women? *J Clin Endocrinol Metab* 1998;83:3920-3924.

Davis SR, McCloud P, Strauss BJ, Burger H. Testosterone enhances estradiol's effects on postmenopausal bone density and sexuality. *Maturitas* 1995;21:227-236.

Executive summary: Stages of Reproductive Aging Workshop (STRAW): Park City, Utah, July 2001. *Menopause* 2001;8:402-407.

Graves G, Lea R, Bourgeois-Law G. Menopause and sexual function: Canadian consensus on menopause and osteoporosis. *J SOGC* 2001;23:849-852.

Judd HL, Lucas WE, Yen SS. Effect of oophorectomy on circulating testosterone and androstenedione levels in patients with endometrial cancer. *Am J Obstet Gynecol* 1974;118:793-798.

Laumann EO, Paik A, Rosen RC. Sexual dysfunction in the United States: prevalence and predictors. *JAMA* 1999;281:537-544.

Lobo RA. Androgens in postmenopausal women: production, possible role, and replacement options. *Obstet Gynecol Survey* 2001;56:361-376.

Morales AJ, Nolan JJ, Nelson JC, Yen SS. Effects of replacement dose of dehydroepiandrosterone in men and women of advancing age. *J Clin Endocrinol Metab* 1994;78:1360-1367.

Nathorst-Boos J, von Schoultz B. Psychological reactions and sexual life after hysterectomy with and without oophorectomy. *Gynecol Obstet Invest* 1992;4:97-101.

Raisz LG, Wiita B, Artis A, et al. Comparison of the effects of estrogen alone and estrogen plus androgen on biochemical markers of bone formation and resorption in postmenopausal women. *J Clin Endocrinol Metab* 1996;81:37-43.

Rannevik G, Jeppsson S, Johnell O, Bjerre B, Laurell-Borulf Y, Svanberg L. A longitudinal study of the perimenopausal transition: altered profiles of steroid and pituitary hormones, SHBG and bone mineral density. *Maturitas* 1995;21:103-113.

Sarrel P, Dobay B, Wiita B. Estrogen and estrogen-androgen replacement in postmenopausal women dissatisfied with estrogen-only therapy. *J Reprod Med* 1998;43:847-856.

Sherwin BB, Gelfand MM, Brender W. Androgen enhances sexual motivation in females: a prospective, crossover study of sex steroid administration in the surgical menopause. *Psychosom Med* 1985;47:339-351.

Shifren JL, Braunstein GD, Simon JA, et al. Transdermal testosterone treatment in women with impaired sexual function after oophorectomy. *N Engl J Med* 2000;343:682-688.

H.04. Osteoporosis agents

In addition to estrogen, other prescription drugs provide options for osteoporosis therapy. These include selective estrogen-receptor modulators (SERMs) and the bone-specific agents, bisphosphonates and calcitonin. Like estrogen, these agents require adequate calcium and vitamin D intake for optimal efficacy. All these agents, including estrogen, inhibit osteoclastic bone resorption and preserve or increase bone density. However, these drugs do not rebuild damaged skeletal architecture. They should be considered agents that prevent the progression of osteoporosis. All these alternatives to ERT/HRT have been demonstrated to reduce fracture risk.

H.04.a. Bisphosphonates

Bisphosphonates reduce bone resorption through inhibition of osteoclast activity by impeding the differentiation of new osteoclasts, inhibiting the activity of osteoclasts that are present, and hastening osteoclast cell death. These oral therapies act specifically on bone; they do not provide other benefits.

In North America, three bisphosphonates are approved for the management of postmenopausal osteoporosis prevention and treatment: alendronate, risedronate, and etidronate.

Alendronate. Alendronate (Fosamax) is a potent bisphosphonate approved for postmenopausal osteoporosis prevention and treatment in both the United States and Canada. Several large clinical trials with alendronate (oral tablets) have documented its ability to increase BMD and, in women with osteoporosis, to reduce fracture risk in women with osteoporosis.

For women in early postmenopause, 2 to 4 years of alendronate therapy (≥5 mg daily) increased BMD at the spine and hip by 1% to 4% compared with baseline, while women who received placebo experienced declines of 2% to 4%. The effect on BMD with alendronate was similar to that seen in women who took hormone therapy in a trial comparing the two treatments. In older women with low bone density or previous vertebral fractures, alendronate (5 mg daily) increased BMD in the spine and hip by 4% to 10% after treatment for 3 to 7 years.

Decreases in fracture risk have been demonstrated in postmenopausal women with established osteoporosis. In this population, alendronate therapy reduced the risk of fracture at the hip and spine by about 50% and reduced the occurrence of multiple vertebral fracture by about 90%. In the Fracture Efficacy Trial (FIT), postmenopausal women with either osteoporosis or vertebral fracture had significant reductions of 84% for symptomatic vertebral fracture and 42% in overall symptomatic fracture during 4 years of follow-up. Risk reduction reached statistical significance after 6 months. Decreased fracture risk has not been demonstrated in women who do not have low bone mass.

Therapy for up to 7 years has not been associated with untoward skeletal effects. However, bone resorption remains suppressed for up to 2 years when alendronate is discontinued after 5 years of treatment. These data suggest that alendronate therapy may be discontinued after 5 years of treatment, at least in women at relatively low risk of fracture.

Recommended doses of alendronate are 5 mg daily for osteoporosis prevention and 10 mg daily for treatment. Alendronate is also approved in a dose of 5 or 10 mg daily for the management of women receiving glucocorticoids. Administering the full week's dose (35 mg or 70 mg) as a single dose is as effective as the equivalent daily dose, and the weekly dosing regimen is approved for both prevention and treatment.

No significant side effects have been observed with alendronate therapy during placebo-controlled trials. However, in clinical practice, alendronate has been associated with gastrointestinal (GI) intolerance, characterized by heartburn or abdominal pain. Rarely, esophagitis or upper GI bleeding has occurred. No difference in symptoms has been noted between the daily and weekly dosing regimens.

To minimize these symptoms, women should take each dose with a full glass of plain water (not mineral water) to facilitate delivery to the stomach, and should remain upright for 30 minutes. This drug should be taken on an empty stomach, first thing in the morning, to avoid inhibition of absorption by food, beverages, or other medicines. Other than GI disorders, the side effects of alendronate are relatively minor and infrequent.

Etidronate. Etidronate (Didronel) was the first bisphosphonate that received FDA approval; however, it is indicated only for treatment of Paget's disease, not for osteoporosis prevention or treatment, and the dose approved for Paget's is considerably higher than that used in osteoporosis therapy. Etidronate is approved in Canada for osteoporosis prevention and treatment in postmenopausal women as well as the prevention of glucocorticoid-induced osteoporosis. In Canada, etidronate is packaged with calcium tablets and marketed in a "dose pack" as Didrocal.

Treatment with cyclic etidronate and calcium (cycles of 400 mg/day etidronate for 14 days followed by 500 mg/day elemental calcium the remainder of each 3-month cycle) increases BMD 1% to 8% in the spine and hip, and reduces the incidence of vertebral fracture in older women with established osteoporosis. No effect on nonvertebral fracture has been observed in randomized clinical trials.

Therapy in younger postmenopausal women preserves or increases BMD, but an effect on fracture reduction has not been documented.

For osteoporosis, etidronate and calcium can be administered in cycles of 400 mg/day etidronate for 14 days followed by 500 mg elemental calcium per day for the remainder of each 3-month cycle. Administration is cyclic because daily use may cause osteomalacia (abnormalities in bone mineralization). Mild diarrhea is the most common side effect.

Risedronate. Risedronate (Actonel) was originally FDA-approved for Paget's disease. It is now also approved for the prevention and treatment of postmenopausal osteoporosis (as well as glucocorticoid-induced osteoporosis). Risedronate is available in the United States and Canada in strengths of 5 and 35 mg.

Risedronate has demonstrated antiresorptive activity when administered orally. In postmenopausal women, risedronate (5 mg/day for 3 years) suppressed bone turnover and increased bone density in the spine and hip by 3% to 6%. In women with previous vertebral fractures, risedronate therapy reduced subsequent vertebral fracture rates by 40% to 50%. This effect was observed as early as 1 year after starting treatment. After 3 years, the risk of multiple vertebral fractures was reduced by about 90% and nonvertebral fracture incidence decreased by 30% to 40%. In a study designed to evaluate the effect of risedronate on hip fracture risk, treatment for 3 years decreased risk by 40% in women aged 70 to 79 years with established osteoporosis. However, risedronate's effect on hip fracture risk was not observed in older women (≥80 years) who were identified primarily on the basis of fall-related risk factors for hip fracture.

The recommended dose for prevention and treatment of postmenopausal osteoporosis is 5 mg/day or 35 mg/wk. In clinical trials, the incidence of GI side effects has not been significantly different from that of placebo; yet dosage instructions are the same as with alendronate. Whether there is a difference in the GI tolerability between alendronate and risedronate is unclear. In Canada, taking the drug at least 2 hours before and after a meal is an approved alternative dosing schedule.

H.04.b. SERMs

Selective estrogen-receptor modulators (SERMs) are estrogen-like compounds that act as weak estrogen agonists in some organ systems and as estrogen antagonists in others. The goal of SERM therapy is to provide the bone benefits of estrogen without an adverse effect on the endometrium or breast. Because of this, they are sometimes referred to as "designer estrogens." This term, however, has caused some women to mistakenly believe that SERMs provide all the benefits of estrogen without any of the risks.

Tamoxifen. The first SERM available in the United States and Canada — tamoxifen (Nolvadex) — was approved for breast cancer therapy. Later, it was found to also increase bone density in the spine. Fractures of the spine, hip, and wrist were reduced by about 35% in the tamoxifen-treated group compared with the placebo group in the NSABP Breast Cancer Prevention Trial, which involved more than 13,000 women at high risk of developing breast cancer. A subgroup of those women taking tamoxifen oral tablets demonstrated an approximate 2% increase in BMD. The effect of tamoxifen on fracture risk is unclear. The increase in BMD associated with tamoxifen use is a function of the drug's antiresorptive action in bone, a property shared with estrogen. Tamoxifen, however, is not approved (or typically used) for osteoporosis prevention or treatment.

Raloxifene. The SERM raloxifene (Evista), the first SERM approved for postmenopausal osteoporosis prevention and treatment, is marketed in both the United States and Canada. In postmenopausal women, raloxifene reduces serum and urinary markers of bone turnover and produces modest (1%-3%) increases in BMD in the spine, hip, and wrist.

In the Multiple Outcomes of Raloxifene (MORE) trial, a randomized, controlled study, raloxifene significantly reduced the risk of new clinical vertebral fracture in women with osteoporosis. For those women with an existing vertebral fracture, reductions of 66% to 79% were seen at year 1, 46% to 65% at year 2, and 41% to 52% at year 3 for 60 and 120 mg/day doses, respectively. In another large clinical trial, raloxifene reduced the risk of vertebral fracture in postmenopausal women with osteoporosis by 35% to 50%. Reduction in fracture risk at other sites has not demonstrated. The approved dose is 60 mg (oral tablet) daily, administered at any time of the day.

A frequent side effect of raloxifene is the accentuation of vasomotor symptoms. Leg cramps occur more frequently in raloxifene-treated women than in those receiving placebo.

The effect of raloxifene on cardiovascular risk is unknown. Raloxifene lowers total and low-density lipoprotein cholesterol levels. It does not raise high-density lipoprotein cholesterol or triglyceride concentrations. Raloxifene carries the same risk as ERT/HRT and tamoxifen of venous thromboembolic events, such as deep vein thrombosis, but such events are rare. However, these drugs should not be given during periods of prolonged immobilization or to those with a history of clotting disorders.

In a randomized, controlled, 6-month trial of 390 healthy postmenopausal women, raloxifene (60 and 120 mg/day) significantly lowered serum levels of homocysteine (by 8% and 6%, respectively), similar to the 7% reduction obtained with HRT (daily therapy of 0.625 mg CEE and 2.5 mg MPA). In this study, HRT increased C-reactive protein levels by 84%, whereas raloxifene had no significant effect. A randomized, controlled trial (RUTH) is currently being conducted to determine the effect of raloxifene on cardiovascular risk.

Raloxifene does not adversely affect the endometrium. Preliminary trials have found that raloxifene may offer protection against some types of breast cancer. It is hoped that the ongoing Study of Tamoxifen and Raloxifene (STAR) will provide some insight.

H.04.c. Calcitonin

Salmon calcitonin is a potent inhibitor of osteoclast activity in vitro. In clinical settings, calcitonin has very modest effects on BMD, with values in the hip and spine increasing by 1% to 3% after 3 to 5 years of treatment. Originally given by subcutaneous injection (Miacalcin, Calcimar), calcitonin is most often administered as a nasal spray (Miacalcin), and this formulation is approved in both Canada and the United States for treatment of postmenopausal osteoporosis. The drug is not approved for osteoporosis prevention.

In women with established osteoporosis, therapy with nasal calcitonin (200 IU daily for 5 years) has been shown to reduce the risk of new vertebral fractures by 36%. No effect on spine fractures was seen with higher or lower doses, and no effect on nonvertebral fracture risk was observed at any dose.

Small studies suggest that calcitonin may hasten the improvement of bone pain following acute vertebral fractures, but the drug is not approved for this indication.

The drug is dosed as 200 IU (1 spray) administered daily in alternating nostrils. Although it is a hormone, calcitonin has none of the effects of ERT/HRT on menopause symptoms, and it does not affect tissue in the breast or uterus. Calcitonin has few adverse effects other than local nasal irritation with the nasal spray formulation.

Because calcitonin is a less potent agent than other pharmacologic therapies for osteoporosis, it is reserved as an alternative for women who cannot or choose not to take one of the other agents. It is recommended for use in women who are at least 5 years beyond menopause because efficacy has not been observed in the early postmenopausal period.

H.04.d. Others

Other marketed treatments have been studied for their effects on bone, but they are not FDA-approved for osteoporosis.

Sodium fluoride. Treatment with sodium fluoride has been shown to increase trabecular bone mass, especially in the spine. However, bone formed during therapy is not of normal quality, and fracture rates may actually increase. With the availability of proven effective agents, sodium fluoride is no longer an appropriate option to treat osteoporosis.

Anabolic steroids. An osteoporosis therapy used for many years is anabolic steroids (eg, IM nandrolone decanoate). Efficacy has not been documented, and side effects and safety are concerns.

Progestogens. Progestogen alone may have some effect on bone, although various compounds have different qualities. For example, studies suggest that norethisterone acetate and norethindrone may have a beneficial effect, whereas medroxyprogesterone acetate may slow the rate of bone loss in the spine but not in other sites. Topical progesterone is often promoted as a therapy for osteoporosis, but a randomized, prospective trial showed no effect on bone turnover or BMD.

Thiazides. Thiazide therapy improves calcium balance by inhibiting urinary calcium loss. Prospective studies demonstrate a slowing of bone loss, while observational studies suggest that thiazide therapy reduces fracture risk. Currently, thiazides should not be considered an effective therapy for osteoporosis.

Statins. The observation that bisphosphonates inhibit a step in the cholesterol synthesis pathway raised interest in the possibility that hydroxymethylglutaryl-coenzyme A (HMG-CoA) reductase inhibitors, also known as statins, could also inhibit bone resorption. The effects of statins on fracture risks in several case-control, observational studies have been inconsistent, with no effects noted in the largest studies. In animal studies, statins increase bone formation. Randomized trials are underway to evaluate the effects of statins on human BMD.

Phytoestrogens. Phytoestrogens (whole foods and supplements) offer promise, but no clinical trial has yet demonstrated an effect on fracture reduction. (For more, see Section I.05.b.2.)

Custom-compounded formulations. Some clinicians prescribe custom-compounded formulations of estriol or oral micronized progesterone for bone benefits; however, more research is needed to document the efficacy and safety of these non-FDA-approved products.

Investigational therapies. A number of new therapies are under investigation, including the following.

- *Parathyroid hormone.* Recombinant human parathyroid hormone (rhPTH or simply PTH) is an 84-amino acid, nonestrogen, hormonal peptide that regulates calcium balance. Unlike all the marketed options, PTH is a true growth-promoting (anabolic) drug.

Daily subcutaneous injections of PTH activate bone formation and result in substantial increases in trabecular bone density and connectivity in women with postmenopausal osteoporosis, regardless of whether they are receiving ERT. In postmenopausal women with prior vertebral fracture, 19 months of PTH (20 or 40 µg daily) reduced the incidence of new vertebral fractures by 65% and 69%, respectively, and new nonvertebral fractures by 53% and 54%. The effect of PTH on hip fracture risk is not known.

Dose-related hypercalcemia and related symptoms (eg, nausea, headache) are the most common side effects observed with PTH, but they occur infrequently and transiently at the appropriate dose. The need for daily injections of the hormone with a pen-like device, as used for insulin, may be considered a nuisance by some women.

It is unclear whether PTH should be administered alone or in combination with an antiresorptive agent, or whether antiresorptive treatment should be initiated when PTH therapy is stopped, to prevent subsequent loss of bone. The BMD response to PTH when administered with ERT may be greater than with PTH alone, but whether this results in improved fracture reduction is undetermined.

FDA approval of teriparatide, the N-terminal fragment rhPTH(1-34), for postmenopausal osteoporosis is anticipated; the brand name is Forteo.

- *Tibolone.* This synthetic steroid has estrogenic, androgenic, and progestogenic properties. At a dose of 2.5 mg/day for 2 years, tibolone has been shown to be effective in preventing bone loss in postmenopausal women and increasing BMD in women with established osteoporosis. A more recent study showed that lower doses (0.625 and 1.25 mg/day) are effective for preventing postmenopausal bone loss. Tibolone (2.5 mg/day) has also been shown to be effective in treating menopause symptoms, such as hot flashes. Tibolone is available in many countries as Livial, but this drug is not approved in the United States or Canada.

- *Zoledronic acid.* In 2002, a randomized, placebo-controlled clinical trial using an IV bisphosphonate formulation, zoledronic acid, found that a single annual dose in postmenopausal women with osteoporosis provided 1-year beneficial effects on BMD and bone turnover similar to those seen with daily or weekly oral formulations. No significant adverse effects, including GI upset, were observed.

However, additional documentation regarding fracture risk reduction and the long-term side effect profile are needed. Zoledronic acid may prove to be an effective option to avoid problems with oral dosing, including GI intolerance and poor adherence to therapy. Zoledronic acid may be marketed in the future as Zometa.

H.04.e. Combining therapies

Combining ERT/HRT with other prescription therapies for osteoporosis has not been widely studied, yet it is common in clinical practice.

Combining a bisphosphonate and ERT has been shown to produce small but significantly greater gains in BMD than either ERT or bisphosphonate alone at the lumbar spine (8.1% vs 6%) and hip trochanter (3.5% vs 0.5%) in postmenopausal women with osteoporosis. In a study of combined cyclic etidronate and HRT therapy, BMD gains were 3% higher at the spine and 2% higher at the hip over gains made with HRT alone. Similarly, combining raloxifene and alendronate results in somewhat greater increase in BMD than was observed with either drug alone.

Whether these small changes in BMD result in added fracture protection is not known. Combining therapies increases cost and the potential for side effects, and the long-term safety of combined therapies has not yet been determined. Clinicians are advised to use combination antiresorptive therapy with caution.

Bibliography

Abdalla HI, Hart DM, Lindsay R, et al. Prevention of bone mineral loss in postmenopausal women by norethisterone. *Obstet Gynecol* 1985;66:789-792.

Albertazzi P, Di Micco R, Zanardi E. Tibolone: a review. *Maturitas* 1998;30:295-305.

Black DM, Cummings SR, Karpf DB, et al. Randomized trial of effect of alendronate on risk of fracture in women with existing vertebral fractures. Fracture Intervention Trial Research Group. *Lancet* 1996;348;1535-1541.

Bone HG, Greenspan SL, McKeever C, et al for the Alendronate/Estrogen Study Group. Alendronate and estrogen effect in postmenopausal women with low bone mineral density. *J Clin Endocr Metab* 2000;85:720-726.

Cauley JA, Seeley DG, Ensrud K, et al. Estrogen replacement therapy and fractures in older women. Study of the Osteoporotic Fractures Research Group. *Ann Intern Men* 1995;122:9-16.

Chan KA, Andrade SE, Boles M, et al. Inhibitors of hydroxymethyl-glutaryl-coenzyme A reductase and risk of fracture among older women. *Lancet* 2000;355:2185-2188.

Chesnut CH, Silverman S, Andriano K, et al. A randomized trial of nasal spray calcitonin in postmenopausal women with established osteoporosis: the Prevent Recurrence of Osteoporotic Fracture Study. PROOF Study Group. *Am J Med* 2000;109:267-276.

Christiansen C. Treatment of osteoporosis. In: Lobo RA, ed. *Treatment of the Postmenopausal Woman: Basic and Clinical Aspects.* 2nd ed. Philadelphia, PA: Lippincott Williams & Wilkins; 1999:315-328.

Cohen JF, Lu Y. Characterization of hot flashes reported by healthy postmenopausal women receiving raloxifene or placebo during osteoporosis prevention trials. *Maturitas* 2000;34:65-73.

Colditz GA, Hankinson SE, Hunter DJ, et al. The use of estrogens and progestins and the risk of breast cancer in postmenopausal women. *N Engl J Med* 1995;332:1589-1593.

Cosman F, Nieves J, Woelfert L, et al. Parathyroid hormone added to established hormone therapy: effects on vertebral fracture and maintenance of bone mass after parathyroid hormone withdrawal. *J Bone Miner Res* 2001;16:925-931.

Cranney A, Guyatt G, Krolicki N, et al. A meta-analysis of etidronate for the treatment of postmenopausal osteoporosis. Osteoporosis Research Advisory Group. *Osteoporos Int* 2001;12:140-151.

Cummings SR, Black DM, Thompson DE, et al. Effect of alendronate on risk of fracture in women with low bone density but without vertebral fractures: results from the Fracture Intervention Trial. *JAMA* 1998;280:2077-2082.

Cummings SR, Eckert S, Krueger KA, et al, for the Multiple Outcomes of Raloxifene Evaluation. The effect of raloxifene on risk of breast cancer in postmenopausal women: results from the MORE randomized trial. *JAMA* 1999;281:2189-2197.

Daly E, Vessey MP, Hawkins MM, et al. Risk of venous thromboembolism in users of hormone replacement therapy. *Lancet* 1996;348:977-980.

Dawson-Hughes B, Harris SS, Krall EA, et al. Rates of bone loss in postmenopausal women randomly assigned to one of two dosages of vitamin D. *Am J Clin Nutr* 1995;61:1140-1145.

Delmas PD, Bjanarson NH, Mitlak BH, et al. Effects of raloxifene on bone mineral density, serum cholesterol concentrations, and uterine endometrium in postmenopausal women. *N Engl J Med* 1997;337:1641-1647.

Dempster DW, Cosman F, Kurland ES, et al. Effects of daily treatment with parathyroid hormone on bone microarchitecture and turnover in patients with osteoporosis: a paired biopsy study. *J Bone Miner Res* 2001;16:1846-1853.

Eastell R. Treatment of postmenopausal osteoporosis. *N Engl J Med* 1998;338:736-746.

Ettinger B, Black DM, Mitlak BH, et al. Reduction of vertebral fracture risk in postmenopausal women with osteoporosis treated with raloxifene. *JAMA* 1999;282:637-645.

Ettinger B, Genant HK, Cann CE. Long-term estrogen replacement therapy prevents bone loss and fractures. *Ann Intern Med* 1985; 102:319-324.

Fisher B, Costantino JP, Wickerham L, et al. Tamoxifen for prevention of breast cancer: report of the National Surgical Adjuvant Breast and Bowel Project P-1 Study. *J Natl Cancer Inst* 1998;90:1371-1378.

Fogelman I, Ribot C, Smith R, et al. Risedronate reverses bone loss in postmenopausal women with low bone mass: results from a multinational, double-blind, placebo-controlled trial. *J Clin Endocrinol Metab* 2000;85:1895-1900.

Gallagher JC, Baylink DJ, Freeman R, McClung M. Prevention of bone loss with tibolone in postmenopausal women: results of two randomized, double-blind, placebo-controlled, dose finding studies. *J Clin Endocrinol Metab* 2001;86:4717-4726.

Gallagher JC, Kable WT, Goldgar D. Effect of progestin therapy on cortical and trabecular bone: comparison with estrogen. *Am J Med* 1991;90:171-178.

Gradishar W, Glusman J, Lu Y, Vogel C, Cohen FJ, Sledge GW Jr. Effects of high dose raloxifene in selected patients with advanced breast carcinoma. *Cancer* 2000;88:2047-2053.

Grady D, Rubin SM, Petitti DB, et al. Hormone therapy to prevent disease and prolong life in postmenopausal women. *Ann Intern Med* 1992;117:1016-1037.

Gruber HE, Ivey JL, Baylink DJ, et al. Long-term calcitonin therapy in postmenopausal osteoporosis. *Metabolism* 1984;33:295-303.

Harris ST, Eriksen EF, Davidson M, et al. Effect of combined risedronate and hormone replacement therapies on bone mineral density in postmenopausal women. *J Clin Endocrinol Metab* 2001;86:1890-1897.

Harris ST, Watts NB, Genant HK, et al. Effects of risedronate treatment on vertebral and nonvertebral fractures in women with postmenopausal osteoporosis: a randomized controlled trial. *JAMA* 1999;282:1344-1352.

Harris ST, Watts NB, Jackson RD, et al. Four-year study of intermittent cyclic etidronate treatment of postmenopausal osteoporosis: three years of blinded therapy followed by one year of open therapy. *Am J Med* 1993;95:557-567.

Harrison JE, Chow R, Dornan J, et al. Evaluation of a program for rehabilitation of osteoporotic patients (PRO): 4-year follow-up. *Osteoporosis Int* 1993;3:13-17.

Heath DA, Bullivant BG, Boiven C, Balena R. The effects of cyclical etidronate on early postmenopausal bone loss: an open, randomized controlled study. *J Clin Densitom* 2000;3:27-33.

Herd RJM, Balena R, Blake GM, et al. The prevention of early postmenopausal bone loss by cyclical etidronate therapy: a 2-year, double-blind, placebo-controlled study. *Am J Med* 1997;103:92-99.

Hodgson SF, Watts NB, Bilezikian JP, et al. American Association of Clinical Endocrinologists 2001 medical guidelines for clinical practice for the prevention and management of postmenopausal osteoporosis. *Endocr Pract* 2001;7:293-312.

Hodsman A, Adachi J, Olszynski W. Use of bisphosphonates in the treatment of osteoporosis. Prevention and management of osteoporosis: consensus statements from the Scientific Advisory Board of the Osteoporosis Society of Canada. *CMAJ* 1996;155:945-948.

Hosking D, Clair ED, Chilvers CE, et al, for the Early Postmenopausal Intervention Cohort Study Group. Prevention of bone loss with alendronate in postmenopausal women under 60 years of age. *N Engl J Med* 1998;338:485-492.

Johnell O, Scheele WH, Lu Y, Reginster J-Y, Need AG, Seeman E. Additive effects of raloxifene and alendronate on bone density and biochemical markers of bone remodeling in postmenopausal women with osteoporosis. *J Clin Endocrinol Metab* 2002;87:985-992.

LaCroix AZ, Ott SM, Ichikawa L, Scholes D, Barlow WE. Low-dose hydrochlorothiazide and preservation of bone mineral density in older adults: a randomized, double-blind, placebo-controlled trial. *Ann Intern Med* 2000;133:516-526.

Leonetti HB, Longo S, Anasti JN. Transdermal progesterone cream for vasomotor symptoms and postmenopausal bone loss. *Obstet Gynecol* 1999;94:225-228.

Levis S, Quandt SA, Thompson D, et al, for the FIT Research Group. Alendronate reduces the risk of multiple symptomatic fractures: results from the Fracture Intervention Trial. *J Am Geriatr Soc* 2002; 50:409-415.

Liberman UA, Weiss SR, Broll J, et al. Effect of oral alendronate on bone mineral density and the incidence of fractures in postmenopausal osteoporosis. The Alendronate Phase III Osteoporosis Treatment Study Group. *N Engl J Med* 1995; 333:1437-1443.

Lindsay R, Cosman F, Lobo RA, et al. Addition of alendronate to ongoing hormone replacement therapy in the treatment of osteoporosis: a randomized, controlled clinical trial. *J Clin Endocrinol Metatab* 1999;84:3076-3081.

Lindsay R, Nieves J, Formica C, et al. Randomized controlled study of the effect of parathyroid hormone on vertebral-bone mass and fracture incidence among postmenopausal women on oestrogen with osteoporosis. *Lancet* 1997;350:550-555.

Lindsay R, Tohme JF. Estrogen treatment of patients with established postmenopausal osteoporosis. *Obstet Gynecol* 1990;76:290-295.

Lippuner K, Haenggi W, Birkhauser MH, Casez JP, Jaeger P. Prevention of postmenopausal bone loss using tibolone or conventional peroral or transdermal hormone replacement therapy with 17beta-estradiol and dydrogesterone. *J Bone Min Res* 1997;12:806-812.

Lufkin EG, Whitaker MD, Nickelsen T, et al. Treatment of established postmenopausal osteoporosis with raloxifene: a randomized trial. *J Bone Miner Res* 1998;13:1747-1754.

Maricic M, Adachi JD, Sarkar S, Wu W, Wong M, Harper K. Early effects of raloxifene on clinical vertebral fractures at 12 months in postmenopausal women with osteoporosis. *Arch Intern Med* 2002;162:1140-1143.

McClung M, Clemmesen B, Daifotis A, et al. Alendronate prevents postmenopausal bone loss in women without osteoporosis: a double-blind, randomized, controlled trial. *Ann Intern Med* 1998; 128:253-261.

McClung MR, Geusens P, Miller PD, et al. Effect of risedronate on the risk of hip fracture in elderly women. *N Engl J Med* 2001; 344:333-340.

Meier CR, Schlienger RG, Krasenzlin ME, Schlegel D, Jick H. HMG-CoA reductase inhibitors and the risk of fractures. *JAMA* 2000;283:3205-3210.

Michaëlsson K, Baron JA, Farahmand BY, et al. Hormone replacement therapy and risk of hip fracture: population based case-control study. The Swedish Hip Fracture Study Group. *BMJ* 1998;316:1858-1863.

Miller PD, Watts NB, Licata AA, et al. Cyclical etidronate in the treatment of postmenopausal osteoporosis: efficacy and safety after seven years of treatment. *Am J Med* 1997;103:468-476.

Mortensen L, Charles P, Bekker PJ, et al. Risedronate increases bone mass in an early postmenopausal population: two years of treatment plus one year of follow-up. *J Clin Endocr Metab* 1998;83:396-402.

Neer RM, Arnaud CD, Zanchetta JR, et al. Effect of parathyroid hormone (1-34) on fractures and bone mineral density in postmenopausal women with osteoporosis. *N Engl J Med* 2001;344:1434-1441.

Nieves JW, Komar L, Cosman F, Lindsay R. Calcium potentiates the effect of estrogen and calcitonin on bone mass: review and analysis. *Am J Clin Nutr* 1998;67:18-24.

The North American Menopause Society. Management of postmenopausal osteoporosis: position statement of The North American Menopause Society. *Menopause* 2002;9:84-101.

The North American Menopause Society. The role of isoflavones in menopausal health: consensus opinion of The North American Menopause Society. *Menopause* 2000;7:215-229.

Overgaard K, Hansen MA, Jensen SB, Christiansen C. Effect of calcitonin given intranasally on bone mass and fracture rates in established osteoporosis: a dose response study. *BMJ* 1992; 305:556-561.

Pun KK, Chan LW. Analgesic effect of intranasal salmon calcitonin in the treatment of osteoporotic vertebral fractures. *Clin Ther* 1989;11:205-209.

Quigley ME, Martin PL, Burner AM, et al. Estrogen therapy arrests bone loss in elderly women. *Am J Obstet Gynecol* 1987;156:1516-1523.

Ravn P, Bidstrup M, Wasnich RD, et al. Alendronate and estrogen-progestin in the long-term prevention of bone loss: four-year results from the early postmenopausal intervention cohort study. *Ann Intern Med* 1999;131:935-942.

Ravn P, Weiss SR, Rodriguez-Portales JA, et al for the Alendronate Osteoporosis Prevention Study Group. Alendronate in early postmenopausal women: effects on bone mass during long-term treatment and after withdrawal. *J Clin Endocrinol Metab* 2000; 85:1492-1497.

Recker RR, Davies KM, Dowd RM, Heaney RP. The effect of low-dose continuous estrogen and progesterone therapy with calcium and vitamin D on bone in elderly women: a randomized, controlled trial. *Ann Intern Med* 1999;130:897-904.

Reeve J, Mitchell A, Tellez M, et al. Treatment with parathyroid peptides and estrogen replacement for severe postmenopausal vertebral osteoporosis: prediction of long-term responses in spine and femur. *J Bone Miner Metab* 2001;19:103-114.

Reginster J-Y, Minne H, Sorensen OH, et al. Randomized trial of the effects of risedronate on vertebral fractures in women with established postmenopausal osteoporosis. *Osteoporos Int* 2000; 11:83-91.

Reid IR, Brown JP, Burckhardt P, et al. Intravenous zoledronic acid in postmenopausal women with low bone mineral density. *N Engl J Med* 2002;346:653-661.

Rittmaster RS, Bolognese M, Ettinger MP, et al. Enhancement of bone mass in osteoporotic women with parathyroid hormone followed by alendronate. *J Clin Endocrinol Metab* 2000;85:2129-2134.

Rymer J, Chapman M, Fogelman I. Tibolone and the prevention of bone loss. *Osteoporos Int* 1994;4:314-319.

Schairer C, Byrne GM, Rosenberg PS, et al. Estrogen replacement therapy and breast cancer survival in a large screening study. *J Natl Cancer Inst* 1999;91:264-270.

Schnitzer T, Bone HG, Crepaldi G, et al. Therapeutic equivalence of alendronate 70 mg once-weekly and alendronate 10 mg daily in the treatment of osteoporosis. *Aging Clin Exp Res* 2000;12:1-12.

Sellers TA, Mink PJ, Cerhan JR, et al. The role of hormone replacement therapy in the risk for breast cancer and total mortality in women with a family history of breast cancer. *Ann Intern Med* 1997;127:973-980.

Storm T, Thamsborg G, Steiniche T, et al. Effect of intermittent cyclical etidronate therapy on bone mass and fracture rate in women with postmenopausal osteoporosis. *N Engl J Med* 1990;322:1265-1271.

Tonino RP, Meunier PJ, Emkey R, et al. Skeletal benefits of alendronate: 7-year treatment of postmenopausal osteoporotic women. *J Clin Endocrinol Metab* 2000;85:3109-3115.

van Staa TP, Wegman S, de Vries F, Leufkens B, Cooper C. Use of statins and risk of fractures. *JAMA* 2001;285:1850-1855.

Walsh BW, Kuller LH, Wild RA, et al. Effects of raloxifene on serum lipids and coagulation factors in healthy postmenopausal women. *JAMA* 1998;279:1445-1451.

Walsh BW, Paul S, Wild RA, et al. The effects of hormone replacement therapy and raloxifene on C-reactive protein and homocysteine in healthy postmenopausal women: a randomized, controlled trial. *J Clin Endocrinol Metab* 2000;85:214-218.

Wang PS, Solomon DH, Mogun H, Avorn J. HMG-CoA reductase inhibitors and the risk of hip fractures in elderly patients. *JAMA* 2000;283:3211-3216.

Wimalawansa SJ. A four-year randomized controlled trial of hormone replacement and bisphosphonate, alone or in combination, in women with postmenopausal osteoporosis. *Am J Med* 1998;104:219-226.

The Writing Group for the PEPI Trial. Effects of hormone replacement therapy on bone mineral density: results from the Postmenopausal Estrogen/Progestin Interventions (PEPI) trial. *JAMA* 1996;276:1389-1396.

Section I: Therapeutic options: Complementary and alternative medicine (CAM)

Complementary and alternative medicine (CAM), also referred to as *integrative* medicine, includes a broad range of healing philosophies, approaches, and therapies that conventional medicine does not commonly use, accept, study, understand, or make available. A therapy is generally called *complementary* when it is used in addition to conventional treatment, whereas it is called *alternative* when it is used instead of conventional treatment.

Conventional therapies are those that are widely accepted and practiced by the mainstream medical community, including holders of MD (medical doctor) or DO (doctor of osteopathy) degrees, some of whom also may practice CAM. Other terms for conventional medicine are allopathic, Western, modern, and mainstream medicine; and biomedicine.

Traditional medicine, on the other hand, refers to historical and indigenous systems of medicine that have been used for centuries or, in the case of Traditional Chinese Medicine (TCM) and Ayurveda, even longer. Therapies used in traditional medicine are sometimes called *natural.* Many CAM therapies are called *holistic,* which generally means they consider the whole person, including physical, mental, emotional, and spiritual aspects.

As reported by the NIH, a national survey conducted in 2000 found that approximately one-third of Americans used complementary and alternative medicine. More than 50% of Canadians use "natural health products," including herbal products, vitamin and mineral supplements, and homeopathic medicines, as well as TCM and Ayurveda.

Many women who choose CAM therapies do so because these healthcare approaches mirror their own values, beliefs, and philosophical orientations toward health and life. Some turn to CAM therapies because of their dissatisfaction with conventional medicine, but most CAM users also use conventional methods. Consumers often believe that "natural" therapies are safe. However, it is unrealistic to believe that a treatment can provide benefit without the potential for negative effects.

Despite the broad use of CAM therapies, healthcare professionals and the public need more substantial scientific information to demonstrate convincingly that CAM practices lead to positive clinical outcomes, improve quality of life, and are effective, safe, and/or beneficial. In 1998, the US Congress established the National Center for Complementary and Alternative Medicine (NCCAM) at the NIH to stimulate, develop, and support research on CAM for the benefit of the public. In 1999, the Office of Natural Health Products was established as a directorate in Health Canada to oversee the regulation, labeling, developing, licensing, monitoring, and research involving natural health products.

NCCAM is an advocate for quality science, rigorous and relevant research, and open and objective inquiry into which CAM practices work, which do not, and why. Its overriding mission is to provide the American public with reliable information about the safety and effectiveness of CAM practices. NCCAM is not a referral agency for alternative medical treatments or individual practitioners. NCCAM can be reached through its consumer clearinghouse (toll-free at 1-888-644-6226) and through its Web site (http://nccam.nih.gov). PubMed (http://www.nlm.nih.gov/hinfo.html) contains bibliographic citations (1966 to present) related to CAM. NCCAM also maintains the Complementary and Alternative Medicine Database of the Combined Health Information Database (http://chid.nih.gov/).

NCCAM groups CAM therapies into five major domains: (1) alternative medical systems, (2) mind-body interventions, (3) manipulative and body-based methods, (4) energy therapies, and (5) biologically based treatment. A brief description of these systems follows.

I.01. Alternative medical systems

Alternative medical systems include complete systems of theory and practice that have evolved independent of and often prior to the conventional biomedical approach. Many are traditional systems of medicine that are practiced by individual cultures throughout the world, including a number of venerable Asian approaches.

I.01.a. Traditional Chinese Medicine

Traditional Chinese Medicine (TCM) emphasizes the proper balance or disturbances of qi (pronounced chi and meaning vital energy) in health and disease. TCM consists of a group of techniques and methods, including acupuncture, herbal medicine, oriental massage, and qi gong.

TCM includes menopause as part of a syndrome that involves an imbalance of body energy. Practitioners of TCM consistently diagnose this imbalance as a spectrum of deficiency of kidney energy. The TCM practitioner may use herbs, meditative or breathing exercises, massage, or diet to balance the energy and, therefore, reduce menopause symptoms. Acupuncture is also used by TCM practitioners in treating menopause, although clinical trials are lacking.

Acupuncture involves stimulating specific anatomic points in the body for therapeutic purposes, usually by puncturing the skin with a needle. Acupuncture is widely practiced in North America. The most common procedures utilize sterile thin, solid, metallic needles that the practitioner inserts into the skin to stimulate acupuncture points. The pins are manipulated either manually or by electrical stimulation to relieve pain or prevent a broad spectrum of other health conditions.

Most studies evaluating the efficacy of acupuncture do not provide comparable results due to problems with design, sample size, and other factors. The results are further complicated by inherent difficulties in the use of appropriate controls, such as sham acupuncture groups.

Some specific uses for acupuncture include pain relief, treatment of organic, mental, and emotional dysfunctions, treatment of energy disturbances, prevention of illness (eg, immune system support), induction of analgesia, treatment of addictions, and performance enhancement.

There is evidence of efficacy of acupuncture or postoperative dental pain. Some evidence exists for efficacy relieving pain associated with menstrual cramps, epicondylitis (tennis elbow), and fibromyalgia. In comparison with the side effects and iatrogenic risks of pharmaceutical therapy usually prescribed for these conditions, acupuncture provides a relatively benign option.

The NIH Consensus Development Panel on Acupuncture stated that acupuncture may be a useful adjunct or alternative therapy and it may be included in a comprehensive management program for a number of conditions including addiction, stroke rehabilitation, headache, menstrual cramps, epicondylitis, fibromyalgia, myofascial pain, osteoarthritis, low back pain, carpal tunnel syndrome, and asthma. Acupuncture has shown efficacy in relieving the nausea and vomiting associated with surgery or chemotherapy, and it is FDA-approved for this purpose.

There is anecdotal evidence supporting the effectiveness of acupuncture in relieving hot flashes in some women. In addition, one study in perimenopausal women demonstrated efficacy of acupuncture in reducing the number of hot flashes and the amount of perspiration generated. More trials are needed to confirm this small study.

I.01.b. Other cultural systems

Ayurveda is India's traditional system of medicine. Ayurvedic medicine (meaning "science of life") is a comprehensive system of medicine that places equal emphasis on body, mind, and spirit, and strives to restore the innate harmony of the individual. Some of the primary Ayurvedic treatments include diet, exercise, meditation, herbs, massage, exposure to sunlight, and controlled breathing.

Other traditional medical systems have been developed by Native American, Aboriginal, African, Middle-Eastern, Tibetan, and Central and South American cultures.

This guidebook does not address how menopause treatment is approached using these systems.

I.01.c. Homeopathic medicine

Homeopathy is an unconventional Western system that is based on the principle that "like cures like" (ie, that the same substance that in large doses produces the symptoms of an illness, in very small doses cures it). Minute doses of specially prepared plant extracts and minerals are used to stimulate the body's defense mechanisms and healing processes to treat illness. The approach focuses on the links among an individual's physical, emotional, and mental symptoms.

For peri- and postmenopausal women, homeopathic remedies include substances that address a group of symptoms and also enhance feelings of well-being. The three most commonly prescribed homeopathic remedies for menopausal symptoms are lachesis (derived from venom of the South American bushmaster snake), pulsatilla (derived from the wildflower *Anemone pulsatilla*), and sepia (derived from cuttlefish ink). Double-blind, placebo-controlled trials have not shown homeopathic remedies to be more effective than placebo, although they are generally quite safe.

I.01.d. Naturopathic medicine

In naturopathic medicine, disease is viewed as a manifestation of alterations in the processes by which the body naturally heals itself, and emphasizes health restoration rather than disease treatment. Naturopathic physicians employ an array of healing practices, including diet and clinical nutrition; homeopathy; acupuncture; herbal medicine; hydrotherapy; spinal and soft-tissue manipulation; physical therapies involving electric currents, ultrasound, and light therapy; therapeutic counseling; and pharmacology.

Naturopathic physicians provide primary care diagnosis and therapy. Formal training for the doctor of naturopathy (ND) degree mirrors the course work of allopathic physicians (MDs and DOs), including such areas as minor surgery, clinical pharmacology, and obstetrics, as well as classroom and clinical instruction in most of the CAM modalities. NDs are not licensed to practice in all 50 US states.

Naturopathic physicians offer a unique service, ranging from integrative medicine to lifestyle education. Individuals may choose NDs as their primary care providers, with allopathic physicians serving as specialist referrals. Most often, naturopathic physicians function as collaborators with internists, family care practitioners, and gynecologists, providing for a responsible medical care continuum. As with other CAM practices, ND services are not covered by all health insurance policies.

Practice guidelines established by the American Association of Naturopathic Physicians (AANP) reflect the posture of other national medical organizations, and obligate the ND to make referrals as requested by the individual or when such action is clearly in the person's best interest. Safety and efficacy of physician practice and treatment are assessed by the AANP and by peer-reviewed journals dedicated to the specific modalities themselves.

Bibliography

Berman BM, Swyers JP, Hartnoll SM, Singh BB, Bausell B. The public debate over alternative medicine: the importance of finding a middle ground. *Altern Ther Health Med* 2000;6:98-101.

Buckman R, Lewith G. What does homeopathy do — and how? *BMJ* 1994;309:103-106.

Dower C, O'Neil EH, Hough HJ. *Profiling the Professions: A Model for Evaluating Emerging Health Professions.* San Francisco, CA: Center for the Health Professions, University of California, San Francisco; 2001.

Ernst E. Is homeopathy a placebo? *Br J Clin Pharmacol* 1990; 30:173-174.

Fugh-Berman A. Complementary medicine: herbs, phytoestrogens, and other treatments. In: Lobo RA, ed. *Treatment of the Postmenopausal Woman: Basic and Clinical Aspects.* 2nd ed. Philadelphia, PA: Lippincott Williams & Wilkins; 1999:453-459.

Hudson T, Northrup C. *Women's Encyclopedia of Natural Medicine.* Los Angeles, CA: Keats Publishing; 1999.

Ikenze I, Akenze A. *Menopause & Homeopathy: A Guide for Women in Midlife.* Berkeley, CA: North Atlantic Books; 1999.

Irvin JH, Friedman R, Zuttermeister PC, et al. The effect of relaxation response training on menopausal symptoms. *J Psychosom Obstet Gynecol* 1996;17:201-207.

Lockie A, Geddes L. *The Woman's Guide to Homeopathy.* London, England: The Penguin Group; 1992.

MacEoin B. *Homeopathy for Menopause.* Rochester, VT: Healing Arts Press; 1997.

Morton M, Morton M. *Five Steps to Selecting the Best Alternative Medicine: A Guide to Complementary and Integrative Health Care.* Novato, CA: New World Library; 1997.

Murray MT, Pizzorno JE, eds. *Encyclopedia of Natural Medicine.* 2nd ed. Rocklin, CA: Prima Publishing; 1998.

National Institutes of Health Office of Alternative Medicine, Practice and Policy Guidelines. Clinical practice guidelines in complementary and alternative medicine: an analysis of opportunities and obstacles. *Arch Fam Med* 1997;6:149-154.

NIH Consensus Development Panel on Acupuncture. Acupuncture. *JAMA* 1998;280:1518-1524.

Reilly DT, Taylor MA, Beattie NG, et al. Is evidence for homeopathy reproducible? *Lancet* 1994;344:1601-1606.

Wyon Y, Lindgren R, Lundeberg T, Hammar M. Effects of acupuncture on climacteric vasomotor symptoms, quality of life, and urinary excretion of neuropeptides among postmenopausal women. *Menopause* 1995;2:3-12.

Zell B, Hirata J, Marcus A, et al. Diagnosis of symptomatic postmenopausal women by traditional Chinese medicine practitioners. *Menopause* 2000;7:129-134.

I.02. Mind-body interventions

Mind-body interventions employ a variety of techniques designed to facilitate the mind's capacity to affect bodily function and symptoms, including hypnosis, dance, music, and art therapy; prayer; and mental healing.

Biofeedback may also be included in this category. Biofeedback techniques have been used to control hot flashes with some success. In addition, studies have shown that women with stress incontinence can reduce the frequency of incontinence episodes by 80% to 90% after bladder-sphincter biofeedback. Complete cures have been noted in nearly one-fourth of the patients. Biofeedback can also be helpful with some types of headaches.

Bibliography

Burns PA, Pranikoff K, Nochajski T, et al. Treatment of stress incontinence with pelvic floor exercises and biofeedback. *J Am Geriatr Soc* 1990;38:341-344.

Cardozo LD, Abrams PD, Stanton SL, et al. Idiopathic bladder instability treated by biofeedback. *Br J Urol* 1978;50:521-523.

I.03. Manipulative and body-based methods

This category includes methods that are based on manipulation and/or movement of the body. For example, chiropractors focus on the relationship between structure (primarily the spine) and function, and how that relationship affects the preservation and restoration of health, using manipulative therapy as an integral treatment tool. Osteopathic physicians who place particular emphasis on the musculoskeletal system (believing that all of the body's systems work together and that disturbances in one system may affect function elsewhere in the body) practice osteopathic manipulation. Massage therapists manipulate the soft tissues of the body to normalize those tissues.

Bibliography

National Center for Complementary and Alternative Medicine Health Information. Accessible at http://www.nccam.nih.gov/health/.

I.04. Energy therapies

Energy therapies focus either on energy fields originating within the body (biofields) or those from other sources (electromagnetic fields).

Biofield therapies are intended to affect the energy fields, whose existence is not yet experimentally proven, that surround and penetrate the human body. Some forms of energy therapy manipulate biofields by applying pressure and/or manipulating the body by placing the hands in, or through, these fields. Examples include qi gong, reiki, and therapeutic touch. *Qi gong* is a component of traditional oriental medicine that combines movement, meditation, and regulation of breathing to enhance the flow of vital energy (qi) in the body, improve blood circulation, and enhance immune function. *Reiki*, the Japanese word representing Universal Life Energy, is based on the belief that by channeling spiritual energy through the practitioner, the spirit is healed and it, in turn, heals the physical body. *Therapeutic touch* is derived from the ancient technique of "laying-on of hands" and is based on the premise that it is the healing force of the therapist that affects the individual's recovery and that healing is promoted when the body's energies are in balance. By passing their hands over the individual, healers identify energy imbalances.

Bioelectromagnetic-based therapies involve the unconventional use of electromagnetic fields to treat disease (eg, asthma, cancer) or manage pain and migraine headaches.

This guidebook does not address how menopause treatment is approached by using these therapies.

Bibliography

National Center for Complementary and Alternative Medicine Health Information. Accessible at http://nccam.nih.gov/health/.

I.05. Biologically based treatment

This category of CAM includes biologically based practices, interventions, and products, many of which overlap with conventional medicine's use of dietary supplements. Included are special dietary, orthomolecular, and individual biological therapies, as well as herbal therapies.

Special diet therapies (eg, those proposed by Drs. Atkins, Ornish, Pritikin, and Weil) are believed to prevent and/or control illness as well as promote health. However, studies on the long-term safety and efficacy of the diets are lacking. Orthomolecular therapies aim to treat disease with varying concentrations of chemicals, such as magnesium, melatonin, and mega-doses of vitamins. Biological therapies include, for example, the use of laetrile and shark cartilage to treat cancer, and bee pollen to treat autoimmune and inflammatory disease. Herbal therapies employ individual or mixtures of herbs for therapeutic value. An herb is a plant or plant part that produces and contains chemical substances that act upon the body. This guidebook covers botanical products used to treat menopause-related conditions.

I.05.a. Government regulation of dietary supplements

Dietary supplements include herbs, vitamins, minerals, amino acids, and other supplements intended for ingestion as an addition to the diet. Dietary supplements are regulated by the government. However, regulations are not well enforced.

Most dietary supplements were first classified by the US government as food. However, in 1990, the US Congress passed the Nutrition Labeling and Education Act, adding "herbs or similar nutritional substances" to its definition of dietary supplements. In 1994, the Dietary Supplement Health and Education Act (DSHEA) was passed, creating a dietary supplement category that is neither drug nor food. The DSHEA defines a dietary supplement as a pill, capsule, tablet, or liquid that contains a "dietary ingredient." These include vitamins, minerals, amino acids, enzymes, organ tissues, herbs, plants in various forms (such as extracts), and combinations.

Regulations regarding whether a dietary supplement is safe are opposite those for prescription drugs. Demonstrating safety is not required before a dietary supplement is approved, and the FDA (not the marketer) has the responsibility of proving a dietary supplement is harmful before it can be removed from the market. Under the current law, the marketer is responsible for ensuring that the labels are truthful and not misleading, that labels contain enough information for consumers to make an informed choice, that the serving size ("dosage") is appropriate, and that all the dietary ingredients in the product are accurately listed and safe. The label must identify the product as a dietary supplement. If a product is suspected of causing harm, the FDA can halt sales and have it analyzed. However, relying on postmarketing surveillance has many deficiencies, particularly when the organization providing oversight is ill-equipped for the responsibility.

As noted in Section G.01., until recently, US marketers of dietary supplements could make "structure and function" health claims (eg, enhances muscles) without prior FDA review, but they could not claim that a product prevents, treats, or cures a disease (eg, prevents heart attacks, cures depression) unless the FDA had approved the claim. In February 2000, the FDA announced its decision to permit dietary supplement marketers to make health claims for "natural conditions" (eg, hot flashes, age-related memory loss) without providing documentation for efficacy or safety. Serious medical conditions (eg, prevents heart attacks, prevents osteoporosis) remain in the disease category under the new ruling.

In Canada, the regulations are similar to those in the United States. Although Health Canada's Office of Natural Health Products was created in 1999 to oversee regulation, labeling, monitoring, and research of natural health products, there is no routine surveillance for product quality. Several hundred herbal product brands have been reviewed and issued Drug Identification Numbers (DIN) or General Public numbers (GP) by the Therapeutic Products Program of Health Canada; however, this review confirms a product's formulation, labeling, and instructions, not bioactivity or clinical efficacy. The Society of Obstetricians and Gynaecologists of Canada advise Canadian women to purchase only those brands with a DIN or GP.

Botanicals are classified by the FDA as a food, drug, or dietary supplement. There are numerous quality control concerns with botanicals, including misidentification, "underlabeling" (ie, including prescription drugs in OTC products), adulteration, substitution, and contamination. In addition, there is a lack of analytical method standards for many products, leading to difficulty when attempting to asses product quality. Marketers use different methods to determine the levels of "active ingredient" in their products.

Some marketers provide quality products, but the average consumer has difficulty determining which products to choose. In the United States, products designated USP *(United States Pharmacopeia)* or NSF (National Sanitary Foundation) are generally reliable indicators of good quality control. The Society of Obstetricians and Gynaecologists of Canada advise Canadian women to purchase only those brands with a DIN or GP. It is also preferable to choose specific brands that have been used in clinical trials.

Bibliography

Chandler F, ed. *Herbs: Everyday Reference for Health Professionals.* Ottawa, ON, Canada: Canadian Pharmacists Association and the Canadian Medical Association; 2000.

National Center for Complementary and Alternative Medicine Health Information. Accessible at http://www.nccam.nih.gov/health/.

US Food and Drug Administration Center for Food Safety and Applied Nutrition. *Dietary Supplement Health and Education Act of 1994.* Accessible at http://www.vm.cfsan.fda.gov/~dms/dietsupp.html.

I.05.b. Botanical therapies

Unlike modern plant-derived drugs, botanical therapies are complex mixtures of preparations made from the whole plant or plant part, such as root, leaves, gum, resin, or essential oil. Most botanical therapies are herbs.

Herbal therapies are administered in a variety of ways, including the following ways that are intended for ingestion:

- tea infusions (soft, aromatic parts of the plant are steeped, not boiled, in water),

- tea decoctions (barks and roots, boiled in water),

- essential oils (highly concentrated),

- tinctures and fluid extracts (herb macerated into water-alcohol mixture),

- dried standardized extracts (which typically contains part of a plant, but can contain the whole plant; extracts are standardized to one ingredient only), and

- homeopathic preparations (extremely diluted).

Herbal therapies are also available in supplements that are standardized to one ingredient or, in the case of mixtures, to more than one ingredient. However, the content and biological activity of the herbal therapies offered in supplement form may vary according to the production process. Because of the different ways that herbal therapies are available, "recommended doses" are not provided for many of the herbs mentioned in this guidebook. For more, consult the following texts:

Blumenthal M Sr. *The Complete Commission E Monographs: Therapeutic Guide to Herbal Medicines*. Austin, TX: American Botanical Council; 1998.

Blumenthal M, Goldberg A, Brinckmann J, eds. *Herbal Medicine: Expanded Commission E Monographs*. Newton, MA: Integrative Medicine Communications; 2000.

Robbers JE, Tyler VE. *Tyler's Herbs of Choice: The Therapeutic Use of Phytomedicinals*. 2nd ed. Binghamptom, NY: The Haworth Herbal Press; 1999.

Many herbal drugs were included in the *United States Pharmacopeia* (USP) from the first edition published in 1820 until the 1930s, when most of the herbal ingredients were deleted due to a "lack of general use." Yet, herb products have been available, mostly as teas and, since the 1970s, as capsules, tablets, and extracts. Many herbs were also found in over-the-counter (OTC) products. However, in 1972, the OTC Review at the FDA evaluated all ingredients used in OTC products, requiring a higher standard of evidence (ie, controlled clinical trials) for determining safety and efficacy. Most herbs had not been subjected to clinical investigation in the US and the FDA's OTC expert panels did not seek data from foreign studies. Thus, most of these herbal ingredients were deemed to be Category III (ie, not enough information to determine safety or efficacy) and were eventually moved to Category II (ie, banned because the ingredient was either unsafe or ineffective) because the government could not allow an ingredient of undetermined safety or efficacy to be continued on the market in OTC drug products.

Nevertheless, there was increased demand for herbal medicines in the United States. By passing the Dietary Supplement Health and Education Act of 1994 (DSHEA), the US Congress acknowledged public support for consumers' rights to maintain full access to vitamins, minerals, herbs, and other dietary supplements, as well as information on the responsible use of these products.

There are a few herbs that are still FDA-approved as safe and effective ingredients in OTC drugs (eg, aloe, capsicum, cascara, ipecac, psyllium, witch hazel). Little US governmental recognition has been given to other herbs, some of which are clinically tested and are approved as OTC medicines in other Western industrialized nations. However, the Office of Dietary Supplements (ODS), in collaboration with the National Center for Complementary and Alternative Medicine (NCCAM) — two components of the National Institutes of Health (NIH) — have established several Centers for Dietary Supplement Research with an emphasis on botanicals.

I.05.b.1. General precautions

No therapy is without risk, even so-called "natural" therapies, such as botanicals. Botanical therapies may interact with prescription drugs, resulting in enhanced or diminished effects of the herb, the drug, or both. A new effect may be observed that is not seen with either substance taken alone. However, the accuracy of many reported adverse herb-drug interactions is questionable, as some products were not tested for purity.

Pharmacokinetic interactions may occur. Mucilage-rich herbs may interfere with drug absorption. St. John's wort, an inducer of the CYP3A4, has been shown to decrease the rate of metabolism of a number of drugs. Diuretic herbs that alter sodium reabsorption in the renal tubule can increase plasma levels of many drugs, including lithium; women who use lithium should be asked if they are using any "slimming therapies" purchased OTC.

Pharmacodynamic interactions between agonists and antagonists at receptor sites are also possible, resulting in an inhibitory or additive effect.

Dramatic quantitative and qualitative differences in drug effects may result from genetic variability in metabolizing drugs and/or herbs.

Although many drug-herb interactions are not likely to be clinically significant, caution should be exercised, particularly when prescribing drugs that have a narrow therapeutic index and serious toxicity (eg, warfarin), and when the medication is necessary for life (eg, cyclosporine). Women with a disease that can be fatal if undertreated (eg, epilepsy) also require close observation.

Many herbs have hypoglycemic activity. Women who are taking insulin or oral hypoglycemics should closely monitor blood glucose when adding new herbal therapies, and drug doses adjusted, when appropriate.

A number of herbs have been found to inhibit platelet aggregation, including dong quai, evening primrose oil, ginkgo, ginseng, ginger, garlic, and feverfew (among others). Combining these with another anticoagulant, such as warfarin (Coumadin), aspirin (including low-dose aspirin for cardiovascular benefits), or vitamin E, is not recommended. Women using warfarin should be told about this effect. If a woman insists on continuing herbal therapy, extra blood draws are advised, with adjustment of drug dose, when indicated. These botanicals should be avoided in women experiencing abnormal uterine bleeding. To be safe, healthcare providers should advise all women to discontinue all herbal therapy (and all OTC therapies) 7 to 10 days before surgery; botanicals can usually be resumed when back at home.

I.05.b.2. Phytoestrogens

The most studied of the botanicals for menopause-related conditions are phytoestrogens, plant compounds that have estrogen-like biologic activity and a chemical structure similar to that of estrogen. There are three principal varieties of phytoestrogens: isoflavones, coumestans, and lignans.

Isoflavones comprise the most widely used phytoestrogen for menopause. Isoflavones are a class of phytochemicals, a broad group of nonsteroidal compounds of diverse structure that bind to estrogen receptors in animals and human beings. The isoflavones include the biochemicals genistein, daidzein, glycitein, biochanin A, and formononetin. Genistein and daidzein are found in high amounts in soybeans and soy products as well as in red clover.

Peri- and postmenopausal women are confronted with numerous foods and supplements referred to by a variety of terms such as phytoestrogens or plant estrogens, soy, soy protein, and isoflavones. Unfortunately, the terms are often used interchangeably.

Soy is the most widely used isoflavone-containing food. The term soy usually refers to a product derived from the whole soy (or soya) bean. Soy protein refers to a product derived by extracting the protein out of the whole bean.

The common soy foods and their isoflavone content are listed in Table 1. The isoflavone content of each soy food can vary considerably depending on growing conditions and processing. In Southeast Asia, many soy foods are manufactured from fermentation of soy beans (eg, miso and tempeh). This process tends to concentrate the isoflavones. Other processing to remove fats, taste, and color tends to remove isoflavones.

Soy and other isoflavone supplements are regulated as dietary supplements; thus, they are not monitored for purity, amount of active ingredient, or health claims (see Section G.01).

Table 1. Isoflavone content of foods

Food	Mean mg isoflavone per 100 g food
Soybeans, green, raw	151.17
Soy flour	148.61
Soy protein isolate	97.43
Miso soup	60.39
Tempeh	43.52
Soybeans, spouted, raw	40.71
Tofu, silken	27.91
Tofu yogurt	16.30
Soy hot dog	15.00
Soy milk	9.65
Soy sauce, shoyu	1.64

Functionally, isoflavones can exert both estrogenic and antiestrogenic effects, depending on their concentration, the concentration of endogenous sex hormones, and the specific end organ involved. Some effects of these molecules may result from interactions with pathways of cellular activity that do not involve the estrogen receptor. In addition, it is not clear whether the observed health effects in human beings are attributable to isoflavones alone or to isoflavones plus other components in whole foods.

The most convincing health effects have been attributed to the actions of soy protein supplements on plasma lipid concentrations. Studies have associated soy supplements with statistically significant reductions in low-density lipoproteins (LDL) and triglycerides and increases in high-density lipoproteins (HDL). A meta-analysis of 38 published controlled clinical trials of soy protein consumption (47 g/day on average) concluded that soy protein was associated with a mean 9.3% reduction in total cholesterol, 12.9% reduction in LDL, and 10.5% reduction in triglycerides, with no change in HDL. This cholesterol-lowering effect was confined to subjects with elevated baseline cholesterol levels. On average, those with hypercholesterolemia achieved a 10% reduction in cholesterol levels in response to approximately 25 g per day of soy protein.

In 1999, the FDA approved the health claim that "25 grams per day of soy protein, as part of a diet low in saturated fat and cholesterol, may reduce the risk of heart disease." Based on current study findings, the recommendation appears sound, especially if combined with a healthy lifestyle. The FDA concluded that there was insufficient evidence to stipulate an amount of isoflavones that should be contained in the 25 g of soy protein.

In studies in peri- and postmenopausal women, these cholesterol-lowering effects were seen in participants with either normal or elevated levels of cholesterol, in addition to a beneficial effect on HDL-cholesterol. In one study of 42 postmenopausal women with normal cholesterol levels, subjects consuming daily servings of whole soy foods containing approximately 60 mg of isoflavones for 12 consecutive weeks had significant increases in HDL and decreases in the total cholesterol to HDL ratio. Similar effects were seen in another 12-week study of 50 symptomatic perimenopausal women given 20 g/day of soy protein containing 34 mg isoflavones. A third study of 18 postmenopausal women found that a high isoflavone diet (132 mg/day) was more effective than low and very low isoflavone diets (65 mg/day and 7 mg/day, respectively) in reducing LDL levels and the LDL to HDL ratio.

While high soy protein diets seem to have positive effects on the serum lipids in peri- and postmenopausal women, isoflavones extracted from soy or red clover do not seem to have the same short-term effect. In five short-duration studies using extracts of soy (three studies) or red clover (two studies) in peri- and postmenopausal women, there was no significant change in any of the serum lipid parameters. Daily isoflavone doses ranged from 40 to 80 mg and treatment duration ranged from 8 to 12 weeks. However, in a 6-month study, administration of red clover isoflavones *did* result in a significant rise in HDL levels and a significant decrease in lipoprotein B levels. These changes were not evident at 3 months. The magnitude of the response at 6 months, however, was independent of the three doses used (28.5 mg, 57 mg, or 85.5 mg).

These results suggest that longer treatment courses with isoflavones supplements are necessary to obtain measurable changes in lipoproteins compared with dietary soy protein. It is possible that lipid changes are slower with the use of isoflavone supplements because of the lack of intake of other cholesterol-lowering compounds, such as saponins, amino acids, and phytic acid found in soy protein and the lack of other dietary modifications such as a reduction in animal fat and protein.

There is uncertainty about the importance of isoflavones as a part of the soy protein matrix. Three studies in human subjects suggest that soy protein with higher levels of isoflavones might have more robust effects on lowering LDL concentrations than soy protein with lower isoflavone amounts. In a study of both men and women, there was an increasing reduction in LDL concentrations with increasing isoflavone content (from 3 to 62 mg) in 25 mg of soy protein. In a study in normocholesterolemic premenopausal women, soy protein (53 g/day) with the highest isoflavone content (129 mg) had a more robust effect on lowering LDL concentrations than the same amount of soy protein with about one-half the isoflavone content (65 mg). In postmenopausal women, consumption of soy protein (63 mg/day) with 132 mg isoflavones lowered LDL more than the same amount of soy protein with about 65 mg isoflavones.

Clinical studies have tended to support the conclusion of little or no cardiovascular benefits of administering soy isoflavone extracts. In a study of peri- and postmenopausal women, treatment for 5 weeks with 80 mg per day of soy isoflavone extract improved systemic arterial compliance, an indicator of vascular elasticity; however, there was no effect on endothelium-dependent flow mediated dilation or on plasma concentrations of HDL or LDL. The lack of effect of soy isoflavones extracts on flow-mediated dilation and plasma lipoprotein concentrations was confirmed in a recent study.

The effect of soy protein or isoflavone supplement intake on bone metabolism during peri- or postmenopause is under investigation; however, the effects seem to be very small. Based on current evidence, soy protein supplements or isoflavone extracts taken alone will not prevent postmenopausal bone loss. Estrogen benefits for bone metabolism are mediated primarily by way of estrogen-receptor alpha (ER-α). Isoflavones, while having relatively high affinity for estrogen-receptor beta (ER-β), have minimal affinity for ER-α. However, clinical trials demonstrate bone formation with the synthetic isoflavone, ipriflavone, which is available OTC in the United States in doses ranging from 200 to 600 mg.

Both soy protein supplements and isoflavone extracts are moderately effective in reducing the numbers of hot flashes, but most studies found comparable improvements in placebo recipients. Randomized controlled clinical trials have shown that, in general, hot flashes are only slightly reduced in women consuming soy or isoflavones as compared with control subjects. Generally, there is approximately a 45% reduction in numbers of hot flashes (about 15% better effect than placebo).

There is no credible evidence that either soy protein or soy isoflavone extracts reduce vaginal dryness. The lack of effect is now understood. During the menopause transition, women lose ER-β receptors from the vaginal walls with only ER-α receptors remaining. Given the very low affinity of isoflavones for ER-α, there is not a cellular mechanism for improving vaginal dryness.

Inadequate data exist to draw conclusions about the value of either soy protein or isoflavones in reducing breast cancer risk. Although epidemiological data suggest that isoflavone consumption is associated with a decreased risk of breast cancer, some short-term data suggest that isoflavone consumption may increase breast tissue proliferation. Therefore, soy foods cannot be recommended as part of a breast cancer prevention strategy. Whether breast cancer survivors should be advised to avoid soy/phytoestrogens is unknown.

The role of soy or isoflavones in the prevention of endometrial cancer is unknown. In moderate doses, isoflavones do not appear to alter endometrial proliferation in either peri- or postmenopausal women.

In its consensus opinion on the role of isoflavones in menopausal health, published in 2000, NAMS concluded the following. Although the observed health effects in humans cannot be attributed to isoflavones alone, it is clear that foods or supplements that contain isoflavones have some physiologic effects. Clinicians may recommend that menopausal women consume whole foods that contain isoflavones, especially for the cardiovascular benefit of these foods; however, a level of caution needs to be observed in making these recommendations. Additional trials are needed before specific recommendations can be made regarding increased consumption of foods or supplements that contain high amounts of isoflavones.

Bibliography

Adlercreutz H. Epidemiology of phytoestrogens. *Baillieres Clin Endocrinol Metab* 1998;12:605-623.

Albertazzi P, Pansini F, Bonaccorsi G, Zanotti L, Forini E, de Aloysio D. The effect of dietary soy supplementation on hot flushes. *Obstet Gynecol* 1998;91:6-11.

Anderson JW, Johnstone BM, Cook-Newell ML. Meta-analysis of the effects of soy protein intake on serum lipids. *N Engl J Med* 1995;333:276-282.

Baird DD, Umbach DM, Lansdell L, et al. Dietary intervention study to assess estrogenicity of dietary soy among postmenopausal women. *J Clin Endocrinol Metab* 1995;80:1685-1690.

Bakhit RM, Klein BP, Essex-Sorlie D, Ham JO, Erdman JW Jr, Potter SM. Intake of 25 g of soybean protein with or without soybean fiber alters plasma lipids in men with elevated cholesterol concentrations. *J Nutr* 1994;124:213-222.

Bazzano LA, He J, Ogden LG, et al. Legume consumption and risk of coronary heart disease in US men and women: NHANES I epidemiologic follow-up study. *Arch Intern Med* 2001;161:2573-2578.

Brzezinski A, Adlercreutz H, Shaoul R, et al. Short-term effects of phytoestrogen-rich diet on postmenopausal women. *Menopause* 1997;4:89-94.

Chen GD, Oliver RH, Leung BS, Lin LY, Yeh J. Estrogen receptor and expression in the vaginal walls and uterosacral ligaments of premenopausal and postmenopausal women. *Fertil Steril* 1999;71:1099-1102.

Crouse JR, Morgan TM, Terry JG, Ellis J, Vitolins M, Burke GL. A randomized trial comparing the effect of casein with that of soy protein containing varying amounts of isoflavones on plasma concentrations of lipids and lipoproteins. *Arch Intern Med* 1999; 159:2070-2076.

Dalais FS, Rice GE, Wahlquist ML. Effects of dietary phytoestrogens in postmenopausal women. *Climacteric* 1998;1:124-129.

Fugh-Berman A, Kronenberg F. Red clover *(Trifolium pretense)* for menopausal women: current state of knowledge. *Menopause* 2001;8:333-357.

Hale GE, Hughes CL, Robboy SJ, Agarwal SK, Bievre M. A double-blind randomized study on the effects of red clover isoflavones on the endometrium. *Menopause* 2001;8:338-346.

Hargreaves DF, Potten CS, Harding C, et al. Two-week dietary soy supplementation has an estrogenic effect on normal premenopausal breast. *J Clin Endocrinol Metab* 1999;84:4017-4024.

Hodgson JM, Puddey IB, Croft KD, Mori TA, Rivera J, Beilin LJ. Isoflavonoids do not inhibit in vivo lipid peroxidation in subjects with high-normal blood pressure. *Atherosclerosis* 1999;145:167-172.

Howes JB, Sullivan D, Lai N, et al. The effects of dietary supplementation with isoflavones from red clover on the lipoprotein profiles of post menopausal women with mild to moderate hypercholesterolaemia. *Atherosclerosis* 2000;152:143-147.

Hudson T, Northrup C. *Women's Encyclopedia of Natural Medicine.* Los Angeles, CA: Keats Publishing; 1999.

Ingram D, Sanders K, Kolybaba M, Lopez D. Case-control study of phyto-oestrogens and breast cancer. *Lancet* 1997;350:990-994.

Knight DC, Howes JB, Eden JA. The effect of Promensil, an isoflavone extract, on menopausal symptoms. *Climacteric* 1999;2:79-84.

Kuiper GG, Lemmen JG, Carlsson B, et al. Interaction of estrogenic chemicals and phytoestrogens with estrogen receptor beta. *Endocrinology* 1998;139:4252-4263.

Martin PM, Horwitz KB, Ryan DS, McGuire WL. Phytoestrogen interaction with estrogen receptors in human breast cells. *Endocrinology* 1978;103:1860-1867.

McMichael-Phillips DF, Harding C, Morton M, et al. Effects of soy-protein supplementation on epithelial proliferation in the histologically normal human breast. *Am J Clin Nutr* 1998; 68(6 suppl):1431S-1435S.

Mei J, Yeung SSC, Kung AWC. High dietary phytoestrogens intake is associated with higher bone mineral density in postmenopausal but not premenopausal women. *J Clin Endocrinol Metab* 2001; 86:5217-5221.

Merz-Demlow BE, Duncan AM, Wangen KE, et al. Soy isoflavones improve plasma lipids in normocholesterolemic, premenopausal women. *Am J Clin Nutr* 2000;71:1462-1469.

Messina M. Soy, soy phytoestrogens (isoflavones), and breast cancer. *Am J Clin Nutr* 1999;70:574-575.

Murkies AL, Lombard C, Strauss BJG, Wilcox G, Burger HG, Morton MS. Dietary flour supplementation decreases postmenopausal hot flushes: effect of soy and wheat. *Maturitas* 1994;21:189-195.

Nestel PJ, Yamashita T, Sasahara T, et al. Soy isoflavones improve systemic arterial compliance but not plasma lipids in menopausal and perimenopausal women. *Arterioscler Thromb Vasc Biol* 1997; 17:3392-3398.

The North American Menopause Society. The role of isoflavones in menopausal health: consensus opinion of The North American Menopause Society. *Menopause* 2000;7:215-229.

Peterson G, Barnes S. Genistein inhibits both estrogen and growth factor-stimulated proliferation of human breast cancer cells. *Cell Growth Differ* 1996;7:1345-1351.

Potter SM, Baum JA, Teng H, Stillman RJ, Shay NF, Erdman JW. Soy protein and isoflavones: their effects on blood lipids and bone density in postmenopausal women. *Am J Clin Nutr* 1998; 689(suppl):1375S-1379S.

Samman S, Wall PML, Chan GSM, Smith SJ, Petocz P. The effect of supplementation with isoflavones on plasma lipids and oxidisability of low density lipoprotein in premenopausal women. *Atherosclerosis* 1999;147:277-283.

Scambia G, Mango D, Signorile PG, et al. Clinical effects of a standardized soy extract in postmenopausal women: a pilot study. *Menopause* 2000;7:105-111.

Scheiber MD, Liu JH, Sabbiah MTR, Rebar RW, Setchell KDR. Dietary inclusion of whole soy foods results in significant reductions in clinical risk factors for osteoporosis and cardiovascular disease in normal postmenopausal women: NAMS fellowship findings. *Menopause* 2001;5:384-392.

Simons LA, von Konigsmark M, Simons J, Celermajer DS. Phytoestrogens do not influence lipoprotein levels or endothelial function in healthy, postmenopausal women. *Am J Cardiol* 2000;85:1297-1301.

St. Germain A, Peterson CT, Robinson JG, Alekel DL. Isoflavone-rich or isoflavone-poor soy protein does not reduce menopausal symptoms during 24 weeks of treatment. *Menopause* 2001;1:17-26.

Upmalis DH, Lobo R, Bradley L, Warren M, Cone FL, Lamia CA. Vasomotor symptom relief by soy isoflavone extract tablets in postmenopausal women: a multicenter, double-blind, randomized, placebo-controlled study. *Menopause* 2000;7:236-242.

Wangen KE, Duncan AM, Xu X, Kurzer MS. Soy isoflavones improve plasma lipids in normocholesterolemic and mildly hypercholesterolemic postmenopausal women. *Am J Clin Nutr* 2001;73:225-231.

Wiseman H, O'Reilly JD, Adlercreutz H, et al. Isoflavone phytoestrogens consumed in soy decrease F2-isoprostane concentrations and increase resistance of low density lipoprotein to oxidation in humans. *Am J Clin Nutr* 2000;72:395-400.

I.05.b.3. Herbs

A number of herbs have been used to treat acute menopause-related symptoms, including black cohosh and dong quai, plus a wide variety of multiherb products. Herbs are not usually considered for the prevention or treatment of serious diseases, such as osteoporosis.

Many OTC products contain mixtures of various herbs that are advertised for relief of menopause-related symptoms. Although anecdotal evidence may support efficacy, no clinical trial data document safety and efficacy of these mixtures. Individualized mixtures prepared by Chinese herbalists may be more reliable, although trial data are also limited for these products.

Many women and some healthcare providers believe that herbal therapies are safer than prescription drugs because they are "natural" — but herbs can have pharmacologic effects and side effects. With these therapies, it is prudent to exercise caution. Randomized trials are needed to document the safety and efficacy of these products. In addition, there are no studies regarding concomitant use with ERT/HRT or bone-specific agents.

Marketed herb products are regulated as dietary supplements. They are not monitored for purity, amount of active ingredient, or health claims (see Section I.05.a).

The following sections present information on some of the more commonly used herbs for treating peri- and postmenopausal women. The individual herbs are listed alphabetically.

Black cohosh

Preparations made from the rhizomes (underground stems) of black cohosh (botanical name *Cimicifuga racemosa* or *Actaea racemosa),* also known as black snakeroot and bugbane, have been used by North American Indians for medicinal purposes for hundreds of years. Hence, another name is squaw root. In the 19th century, healthcare practitioners used black cohosh primarily for gynecologic conditions, including menstrual disorders and uterine disorders. This North American plant has been used in European phytotherapy for the treatment of menopausal symptoms for over 50 years. Black cohosh is the most widely studied herb in menopause treatment.

A number of the plant's constituents have been identified but black cohosh's precise mechanism of action in humans is unknown. There are reports of estrogenic action in animal, human, and in vitro studies, providing rationale for describing black cohosh as a phytoestrogen. However, recent studies of an isopropanolic extract of black cohosh (Remifemin) have reported no effect on follicle-stimulating hormone (FSH), vaginal epithelium, or a breast cancer cell line. Explaining these conflicting reports is difficult. A possible reason for the discrepancy is that different extracts and processing techniques may lead to different active ingredients in the final product. Additionally, the studies are not directly comparable because different testing models were used.

The isopropanolic preparation marketed as Remifemin is the most widely studied product. Remifemin was developed and produced by Schaper & Brümmer, Germany; it is marketed in the United States by GlaxoSmithKline Consumer Healthcare. (Exact information is provided to distinguish the tested herbal formulas from untested brands; however, this does not imply that these brands are better than other brands.)

Each tablet contains 20 mg of black cohosh extract, which has 1 mg triterpenes (standardized to triterpene glycoside 27-deoxyactein). The formulation and strength have changed during the past 40 years, so studies performed with earlier versions may not be applicable to the currently marketed preparation.

In 1989, the German Federal Institute for Drugs and Medical Devices approved black cohosh for menopause-related complaints (as well as premenstrual syndrome and dysmenorrhea).

In clinical trials, women reported improvements in hot flashes with black cohosh (Remifemin) that were superior to placebo, although the study populations were small. No vaginal bleeding was reported in study periods of up to 6 months, and no endometrial thickening was observed after 12 weeks of treatment. Longer trials are required to assure endometrial safety. Several uncontrolled trials showed improvement in depression and measures of well-being among menopausal women using black cohosh.

A clinical trial over a 24-week period that evaluated the reproductive hormone and vaginal cytology effects of black cohosh (an isopropanolic extract at the standard 39.0 mg/day dose or at the higher 127.3 mg/day dose) found that its benefit in relieving hot flashes was not associated with systemic estrogen-agonistic effects. While the specific product (Remifemin) appears to have little or no estrogenic activity, the overall effect on breast cancer is unknown.

Critics contend that the evidence base for the efficacy of black cohosh is poor. Many studies are small, brief, uncontrolled, and unrandomized, and few defined their participants' hormonal status before treatment. Large, randomized trials are needed to confirm efficacy.

The incidence of adverse events with black cohosh is low, particularly with single-agent supplements. Side effects include occasional gastric discomfort, nausea, vomiting, dizziness, frontal headache, and bradycardia. The gastrointestinal disturbances are primarily with first use.

With the supplement Remifemin, a daily dose of 40 mg is considered the recommended dose. Results should be evident within 8 to 12 weeks. Black cohosh traditionally has not been used for long periods of time, and no published studies have followed women for more than 6 months. In the United States, Remifemin and other supplements containing black cohosh are marketed and regulated as a dietary supplement.

Cranberry

The juice of cranberries *(Vaccinia macrocarpon)* has been used as a home remedy for acidifying the urine. It has also been found to decrease bacterial adherence. In a study of elderly women (mean age, 78.5 years), cranberry juice recipients had significantly lower odds of having bacteria with pyuria than they did when they received the placebo (42% vs 27%). Another study found that regular drinking of cranberry juice could reduce the recurrence of urinary tract infections.

Dong quai

Dong quai *(Angelica sinensis)* is an aromatic herb that is sometimes called Chinese angelica, tang kuei, and dang gui. Among Chinese therapies, it is the most extensively used herb in treating gynecologic conditions. It is also used as a blood tonic for men and women, and it is stimulating (and warming) to the circulation. It has been used in China for at least 1,200 years.

Different effects are observed when the root is extracted into different media. Water extracts have been observed to first stimulate the uterus then relax it, whereas alcohol extracts (tinctures) will only be relaxing. Dong quai should not be used during heavy menstrual flow, as it will tend to increase the flow.

Efficacy for relief of hot flashes has not been confirmed in controlled clinical trials. The only double-blind, randomized, placebo-controlled trial to date found that 4.5 g/day of dong quai used for 12 weeks (71 women) was no more helpful than placebo in relieving hot flashes. It did not affect estrogenization of vaginal epithelial cells or endometrial thickness, as measured by transvaginal ultrasound. Chinese herbalists counter that dong quai is not meant to be used alone, but within an individually tailored mixture of herbs. More research is needed to determine its efficacy and safety.

Side effects include photosensitivity and anticoagulation. Dong quai can trigger heavy uterine bleeding and should never be used in women who have fibroids, hemophilia, or other blood clotting problems. Nor should it be used by those who are taking anticoagulants (see Section I.05.b.1).

Evening primrose oil

Evening primrose *(Oenethera biennis)* produces seeds that are rich in oils containing linoleic acid. Preparations made from the oils are reported to improve atopic eczema, reduce hypercholesterolemia, and relieve mastalgia (breast pain).

Evening primrose oil is also promoted to relieve hot flashes; however, a randomized, double-blind, placebo-controlled study of 56 women with menopause-related hot flashes found no benefit over placebo.

The usual dose of evening primrose oil in supplement form is 1,500 to 3,000 mg daily. Reported side effects include inflammation, thrombosis, immunosuppression, nausea, and diarrhea. Contraindications are epilepsy and mania. Evening primrose oil should not be used with anticoagulants (see Section I.05.b.1) or the psychotherapeutic agents, phenothiazines.

Ginkgo

The medicinal uses of ginkgo (botanical name *Ginkgo biloba*) go back to about 3000 BC. Preparations made from the leaf of the ginkgo tree are used as a circulatory tonic and hypotensive. Conditions treated by ginkgo include vertigo, tinnitus, intermittent claudication, short-term memory loss, macular degeneration, and asthma. Ginkgo is reputed to increase blood flow through small vessels, including cerebral arteries. It acts as an antioxidant and as a blood thinner.

Ginkgo has also been shown to stabilize and/or improve cognitive performance and the social functioning of patients with dementia. In a 52-week, randomized, double-blind, placebo-controlled, multicenter study with a particular extract of ginkgo (EGb 761), 120 mg/day was safe and appeared capable of stabilizing and, in a substantial number of cases, improving the cognitive performance and the social functioning of mild to severely demented outpatients with Alzheimer's disease or multi-infarct dementia for 6 months to 1 year.

There is less evidence for reducing severe memory problems. In a study of individuals older than 50 with mild to moderate memory impairment, ginkgo recipients had improvements in some cognitive functions (digit copying, speed of response in a classification task).

A meta-analysis of 40 controlled trials for "cerebral insufficiency"— a syndrome not recognized in the United States that includes memory and concentration problems, confusion, fatigue, depression, tinnitus, and headache — found that, in 26 studies, the groups receiving ginkgo did significantly better than the control groups. Most of the studies, however, were deemed to be of poor methodologic quality. Of the eight well-controlled trials, all showed a significant benefit for the ginkgo group.

The most serious side effect with ginkgo is bleeding. Ginkgo should not be used by women with bleeding problems or who are on anticoagulants, as ginkgo inhibits platelet function. Subdural hematoma and other bleeding complications have been reported, usually in patients on anticoagulant therapies. (For more, see Section I.05.b.1.)

The most common side effects are gastrointestinal distress and headache. Large doses may cause restlessness, anxiety, allergic skin reactions, sleep disturbances, and gastrointestinal upset, including diarrhea, nausea, and vomiting.

The extracts used in most clinical trials are standardized to contain 24% flavonoids and 6% terpenes. The usual dose is 40 to 80 mg standardized extract capsules three times daily. Treatment should be continued for at least 6 weeks to evaluate therapeutic effect. Among ginkgo supplements, the specific brands reported to have been used in most clinical trials are Tebonin (manufactured by Schwabe, and marketed in the United States by Nature's Way as Ginkgold and by Pharmaton as Ginkoba) and Kaveri (manufactured by Lichtwer, and marketed in the United States by Abkit as Ginkai). (Exact information is provided to distinguish the tested herbal formulas from untested brands; however, this does not imply that these brands are better than other brands.)

Ginseng

The most common types of ginseng are Chinese (or Korean or Oriental) ginseng *(Panax ginseng)*, American ginseng *(Panax quinquefolius)*, and Siberian "ginseng" *(Eleutherococcus senticosus)*, with the latter not being true ginseng, but in the same family. The various types of ginseng exhibit different effects. It is the multi-branched root of these perennial, shade-loving plants that is used in botanical medicine.

Preparations of Oriental ginseng root have been an important tonic and remedy in Traditional Chinese Medicine for thousands of years. More recently, marketers of ginseng supplements promote the products for women and men to build stamina and resistance to disease, although there is no strong documentation for these claims.

Ginseng contains over a dozen terpenoids, especially a group of compounds called ginsenosides. Ginseng can cause estrogenic effects, although the plant does not actually contain phytoestrogens.

It has been reported that the most clinical trials have been conducted on the ginseng supplement with the trade name Ginsana, manufactured and marketed by Pharmaton. (Exact information is provided to distinguish the tested herbal formulas from untested brands; however, this does not imply that these brands are better than other brands.)

Ginseng has been studied for menopause-related complaints. The largest placebo-controlled trial of postmenopausal women found that a ginseng extract had no overall effect on vasomotor symptoms, serum levels of estrogen or follicle-stimulating hormones, or endometrial thickness. Also, overall quality of life was not improved, although there was improvement in subsets involving depression, general health, and well-being. The estrogenic effects of ginseng are suspected as a result of case reports of uterine bleeding occurring after ingesting ginseng or using a face cream containing ginseng.

Side effects associated with ginseng that indicate discontinuation include postmenopausal uterine bleeding, worsening of menopausal symptoms, hypertension, headaches, aggressive behavior, anxiety, agitation, depression, and insomnia. It is contraindicated for use during pregnancy or lactation because of an association with neonatal androgenization. Other side effects include nervousness, insomnia, dizziness, and hypertension. Mastalgia with diffuse breast nodularity also has been reported.

Ginseng can raise blood pressure or produce low glucose levels. Ginseng should be used with caution by those with cardiovascular disease, diabetes, or bipolar disorder. Contrary to previous reports, ginseng has no effect on the activity of warfarin. However, ginseng does have antiplatelet effects that may lengthen bleeding time, and it should not be taken with anticoagulants (see Section I.05.b.1). Ginseng also should not be taken with antihypertensives or stimulants, including diet remedies containing ma huang, ephedrine, or guarana.

Kava

Kava *(Piper methysticum)* is used for soothing mild anxiety, hot flashes, and sleep disruption. It is sometimes called kava kava, ava, awa, intoxicating pepper, kew, rauschpfeffer, sakau, tonga, wulzelstock, and yangona.

The kava used in medicinal treatments comes from the rhizome of the kava shrub. Active constituents in kava are the kavalactones (also called kavapyrones). Kava is ingested as teas or as dietary supplements. In studies of kava in postmenopausal women, significant improvements were seen in symptoms on several scales, including the Kupperman Index and the Depression Status Inventory (DSI).

Laitain is the brand of kava supplements that has been tested in clinical studies. This product is manufactured by Schwabe, but not imported into the United States. (Exact information is provided to distinguish the tested herbal formulas from untested brands; however, this does not imply that these brands are better than other brands.)

Recently, kava has come under considerable scrutiny, where it has been linked with severe hepatotoxicity. Several cases of active liver failure, cholestatic hepatitis, and cirrhosis of the liver have been reported. Health authorities around the world have taken action. Some countries in Europe have banned kava supplements. In January 2002, Health Canada issued a warning advising the public not to consume any products containing kava until a review of its safety and efficacy is completed. In the United States, the FDA issued a warning on March 26, 2002, recommending that kava products not be used before consulting a physician. The FDA has not concluded if kava has a causal relationship to liver disease.

Kava should be avoided by anyone who has or had liver disease, frequently uses alcoholic beverages, or takes prescription medications. It is recommended that a blood test be performed to check liver function before taking kava, and then repeated twice yearly. Use should be stopped if any symptoms develop that may signal liver problems, such as unexplained fatigue, abdominal pain, loss of appetite, fever, vomiting, dark urine, pale stools, or yellow eyes or skin.

Additional caution is advised with kava use, as it is addictive. Kava should not be used with any psychotropic medication, alcohol, antihistamines, or any substance that may cause sleepiness or confusion. Reported side effects include minor gastrointestinal upset, headache, sedation, or restlessness in a small percentage or users.

Extremely heavy, chronic use of kava may cause yellowing of the skin and an ichtyosiform (fish scale-like) eruption known as kava dermopathy, often accompanied by eye irritation. Given the hepatotoxicity concerns, it may be advisable to avoid use altogether until more is known.

Licorice

Licorice root *(Glycyrrhiza glabra)* contains coumarins, flavonoids, and terpenoids. The most well-known ingredients of licorice are glycyrrhizinic acid and its derivatives.

Although mostly used for its anti-inflammatory, antibacterial, antiviral, and expectorant properties, some licorice is used in Traditional Chinese Medicine (TCM) for postmenopausal women. This use may depends on its estrogenic activity, which is probably due to the presence of β-sitosterol. No trial data are available.

Licorice root tinctures, extracts, capsules, and lozenges are available for herbal medicine. Licorice candy may not contain licorice root. Most licorice candies manufactured in the United States do not contain licorice but are flavored with anise, whereas imported candies usually contain real licorice. In TCM, licorice is always used as part of a mixture, and the synergistic effects of mixtures, and perhaps dose limitations, may prevent side effects. All of the reported cases of licorice-induced adverse events have been from licorice-containing candies, gums, laxatives, or chewing tobacco, not from the use of licorice as herbal medicine.

Large chronic doses may result in pseudoprimary aldosteronism with symptoms that may include edema, hypertension, and hypokalemia. Cardiac arrhythmias and cardiac arrest, including two deaths, have occurred in users of licorice products. Cardiomyopathy, hypokalemic myopathy, and pulmonary edema have been reported. Hypokalemia due to licorice may be potentiated by the use of diuretics, and the side effects of systemic steroids and licorice probably are additive. Thus, licorice should not be used with diuretics or with systemic steroids.

Licorice is a potent herb. It is recommended that it be prescribed only by a TCM practitioner.

Sage

Sage *(Salvia officinalis)* is used by some women to help with hot flashes and night sweats. However, it is not recommended due to the toxicity of at least one of its components — a volatile oil called thujone — which can cause seizures or other neurological symptoms.

St. John's wort

Women take preparations made from the perennial St. John's wort to ease mild to moderate depression. St. John's wort *(Hypericum perforatum)* is the most popular antidepressant in Germany for mild to moderate depression. Many European (primarily German) clinical trials have been conducted on this herb. The leaves and flowering tops are used for their medicinal properties. Its mechanism of action is unknown, although some studies suggest that it may be similar to conventional antidepressant medications. Hyperforin is the most frequently cited constituent, as it is known to exhibit sedative effects.

In a database review by the Cochrane group, 27 trials using St. John's wort to treat mild to moderately severe depressive disorders involving 2,291 patients were identified (17 placebo-controlled). Most trials were 4 to 6 weeks long. The data indicate that St. John's wort was superior to placebo and was as effective as standard antidepressants. Side effects were reported by 26.3% of those on St. John's wort compared with 44.7% on antidepressants.

St. John's wort has not been found effective for treating major depression. There are ongoing trials comparing St. John's wort with the selective serotonin reuptake inhibitors (SSRIs), such as fluoxetine (Prozac), which are FDA-approved for the treatment of depression.

It has been reported that the brands of St. John's wort supplements that have been used in most clinical trials include Jarsin (manufactured by Lichtwer and marketed in the United States by Abkit as Kira), Neuroplant (manufactured by Schwabe and marketed in the United States by Nature's Way as Perika and by Pharmaton as Movana), and Remotiv (manufactured by Bayer and marketed in the United States as St. John's wort by GNC). (Exact information is provided to distinguish the tested herbal formulas from untested brands; however, this does not imply that these brands are better than other brands.)

The usual dose of St. John's wort in supplement form is 300 mg (standardized to contain 5% hyperforin, 0.3% hypericin, or both) 3 times daily. Onset of action occurs in 2 to 4 weeks. The dose may be increased to 1,800 mg/day, if necessary, and decreased to 300 to 600 mg daily for maintenance. Many CAM practitioners avoid using this herb longer than 2 years.

Gastrointestinal side effects have been reported with St. John's wort, although dosing with foods minimizes upset. Fatigue is also associated with St. John's wort and, in rare cases, it can increase sensitivity to sunlight. Combined with sunlight, it can also contribute to cataract formation. Those using St. John's wort should avoid sunbathing and should wear sun block, a hat, and wraparound sunglasses.

St. John's wort should not be used concomitantly with psychotropic medications. Taken with SSRIs, it can result in too much serotonin (called "serotonin syndrome"), causing dizziness, restlessness, and muscle twitching. St. John's wort may decrease the activity or serum levels of warfarin, digoxin, theophyllin, indinavir, cyclosporin, and phenprocoumon. Breakthrough bleeding has occurred when St. John's wort is used with the oral contraceptive containing ethinyl estradiol and desogestrel.

Valerian

Valerian preparations are made from the roots and underground plant parts of *Valeriana officinalis.* It is used for its sedative effects to treat nervousness and insomnia. In controlled clinical trials, it improved sleep quality without serious effects on reaction time, alertness, or concentration after 2 weeks of use.

Valerian is approved in Germany to treat nervousness and insomnia. It is not related to the antidepressant drug diazepam, which has a tradename (Valium) that is similar to valerian.

It has been reported that the brand of valerian supplement tested in clinical studies is Sedonium (manufactured by Lichtwer and marketed in the United States under the same name by Abkit). (Exact information is provided to distinguish the tested herbal formulas from untested brands; however, this does not imply that these brands are better than other brands.)

No substantial side effects of valerian have been noted with recommended dosages, although long-term administration has been associated with headache, restlessness, sleeplessness, and cardiac disorders. Unlike other sedatives, it does not appear to interact with alcohol to intensify drowsiness.

Valerian has been used as a bath additive; however, this method of use has not been proven to be effective and may cause severe side effects, especially in women with skin injuries or infections.

Valerian acts immediately and can be used for as long as is required to develop better sleep patterns. However, if the woman suffers from stress or chronic insomnia, the underlying factors should be examined and resolved.

Vitex

Vitex (*Vitex agnus castus*) contains flavonoids and an alkaloid called viticin. Although there have been no clinical studies on its effect on menopausal symptoms, it may have profound hormonal effects. Some herbalists believe that it "balances hormone levels."

In a double-blind, placebo-controlled trial in reproductive-aged women, vitex reduced prolactin levels, normalized the length of luteal phases, and normalized luteal phase progesterone levels. It is believed to cause a progesterone-like effect. A case of ovarian hyperstimulation in a premenopausal woman apparently caused by ingestion of vitex has been reported.

Some CAM practitioners recommend vitex to normalize and regulate the menstrual cycle, including regulating heavy uterine bleeding during perimenopause. Vitex is approved in Germany for treatment of premenstrual syndrome and menopausal complaints.

Vitex is reputed to have a libido-reducing effect in both women and men— and this effect is responsible for its other names: chaste-tree berry (or chasteberry) and monk's pepper. Although clinicians who recommend vitex indicate that this effect is rare, they advise that women with low libido should not be given this herb.

Bibliography

Amato P, Christophe S, Mellon PL. Estrogenic activity of herbs commonly used as remedies for menopausal symptoms. *Menopause* 2002;9:145-150.

Avorn J, Monane M, Gurwitz JH, Glynn RJ, Choodnovskiy I, Lipsitz LA. Reduction of bacteriuria and pyuria after ingestion of cranberry juice. *JAMA* 1994;271:751-754.

Blumenthal M Sr, ed. *The Complete Commission E Monographs: Therapeutic Guide to Herbal Medicines.* Austin, TX: American Botanical Council, 1998.

Blumenthal M, Goldberg A, Brinckmann J, eds. *Herbal Medicine: Expanded Commission E Monographs.* Newton, MA: Integrative Medicine Communications; 2000.

Chenoy R, Hussain S, Tayob Y, et al. Effect of oral gamolenic acid from evening primrose oil on menopausal flushing. *BMJ* 1994;308:501-503.

David E, Morris D. Medicinal uses of licorice through the millennia: the good and plenty of it. *Mol Cell Endocrinol* 1991;78:1-6.

Duker E-M, Kopanski L, Jarry H, Wuttke W. Effects of extracts from Cimicifuga racemosa on gonadotropin release in menopausal women and ovariectomized rats. *Planta Med* 1991;57:420-424.

Flucker MR, Montemuro S. Complementary approaches. *J Obstet Gynaecol Can* 2001;23:1204-1213.

Fugh-Berman A. Complementary medicine: herbs, phytoestrogens, and other treatments. In: Lobo RA, ed. *Treatment of the Postmenopausal Woman: Basic and Clinical Aspects.* 2nd ed. Philadelphia, PA: Lippincott Williams & Wilkins; 1999:453-459.

Hirata JD, Swiersz LM, Zell B, Small R, Ettinger B. Does dong quai have estrogenic effects in postmenopausal women? A double-blind, placebo-controlled trial. *Fertil Steril* 1997;68:981-986.

Hopkins MP, Androff L, Benninghoff AS. Ginseng face cream and unexplained vaginal bleeding. *Am J Obstet Gynecol* 1988;159: 1121-1122.

Hudson T, Northup C. *Women's Encyclopedia of Natural Medicine.* Los Angeles, CA: Keats Publishing; 1999.

Israel D, Youngkin E. Herbal therapies for perimenopausal and menopausal complaints. *Pharmacotherapy* 1997;17:970-984.

Jacobson JS, Troxel AB, Evans J, et al. Randomized trial of black cohosh for the treatment of hot flashes among women with a history of breast cancer. *J Clin Oncol* 2001;19:2739-2745.

Kanowski S, Herrmann WM, Stephan K, Wierich W, Horr P. Proof of efficacy of ginkgo biloba special extract EGb 761 in outpatient suffering from mild to moderate primary degenerative dementia of the Alzheimer type or multi-infarct dementia. *Pharmacopsychiatry* 1996;29:47-56.

Kim HL, Streltzer J, Goebert D. St. John's wort for depression: a meta-analysis of well-defined clinical trials. *J Nerv Ment Dis* 1999;187:532-538.

Kleijnen J, Knipschild P. Ginkgo biloba. *Lancet* 1992;340:1136-1139.

Kleijnen J, Knipschild P. Ginkgo biloba for cerebral insufficiency. *Br J Clin Pharmacol* 1992;34:352-358.

Kontiokari T, Sundqvist K, Nuutinen M, Pokka T, Koskela M, Uhari M. Randomised trial of cranberry-lingonberry juice and Lactobacillus GG drink for the prevention of urinary tract infections in women. *BMJ* 2001;322:1571.

Kuhlmann J, Berger W, Podzuweit H, Schmidt U. The influence of valerian treatment on "reaction time, alertness and concentration" in volunteers. *Pharmacopsychiatry* 1999;32:235-241.

Le Bars PL, Katz MM, Berman N, Itil TM, Freedman AM, Schatzberg AF. A placebo-controlled, double-blind, randomized trial of an extract of Ginkgo biloba for dementia. North American EGb Study Group. *JAMA* 1997;278:1327-1332.

Lieberman S. A review of the effectiveness of cimicifuga racemosa (black cohosh) for the symptoms of menopause. *J Womens Health* 1998;7:525-529.

Lindahl O, Lindwall L. Double blind study of a valerian preparation. *Pharmacol Biochem Behav* 1989;32:1065-1066.

Linde K, Mulrow CD. St. John's wort for depression (Cochrane Review). *Cochrane Database Syst Rev* 2000;2:CD000448.

Liske E. Therapeutic efficacy and safety of Cimicifuga racemosa for gynecologic disorders. *Adv Therapy* 1998;15:45-53.

Liske E. Hänggi W, Henneicke-von Zepelin H, Boblitz N, Wüstenberg P, Rahlfs V. Physiologic investigation of a unique extract of black cohosh (cimicifugae racemosae rhizoma): a 6-month clinical study demonstrates no systemic estrogenic effect. *J Womens Health Gend Based Med* 2002;11:163-174.

Nesselhut T, Scheillhase C, Dietrich R, Kuhn W. Studies on mammary carcinoma cells regarding the proliferative potential of herbal medications with estrogen-like effects. *Arch Gynecol Obstet* 1993;258:817-818.

Newall CA, Anderson LA, Phillipson JD. *Herbal Medicines: A Guide for Health Care Professionals.* London, Eng: Pharmaceutical Press; 1996.

Noe J. Angelic sinensis: a monograph. *J Naturopathic Med* 1997;7:66-72.

Page RL 2nd, Lawrence JD. Potentiation of warfarin by dong quai. *Pharmacotherapy* 1999;19:870-876.

PDR for Herbal Medicines. 2nd ed. Montvale, NJ: Medical Economics Co; 2000.

Rai GS, Shovlin C, Wesnes KA. A double-blind, placebo controlled study of Ginkgo biloba extract (tanakan) in elderly out-patients with mild to moderate memory impairments. *Curr Med Res Opin* 1991;12:350-355.

Robbers JE, Tyler VE, eds. *Tyler's Herbs of Choice: The Therapeutic Use of Phytomedicinals.* 2nd ed. Binghamton, NY: The Haworth Herbal Press; 1999.

Rotblatt M, Ziment I. *Evidence-Based Herbal Medicine.* Philidelphia, PA: Haney & Belfus, Inc, 2002.

Seidl MM, Stewart DE. Alternative treatments for menopausal symptoms: qualitative study of women's experiences. *Can Family Physician* 1998;44:1271-1276.

Seidl MM, Stewart DE. Alternative treatments for menopausal symptoms: systematic review of scientific and lay literature. *Can Family Physician* 1998;44:1299-1308.

Shelton RC, Keller MB, Gelenberg A, et al. Effectiveness of St. John's wort in major depression. *JAMA* 2001;285:1978-1986.

Vogler BK, Pittler MH, Ernst E. The efficacy of ginseng: a systematic review of randomised clinical trials. *Eur J Clin Pharmacol* 1999; 55:567-575.

World Health Organization (WHO). Rhizoma cimicifugae racemosae. *WHO Monographs on Selected Medicinal Plants.* Geneva, Switzerland: WHO Publications; 2002.

Wiklund IK, Mattsson LA, Lindgren R, Limoni C. Effects of a standardized ginseng extract on quality of life and physiological parameters in symptomatic postmenopausal women: a double-blind, placebo-controlled trial. Swedish Alternative Medicine Group. *Int J Clin Pharm Res* 1999;19:89-99.

Zava DT, Dollbaum CM, Blen M. Estrogen and progestin bioactivity of foods, herbs, and spices. *Proc Soc Experi Biol Med* 1998;217: 369-378.

Zierau O, Bodinet C, Kolba S, Wulf M, Vollmer G. Antiestrogenic activities of cimicifuga racemosa extracts. *J Steroid Biochem Mol Biol* 2002;80:125-130.

I.06. Other biologically based therapies

This study guide addresses two additional biologically based therapies, SAM-e and glucosamine/chondroitin.

I.06.a. SAM-e

The nonherbal supplement called SAM-e, which contains the naturally produced physiological substance S-adenosylmethionine, is promoted for relief of depression, osteoarthritis, fibromyalgia, and migraines. In some European countries, SAM-e is a prescription drug. In the United States, it is considered a dietary supplement. SAM-e appears to be well-tolerated, with a side effects profile that includes occasional nausea and gastrointestinal upset. There are anecdotal reports of the product reducing estrogen levels. Controlled trials to document efficacy and safety are lacking.

Bibliography

Caruso I, Pietrogrande V. Italian double-blind multicenter study comparing s-adenosylmethionine, Naproxen, and placebo in the treatment of degenerative joint disease. *Am J Med* 1997;83(suppl 5A):S665-S715.

Fava M, Giannelli A, Rapisarda V, Patralia A, Guaraldi GP. Rapidity of onset of the antidepressant effect of parenteral S-adenosyl-L-methionine. *Psych Res* 1995;56:295-297.

Kagan BL, Sultzer DL, Rosenlicht N, Gerner RH. Oral S-adenosylmethionine in depression: a randomized, double-blind, placebo-controlled trial. *Am J Psychiatry* 1990;147:591-595.

I.06.b. Glucosamine/chondroitin

Glucosamine and chondroitin are considered by many to be CAM therapies, although some clinicians believe that their use has reached mainstream.

Recently, a number of studies of individuals with osteoarthritis (OA) have found glucosamine to be effective in reducing pain. Glucosamine is an amino-monosaccharide that is present in almost all human tissues, especially cartilaginous tissues. In animal studies, most of the oral dose is absorbed and incorporated into biologic structures, including the liver, kidneys, and the articular cartilage. Glucosamine has been referred to as chondroprotective because it is a substrate in the pathway in the synthesis of glycoaminoglycans and proteoglycans by articular cartilage. Randomized, placebo-controlled clinical trials in individuals with knee OA have found administration of glucosamine for 3 years prevented articular cartilage destruction.

Another cartilage substrate, chondroitin sulfate, has also been studied in OA. Chondroitin sulfate is one of the main constituents of glycosaminoglycans, which are the basic elements of the extracellular substance of connective tissues including cartilage. In vitro studies suggest that chondroitin may inhibit some of the cartilage-degrading enzymes.

No large, well-designed, placebo-controlled clinical trial has addressed the efficacy of glucosamine or chondroitin in the treatment of OA. However, several small studies have found them effective in reducing joint pain. In addition, a larger, placebo-controlled, 3-year trial of glucosamine found it prevented loss of joint space, a surrogate marker for loss of articular cartilage.

Since OA and musculoskeletal ailments are exceedingly common and will increase as the population ages, many proven and unproven remedies will be used to reduce pain, making use of glucosamine and chondroitin more common. The current recommendations of the Arthritis Foundation and *The Medical Letter* caution against recommending these as treatment for OA given the lack of strong clinical trial data. At present, the National Institutes of Health is funding a large, multicenter, placebo-controlled clinical trial of glucosamine and chondroitin (GAIT Study) evaluating the efficacy of these agents alone and in combination with celecoxib, a selective COX-2 inhibitor that is considered the standard of care for the treatment of painful knee OA. Although there are no clinically proven data that these nutritional supplements will treat OA, a number of women will use them to relieve joint pain.

Bibliography

Arthritis Foundation. *Glucosamine Sulfate and Chondroitin Sulfate.* Atlanta, GA: Arthritis Foundation. Accessible at http://www.arthritis.org/conditions/alttherapies/glucosamine.asp.

Glucosamine for osteoarthritis. *Med Lett Drugs Ther* 1997;39:91-92.

Reginster JY, Deroisy R, Rovati LC, et al. Long-term effects of glucosamine sulphate on osteoarthritis progression: a randomised, placebo-controlled clinical trial. *Lancet* 2001;357:251-256.

This section will address the option for managing various symptoms associated with menopause.

J.01. Vasomotor symptoms

Peri- and early postmenopausal fluctuations in estrogen levels are often accompanied by hot flashes and night sweats. The cause of these vasomotor symptoms is still a matter of speculation and the initiating stimulus is unknown.

Few studies have produced quantitative estimates of the effect of hot flashes on quality of life, even though the potential for hot flashes to disrupt daily activity and sleep quality is widely known.

In almost all women, menopause-related vasomotor symptoms will abate over time without any intervention. When therapy is needed, various pharmacologic and nonpharmacologic options are available (see Table 1). With many of these options, efficacy has not been determined in rigorously controlled trials. There is a relatively high (up to 40%) placebo response with hot flashes in controlled studies.

Table 1. Options to manage vasomotor symptoms

- Get regular exercise to promote better, more restorative sleep

- Keep cool by dressing in layers, using a fan, and sleeping in a cool room

- Reduce stress with paced respiration, meditation, yoga, massage, or a leisurely lukewarm bath

- Avoid hot flash triggers (eg, spicy foods, hot drinks, caffeine, alcohol)

- Consider ERT/HRT or other prescription drugs (eg, progestogens, transdermal clonidine, venlafaxine, selective serotonin-reuptake inhibitors)

- Consider nonprescription therapies (eg, vitamin E, soy foods, black cohosh)

Lifestyle changes, such as moderate exercise and avoidance of potential hot flash triggers (eg, caffeine, spicy foods, alcohol, warm rooms) may prevent some hot flashes. However, only anecdotal data support the efficacy of these measures. Physically active women report fewer and less severe hot flashes than age-matched sedentary controls.

Deep, slow abdominal breathing (ie, paced respiration) has been found to increase relaxation and reduce hot flashes. A randomized, controlled trial evaluated the effect of relaxation response training versus that of reading and attention control. Results showed that the women in the relaxation group experienced significant reductions in hot flash intensity, tension-anxiety, and depression. The reading group experienced significant reductions in trait-anxiety and confusion-bewilderment. There were no significant changes in the control group. Deep breathing exercises that reduce respiratory rate and increase tidal volume reduced hot flash frequency by 39% from pretreatment levels.

The research-proven effective treatment for hot flashes is systemic estrogen (ERT) or, for women with a uterus, estrogen plus progestogen (HRT). All oral and transdermal estrogen formulations are FDA-approved for the treatment of moderate to severe vasomotor symptoms.

A dose-response relationship with ERT/HRT has been observed. The lowest possible dose needed to treat symptoms is recommended. For hot flashes, the most commonly used regimen in the United States is 0.625 mg/day of oral conjugated equine estrogens (CEE), although many other effective and FDA-approved oral and transdermal preparations, in equivalent doses, are also used. Half this standard dose has also been found to be effective. Vaginal estrogen preparations at doses to treat atrophic vaginitis will not deliver ample estrogen to the circulatory system to relieve hot flashes.

With cyclic ERT regimens (estrogen only for 3 weeks followed by 1 week off therapy), hot flashes usually resume by the end of the hormone-free week. This is especially true with 17β-estradiol, due to its rapid clearance from the body. Return of hot flashes is a major contributor to the trend toward continuous daily estrogen use.

When hot flashes are not relieved by the usual doses of oral ERT, the dose may be increased or oral therapy can be switched to transdermal ERT. Transdermal estrogen may provide more stability in the circulating levels of estrogen. For women who are not obtaining symptom relief with once-daily dosing of oral ERT due to the possibility of their metabolizing the hormone more rapidly, twice-daily dosing may be advised. However, there should be no increase in the total daily dose.

Symptoms that persist could be the result of other conditions that may affect absorption, including concomitant medications (eg, antiepileptic drugs). Smoking (>1 pack/day) enhances hepatic metabolism of estrogen, resulting in lower levels of unbound estradiol.

In cases of poor response to ERT, serum estrone levels (not estradiol) can be measured. Estrone levels below 150 pg/mL (550 pmol/L) 4 hours after ingestion of oral ERT suggest abnormal estrogen metabolism.

Some perimenopausal women desire relief from hot flashes and contraception. Standard postmenopausal doses of ERT/HRT will not provide protection from an unwanted pregnancy. A low-dose oral contraceptive (OC) may achieve both goals. One study showed a reduction in the incidence and severity of hot flashes with an OC containing 0.02 mg ethinyl estradiol and 1 mg norethindrone acetate. For women who use OCs and have hot flashes during the placebo week, adding a low dose of supplemental estrogen during this time may provide relief. Other options are to begin the next OC pack on the day of withdrawal bleeding, thus reducing the time on placebo.

When ERT/HRT is discontinued, hot flashes often return in about 4 days, depending on the type and route of estrogen therapy. Conjugated equine estrogens (CEE) can remain active for several weeks after treatment has ended because of storage in adipose tissue. Tapering the dose of ERT/HRT is recommended when discontinuing therapy to avoid rebound hot flashes that may be severe. If hot flashes recur, ERT/HRT may be reinstituted and discontinued at a later time.

Among nonprescription therapies, vitamin E (800 IU/day) is reported anecdotally to help some women with mild hot flashes. Uncontrolled studies in the 1940s and 1950s found that vitamin E was effective for relieving hot flashes, but a more recent placebo-controlled study did not support those findings. Some data support the efficacy of soy foods and isoflavone supplements in reducing the incidence and severity of hot flashes, but in many studies, the control groups had statistically similar results. Supplements of black cohosh may also be helpful with mild hot flashes. With these therapies, it may take many weeks before the effects (if any) are felt. (For more, see Sections G.02.c, I.05.b.2, and I.05.b.3.)

When prescription drug therapy is required to treat hot flashes and estrogen is not an option, such as in breast cancer survivors, the following choices are available:

- Venlafaxine hydrochloride (Effexor SR), a combined serotonin and norepinephrine reuptake inhibitor, has been shown to provide relief of hot flashes at 25 to 150 mg/day. Selective serotonin-reuptake inhibitors (SSRIs), such as paroxetine HCl (Paxil) at 10 mg/day for 1 week, then 20 mg/day for 4 weeks, and fluoxetine HCl (Prozac) at 20 mg/day for 4 weeks, have also demonstrated efficacy in a small number of clinical trials and retrospective reports.

- Progestins, such as oral medroxyprogesterone acetate (MPA), 10 to 20 mg daily, or megestrol acetate, 20 mg twice daily, may be effective in relieving hot flashes. MPA in intramuscular (IM) doses of 50, 100, and 150 mg/month has been found to effectively reduce, in a dose-response fashion, the incidence of hot flashes by more than 90% by week 4, although therapy has been associated with uterine bleeding in nearly half of those using it. Compared with IM MPA, oral MPA (20 mg/day) has fewer side effects but also less efficacy, although one study did report an incidence reduction of 90%. Some clinicians believe that megestrol acetate is a logical choice for women at risk for breast cancer because this drug is FDA-approved to treat breast cancer. Others are concerned about prescribing any hormone for women at risk of breast cancer.

- Progesterone has been shown to improve hot flashes in women who topically applied progesterone cream (20 mg per one-quarter teaspoon or 450 mg/oz progesterone) daily for 12 months. More studies are needed with topical products and other modes of administration that are custom-compounded. Oral micronized progesterone is another option, although studies documenting its efficacy in relieving hot flashes are lacking.

- Transdermal clonidine (Catapres-TTS), delivered at 100 µg/week, may provide some relief.

- Oral clonidine, bromocriptine (Parlodel), and naloxone (Narcan) are only partially effective for treating hot flashes. Higher dosages may provide better relief, but they are also associated with higher levels of side effects.

- Methyldopa (Aldomet, for example), in daily doses of 500 to 1,000 mg, appears to be about twice as effective as placebo.

- The combination tablet of phenobarbital, ergotamine tartrate, and levorotatory alkaloids of belladonna (Bellergal-S), a potent sedative, is reported to provide relief only slightly better than placebo.

- Tibolone — a synthetic steroid with estrogenic, androgenic, and progestogenic properties — is available by prescription in many countries but not in the United States or Canada. This product is used primarily to prevent bone loss, but it is also effective in relieving hot flashes. This product may offer another menopause therapy option to US and Canadian women in the future.

Bibliography

Albertazzi P, Pansini F, Bonaccorsi G, Zanotti L, Forini E, De Aloysio D. The effect of dietary soy supplementation on hot flushes. *Obstet Gynecol* 1998;91:6-11.

Albrecht BH, Schiff I, Tulchinsky D, Ryan KJ. Objective evidence that placebo and oral medroxyprogesterone acetate therapy diminish menopausal vasomotor flushes. *Am J Obstet Gynecol* 1981;139:631-635.

Barton DL, Loprinzi CL, Quella SK, et al. Prospective evaluation of vitamin E for hot flashes in breast cancer survivors. *J Clin Oncol* 1998;16:495-500.

Blatt MHG, Weisbader H, Kupperman HS. Vitamin E and climacteric syndrome. *Arch Intern Med* 1953;91:792-799.

Casper RF, Dodin S, Reid RD. The effect of 20 micrograms ethinyl estradiol/1 mg norethindrone acetate (Minestrin™), a low dose oral contraceptive, on vaginal bleeding patterns, hot flashes and quality of life in symptomatic perimenopausal women. *Menopause* 1997;4:139-147.

Christy CJ. Vitamin E in the menopause. *Am J Obstet Gynecol* 1945;50:84-87.

De Leo V, Lanzetta D, Morgante G, De Palma P, D'Antona D. Inhibition of ovulation with transdermal estradiol and oral progestogens in perimenopausal women. *Contraception* 1997;55:239-243.

Fitzpatrick LA, Good A. Micronized progesterone: clinical indications and comparison with current treatments. *Fertil Steril* 1999;72:389-397.

Freedman RR, Woodward S. Behavioral treatment of menopausal hot flushes: evaluation by ambulatory monitoring. *Am J Obstet Gynecol* 1992;167:436-439.

Goldberg RM, Loprinzi CL, O'Fallen JR, et al. Transdermal clonidine for ameliorating tamoxifen-induced hot flashes. *J Clin Oncol* 1984;12:155-158.

Hammar M, Berg G, Lindgren R. Does physical exercise influence the frequency of postmenopausal hot flashes? *Acta Obstet Gynecol Scand* 1990;69:409-412.

Hlatky MA, Boothroyd D, Vittinghoff E, Sharp P, Whooley MA, for the HERS Research Group. Quality-of-life and depressive symptoms in postmenopausal women after receiving hormone therapy: results from the Heart and Estrogen/Progestin Replacement Study (HERS) trial. *JAMA* 2002;287:591-597.

Jensen JN, Christiansen C, Rodbro R. Cigarette smoking, serum estrogens, and bone loss during hormone-replacement therapy early after menopause. *N Engl J Med* 1985;313:973-975.

Kronenberg F. Hot flashes. In: Lobo RA, ed. *Treatment of the Postmenopausal Woman: Basic and Clinical Aspects.* 2nd ed. Philadelphia, PA: Lippincott Williams & Wilkins; 1999:157-177.

Lebherz TB, French LT. Nonhormonal treatment of the menopausal syndrome. *Obstet Gynecol* 1969;33:795-799.

Leonetti HB, Longo S, Anasti JN. Transdermal progesterone cream for vasomotor symptoms and postmenopausal bone loss. *Obstet Gynecol* 1999;94:225-258.

Lobo RA. Clinical aspects of hormonal replacement: routes of administration. In Lobo RA, ed. *Treatment of the Postmenopausal Woman: Basic and Clinical Aspects.* 2nd ed. Philadelphia, PA: Lippincott Williams & Wilkins; 1999:125-139.

Lobo RA, McCormick W, Singer F, Roy S. Depo-medroxy-progesterone acetate compared with conjugated estrogens for the treatment of postmenopausal women. *Am J Obstet Gynecol* 1984;63:1-5.

Loprinzi CL, Michalak JC, Quella SK, et al. Megestrol acetate for the prevention of hot flashes. *N Engl J Med* 1994;331:347-352.

Loprinzi CL, Pisansky TM, Fonseca R, et al. Pilot evaluation of venlafaxine hydrochloride for the therapy of hot flashes in cancer survivors. *J Clin Oncol* 1998;16:2377-2381.

Loprinzi CL, Sloan JA, Perez EA, et al. Phase III evaluation of fluoxetine for treatment of hot flashes. *J Clin Oncol* 2002;20:1578-1583.

McLaren HC. Vitamin E in the menopause. *BMJ* 1949;2:1378-1382.

Nagamani M, Kelver ME, Smith ER. Treatment of menopausal hot flushes with transdermal administration of clonidine. *Am J Obstet Gynecol* 1987;156:561-565.

Nesheim BI, Saetre T. Reduction of menopausal hot flashes by methyldopa: a double-blind crossover trial. *Eur J Clin Pharmacol* 1981;20:413-416.

The North American Menopause Society. Clinical challenges of perimenopause: consensus opinion of The North American Menopause Society. *Menopause* 2000;7:5-13.

The North American Menopause Society. The role of isoflavones in menopausal health: consensus opinion of The North American Menopause Society. *Menopause* 2000;7:215-229.

Pinkerton JV, Santen R. Alternatives to the use of estrogen in postmenopausal women. *Endocr Rev* 1999;20:308-320.

Schiff I, Tulchinsky D, Cramer D, Ryan KJ. Oral medroxyprogesterone in the treatment of postmenopausal symptoms. *JAMA* 1980;244:1443-1445.

Seidl MM, Stewart DE. Alternative treatments for menopausal symptoms: systematic review of scientific and lay literature. *Can Fam Physician* 1998;44:1299-1308.

Stearns V, Isaacs C, Rowland J, et al. A pilot trial assessing the efficacy of paroxetine hydrochloride (Paxil) in controlling hot flashes in breast cancer survivors. *Ann Oncol* 2000;11:17-22.

Steingold KA, Laufer L, Chetkowski RJ, et al. Treatment of hot flashes with transdermal estradiol administration. *J Clin Endocrinol Metab* 1985;61:627-632.

Utian WH, Shoupe D, Bachmann G, Pinkerton J, Pickar JH. Relief of vasomotor symptoms and vaginal atrophy with lower doses of conjugated equine estrogens and medroxyprogesterone acetate. *Fertil Steril* 2001;75:1065-1079.

J.02. Sleep disturbances

During the menopause transition, women may experience sleep disturbances, especially if hormonal fluctuations provoke vasomotor symptoms during the night. Sleep is considered adequate if one can function in an alert state during desired waking hours. Most adults require between 6 and 9 hours of sleep per night.

The decision to use behavioral and/or drug treatments for insomnia depend on the type of insomnia (acute or chronic, primary or secondary to other conditions), the context of the insomnia (high vasomotor symptoms or life strain), and the severity of daytime consequences.

Behavioral therapies can be used alone or with adjunctive pharmacologic or botanical therapies. Behavioral therapies for people with sustained sleep problems include avoiding behaviors that interfere with sleep and reinforcing those that promote sleep (eg, sleep hygiene measures), ritualizing environmental cues, regularizing the sleep/wake schedule, and relaxing to control tension.

Caffeine, alcohol, and nicotine should be avoided close to bedtime, if sleep induction is difficult. About 15 to 30 minutes are required for caffeine from a cup of coffee (80-115 mg) to affect the brain and up to 7 hours are required to rid the system of caffeine. For some, its stimulant effects have lasted up to 20 hours. Besides coffee, tea, cola drinks, and chocolate, caffeine is also present in OTC pain relievers, premenstrual syndrome remedies, diuretics, alertness and allergy/cold medications, as well as weight-control aids.

Alcohol initially promotes drowsiness, but often results in rebound awakening and fragmented sleep, leading to feeling unrefreshed upon awakening. It also affects breathing and tends to swell oral and nasal mucous membranes which may worsen sleep-related breathing disorders. Illicit drugs, such as marijuana, morphine, and heroin, also disrupt normal sleep patterns. Nicotine is frequently overlooked as contributing to sleep disturbances, but it has been observed to prolong sleep onset and decrease sleep duration.

Although eating a large, heavy meal before bed can interfere with sleep, a snack with protein (to support central nervous system neurochemical production, especially serotonin) and carbohydrates (to promote blood/brain barrier entry) is recommended. Strenuous exercise close to a desired sleep time amplifies arousal making it hard to fall asleep; however, regular daily exercise is beneficial.

Nightly rituals and establishing a sleep-conducive environment (quiet, cool, dark, safe) can "condition" better sleep. Counseling should also include advice to avoid using the bedroom for activities other than sleep and sexual activities. Women who do not fall asleep in 10 to 15 minutes should get up and leave the bedroom to engage in relaxing activities elsewhere until drowsy, then lie down to sleep again. This should be repeated as necessary. Resisting the temptation to check the clock will help educate the body to cease habitual awakenings.

Regularizing the sleep schedule can modify sleep quality. Choosing a consistent time to get up (regardless of time to bed and even on weekends) will maintain synchrony with the light/dark cycle, which is important to sleep quality.

Sleep-restriction therapy is a technique that can help re-establish a quality sleep pattern for someone unable to get quality hours of sleep. Women can be advised to:

- Determine current sleep duration (eg, 4 hours) and select a consistent time to arise (eg, 7 AM);

- Spend time in bed equal to perceived current sleep time (eg, go to bed at 3 AM and arise at 7 AM);

- When able to sleep 95% of this duration for several nights, go to bed 30 minutes earlier (eg, 2:30 AM);

- When sleeping 95% of lengthened time for several nights, go to bed another 30 minutes earlier (eg, 2:00 AM);

- Repeat this procedure until bedtime-to-wake time equals desired duration of sleep.

Learning to use relaxation techniques may help women with insomnia. Several modalities may be suggested to help learn how to enter and adopt a relaxed state, including instructional or mood-inducing tapes, concentration techniques such as meditation or creative imagery, or combining mind with movement techniques, such as yoga or tai chi.

Sleeping pills may be used to break a cycle of insomnia, but they should be prescribed as a last resort. Short-acting nonbenzodiazepine sleeping aids, such as zolpidem tartrate (Ambien, with 4-5 hr duration) or zaleplon (Sonata, with 1-3 hr duration), may be prescribed to help with difficulties falling asleep. Benzodiazepines may be useful for women who have trouble staying asleep. The side effects associated with benzodiazepines, such as next-day sedation, rebound insomnia when the drug is discontinued, tolerance, and dependence, underlie recommendations that they be used periodically at most (a maximum of 3 nights per week).

Some botanical sedatives are reputed to positively affect sleep quality. Valerian is one herb that has been observed to decrease sleep onset and promote deeper sleep (see Section I.05.b.3). German chamomile, lavender, hops, lemon balm, and passion flower are said to be mild sedatives, although few empirical data on them are available.

Some women self-medicate with melatonin, an endogenous pineal gland hormone, but its effects on sleep and behavioral sedation are inconsistent in studies. It is most useful in treating circadian-related sleep disorders or jet lag (see Section G.03.c).

Neither ERT nor HRT is FDA-approved as a treatment for insomnia. However, oral ERT has been shown to improve nighttime restlessness and awakening. HRT appears to affect perceived and polysomnographic sleep positively, mainly in conjunction with reducing hot flash and night sweat activity. Estrogen plus a progestin has been observed to lessen sleep disordered breathing (SDB), although small-sample studies have not confirmed these effects. Using progesterone instead of progestin may improve sleep, as progesterone is a mild soporific. Bedtime dosing is advised.

Referral to sleep centers is warranted for women with SDB manifestations or other sleep-related disorders, such as restless leg syndrome (crawly and strong urge to move sensations), periodic limb movements during sleep (jerky, rhythmic movements of legs), or narcolepsy (uncontrollable sleep bouts during waking hours, loss of muscle tone known as cataplexy, hypnogogic hallucinations, excessive daytime sleepiness, fragmented sleep, and automatic behaviors).

Bibliography

Attele AS, Xie JT, Yuan CS. Treatment of insomnia: an alternative approach. *Altern Med Rev* 2000;5:249-259.

Dockhorn RJ, Dockhorn DW. Zolpidem in the treatment of short-term insomnia: a randomized, double-blind, placebo-controlled clinical trial. *Clin Neuropharmacol* 1996;19:333-340.

Driver HS, Taylor SR. Exercise and Sleep. *Sleep Med Rev* 2000; 4:387-402.

Elie R, Ruther E, Farr I, Emilien G, Salinas E. Sleep latency is shortened during 4 weeks of treatment with zaleplon, a novel nonbenzodiazepine hypnotic. Zaleplon Clinical Study Group. *J Clin Psychiatry* 1999;60:536-544.

Harvey, AG. Sleep hygiene and sleep-onset insomnia. *J Nerv Mental Dis* 2000;188:53-55.

Keefe DL, Watson R, Naftolin F. Hormone replacement therapy may alleviate sleep apnea in menopausal women: a pilot study. *Menopause* 1999;6:196-200.

Landolt HP, Roth C, Dijk DJ, Borbely AA. Late-afternoon ethanol intake affects nocturnal sleep and the sleep EEG in middle-aged men. *J Clin Psychopharmacol* 1996;16:428-436.

Landolt HP, Werth E, Borbely AA, Dijk DJ. Caffeine intake (200 mg) in the morning affects human sleep and EEG power spectra at night. *Brain Res* 1995;675:67-74.

Leathwood PD, Chauffard F, Heck E, Munoz-Box R. Aqueous extract of valerian root (*Valeriana officinalis L.*) improves sleep quality in man. *Pharmacol Biochem Behav* 1982;17:65-71.

Morin CM, Hauri PJ, Espie CA, Spielman AJ, Buysse DJ, Bootzin RR. Nonpharmacologic treatment of chronic insomnia: an American Academy of Sleep Medicine review. *Sleep* 1999;22:1134-1156.

Polo-Kantola P, Erkkola R, Helenius H, Irjala K, Polo O. When does estrogen replacement therapy improve sleep quality? *Am J Obstet Gynecol* 1998;178:1002-1009.

Singh NA, Clements KM, Fiatarone MA. A randomized controlled trial of the effect of exercise on sleep. *Sleep* 1997;20:95-101.

Zhdanova IV, Wurtman RJ, Regan MM, Taylor JA, Shi JP, Leclair OU. Melatonin treatment for age-related insomnia. *J Clin Endocrinol Metab* 2001;86:4727-4730.

J.03. Headache

Headaches are one of the most common problems treated both in primary care and neurology settings. However, about half of all headache sufferers do not seek treatment, and about half of those who seek treatment for tension-type or migraine headaches either do not receive appropriate treatment or are dissatisfied with their treatment.

Most tension-type headaches can be effectively treated with nonprescription analgesics and nonsteroidal anti-inflammatory drugs (eg, aspirin, naproxen, ibuprofen). Nonpharmacologic therapies, including physical therapy, stress management, relaxation therapy, and biofeedback, are also helpful for some people. For women who need prophylactic treatment, tricyclic antidepressants or selective serotonin-reuptake inhibitors (SSRIs) may be helpful. Muscle relaxants have not been found to be effective for tension-type headaches.

Migraine headaches can be more difficult to treat. For mild to moderately painful migraines, OTC preparations, such as aspirin or acetaminophen and caffeine combinations, may be as effective as prescription medications. For more severe migraines, the triptan medications, such as sumatriptan (Imitrex), zolmitriptan (Zomig), and rizatriptan (Maxalt), are very effective. Nonsteroidal anti-inflammatory agents, such as naproxen, are also effective for some migraine sufferers, particularly when used with a triptan. The combination drug of isometheptene mucate, dichloralphenazone, and acetaminophen (Midrin), which is used primarily to treat acute migraines, has been found to be effective in treating mixed tension-type/migraine headaches. It should be used with caution, as it may be habit-forming.

Both over-the-counter and prescription drugs used for acute treatment can result in rebound headaches. Care should be taken to monitor their use, and if headaches occur more than twice a week, preventive medications should be considered. Any preventive medication is about 60% likely to be effective for a given individual. Prescription drugs found to be most effective in preventing migraines include beta blockers such as propanolol (Inderal), tricyclic antidepressants such as amitriptyline (Elavil), and anticonvulsants such as divalproex sodium (Depakote). With a preventive drug, starting doses should be low, then increased slowly. Drugs should be taken for at least 2 months to judge effectiveness.

A variety of trigger factors are thought to produce headaches in susceptible individuals. These triggers vary between people, as well as at different times for the same person. The most commonly identified food triggers include aged cheese and red wine. Research also indicates that fasting or skipping meals, too much or too little sleep, stress, and changes in barometric pressure or altitude are also probably triggers for many migraine sufferers. Caffeine may be helpful in treating some migraines, but it may also be a trigger for some individuals. Using a headache diary to identify (and avoid) triggers can be very helpful in headache management.

Changes in hormone levels, such as those that occur with menses, pregnancy, or during perimenopause, are a common cause of migraines. Women who have experienced migraines during their reproductive years may find that their headaches recur or worsen during the hormonal fluctuations of perimenopause. Sometimes migraines begin at perimenopause. Estrogen replacement therapy (ERT) or combined estrogen/progestogen, either as an oral contraceptive (OC) or as hormone replacement therapy (HRT), may exacerbate migraines in some women. Therapy should be discontinued if this occurs. However, for some women, ERT/HRT or OC therapy may help. Benefit is more likely when avoiding hormonal fluctuations (eg, with OCs, add a low-dose estrogen supplement during the withdrawal phase; use continuous ERT/HRT therapy, not cyclic; choose transdermal estrogen). Some evidence suggests that progestogens can precipitate or aggravate headaches. If headaches are worsened by medroxyprogesterone acetate, switching to micronized progesterone may help. Like other medications taken to alleviate or prevent headaches, ERT/HRT or OCs may require a trial of weeks to months before improvement is seen.

Caution should be used when prescribing OCs or ERT/HRT for a woman who has migraine with aura, as studies suggest that these women have an increased risk of stroke.

For many women, headaches are debilitating and frustrating, greatly interfering with quality of life at a time when career and family responsibilities are already stressful. A supportive relationship between the migraine sufferer and the healthcare provider can be extremely effective in determining the appropriate individual interventions.

Bibliography

Dahlof CG, Dimenas E. Migraine patients experience poorer subjective well-being/quality of life even between attacks. *Cephalalgia* 1995;15:31-36.

Fettes I. Migraine in the menopause. *Neurology* 1999;53 (4 suppl 1):S29-S33.

Goadsby PJ, Lipton RB, Ferrari MD. Migraine — current understanding and treatment. *N Engl J Med* 2002;4:257-270.

MacGregor EA, Barnes D. Migraine in a menopause clinic. *Climacteric* 1999;2:218-223.

Moloney M. Migraines and the perimenopause. *Menopause Management* 2000;9(5):8-15.

Silberstein SD, Lipton, RB. *Headache in Clinical Practice.* Oxford, Eng: Isis Medical Media; 1998.

Walling AD. Drug prophylaxis for migraine headaches [erratum in *Am Fam Phys* 1990;42:1220]. *Am Fam Phys* 1990;42:425-432.

J.04. Psychological symptoms

The psychological disturbances reported most often by perimenopausal women are irritability, blue moods, and anxiety. They can often be relieved through nonpharmacologic approaches.

Healthcare providers may be able to diminish or prevent some psychological symptoms by counseling women on what to expect at menopause, both physically and psychologically. Relaxation and stress-reduction techniques, including lifestyle modification, may help women cope with stress-producing factors in their lives during this time of hormonal fluctuations (see Table 2).

Table 2. Nonpharmacologic methods to cope with stress

- Deep breathing exercises and muscle relaxation training

- Daily exercise (yoga may be particularly helpful)

- Healthy diet (plant-based, low fat, low caffeine and low alcohol)

- Sufficient self-care (eg, time for massage, facials)

- Psychological support/therapy (eg, psychotherapy, menopause support group)

- Creative outlets that enhance quality of life

Some women attempt to self-treat their depression (mild or major) by using over-the-counter products, such as St. John's wort or vitamin B_6. Practitioners should always ask what medications and over-the-counter products women are taking and for what reason.

Some women experience symptoms of depression, such as depressed mood, irritability, poor concentration, and fatigue, due to sleep deprivation resulting from hot flashes and night sweats. These symptoms often improve when hot flashes are treated and sleep improves.

If vasomotor symptoms and psychological disturbances are not alleviated by nonpharmacologic methods, ERT/HRT may help. The administration of estrogen in doses that are conventionally used to treat hot flashes will often reduce or eliminate mood swings, tearfulness, irritability, and feelings of sadness. However, while estrogen may potentially have a positive affect on mood and behavior, it is not an antidepressant and should not be considered as such. FDA-approved product labeling for estrogen products includes a statement that there is no adequate evidence that estrogens are effective for nervous symptoms or depression without associated vasomotor symptoms, and it should not be used to treat these conditions.

There is evidence that estrogen has a positive impact on neural functions involved in the regulation of mood and behavior, which suggests a mood-enhancing effect. Many women using ERT report a feeling of well-being — while its absence has the opposite effect. In prospective, controlled trials in postmenopausal women, ERT has been shown to be consistently effective in relieving dysphoric mood (but not the more severe mood disorders associated with depression). Other studies of ERT use in peri- and postmenopausal women who have generalized complaints of depressive symptoms but not major depression also found improvement in mood associated with ERT. However, in some of these studies, the placebo recipients also showed evidence of improved mood over time, indicating that the significant advantage of ERT over placebo in short-term mood enhancement did not persist long term. It may be that although depressive symptoms naturally improve in perimenopausal women over time, this improvement is hastened by treatment with estrogen.

The potential antidepressant effects of ERT were examined in the Rancho Bernardo Study. In the 50 to 59 age group, women using ERT had higher Beck Depression Inventory scores than non-ERT users. After age 60, the rate of depression increased significantly in non-ERT users, but remained the same for those receiving treatment. In a preliminary study of ERT for the treatment of depression in perimenopausal women, transdermal estradiol therapy effectively treated depression independent of its salutary effects on vasomotor symptoms. However, the findings are not sufficient to suggest that estrogen alone is effective in alleviating the totality of symptoms that constitute a depressive syndrome. Additional clinical trials are needed to confirm these observations.

Some evidence suggests that estrogen potentiates the effect of some antidepressants, allowing clinicians to decrease the dose of the antidepressant. In a similar fashion, some women who have not responded to antidepressants may benefit from the addition of estrogen to their treatment regimen. ERT may also accelerate the antidepressant response. Although many women will respond well to ERT, it may actually worsen mood in some women who are clinically depressed.

Perimenopausal women should be screened for clinical depression. Symptoms such as prolonged tiredness, loss of interest in normal activities, sadness, or irritability can result from disease. Women who have been diagnosed with depression prior to menopause may experience exacerbation of symptoms during perimenopause. Taking a history of depression at other times related to hormonal fluctuations (eg, premenstrually, during pregnancy, or postpartum) or to the use of oral contraceptives may help to determine whether a woman is vulnerable to depressive episodes as a function of changes in hormone levels. Depression also may be a side effect of medications. Only when the exact cause of depression is determined can an appropriate treatment plan be developed.

If a woman is suffering from a major depressive episode, then antidepressant medication, short-term psychotherapy, or combination treatment is indicated — regardless of her decision about ERT.

In addition to depressive disorders, an evaluation of anxiety is needed to differentiate normal day-to-day anxiety from pathological responses that would benefit from pharmacological intervention and/or psychotherapy.

Oral contraceptives or ERT/HRT may provide a stabilizing effect during perimenopause, when hormone levels are erratic. These may be particularly helpful for women whose mood is affected by hormonal fluctuations (such as with premenstrual dysphoric disorder or postpartum depression). In women who do not respond after 1 month of hormone use, a dosage adjustment or a change to an alternative form can be tried before considering psychotropic medications and adjunctive psychotherapy. At any time that a woman meets the criteria for depression, regardless of the hormonal

milieu, it is advisable to treat the depression. Fluoxetine HCl at doses of 20 or 60 mg/day, administered during the luteal phase, is effective in treating premenstrual dysphoric disorder.

Progestogens (particularly progestins) may worsen mood in some women, particularly those with a history of premenstrual syndrome. In these women, clinicians can try switching to another progestin, using a continuous-combined HRT regimen where the dose of progestin is lower than in cyclic therapy, using oral micronized progesterone instead of progestin, or using vaginal progestogen. In the absence of contraindications, a short trial of unopposed estrogen may be considered.

Bibliography

Ballinger CB. Psychiatric aspects of menopause. *Br J Psychiatry* 1990;156:773-787.

Bjorn I, Bixo M, Nojd KS, Nyberg S, Backstrom T. Negative mood changes during hormone replacement therapy: a comparison between two progestogens. *Am J Obstet Gynecol* 2000;183: 1419-1426.

Burt VK, Altshuler LL, Rasgon NL. Depressive symptoms in the perimenopause: prevalence, assessment, and guidelines for treatment. *Harvard Rev Psychiatry* 1998;6:121-132.

Ditkoff LC, Crary WG, Cristo M, Lobo RA. Estrogen improves psychological function in asymptomatic postmenopausal women. *Obstet Gynaecol* 1991;178:991-995.

Halbreich U, Rojansky N, Palter S, Tworek H, Hissin P, Wang K. Estrogen augments serotonergic activity in postmenopausal women. *Biol Psychiatry* 1995;37:434-441.

Henderson VW. *Hormone Therapy and the Brain: A Clinical Perspective on the Role of Estrogen.* New York, NY: Parthenon Publishing Group; 2000.

Landau C, Milan FB. Assessment and treatment of depression during the menopause: a preliminary report. *Menopause* 1996;3:201-207.

The North American Menopause Society. Clinical challenges of perimenopause: consensus opinion of The North American Menopause Society. *Menopause* 2000;7:5-13.

Palinkas L, Barrett-Connor E. Estrogen use and depressive symptoms in postmenopausal women. *Obstet Gynecol* 1992;80:30-36.

Pearce J, Hawton K, Blake F. Psychological and sexual symptoms associated with the menopause and the effects of hormone replacement therapy. *Br J Psychiatry* 1995;167:163-173.

Rasgon NL, Altshuler LL, Fairbanks L. Estrogen-replacement therapy for depression. *Am J Psychiatry* 2000;158:1738.

Rubinow DR, Roca CA, Schmidt PJ. Estrogens and depression in women. In: Lobo RA. *Treatment of the Postmenopausal Woman: Basic and Clinical Aspects.* 2nd ed. Philadelphia, PA: Lippincott Williams & Wilkins; 1999:189-194.

Schmidt PJ, Nieman L, Danaceau MA, Tobin MB, Roca CA, Murphy JH. Estrogen replacement in perimenopause-related depression: a preliminary report. *Am J Obstet Gynecol* 2000;183: 414-420.

Sherwin BB. Affective changes with estrogen and androgen replacement therapy in surgically menopausal women. *J Affect Disord* 1988;14:177-187.

Sherwin BB. Hormones and the brain: Canadian consensus on menopause and osteoporosis. *J SOGC* 2001;23:1102-1104.

Sherwin BB. Impact of the changing hormonal milieu on psychologic functioning. In: Lobo RA, ed. *Treatment of the Postmenopausal Woman: Basic and Clinical Aspects.* 2nd ed. Philadelphia, PA: Lippincott Williams & Wilkins; 1999:179-187.

Soares CN, Almeida OP, Joffe H, Cohen LS. Efficacy of estradiol for the treatment of depressive disorders in perimenopausal women: a double-blind, randomized, placebo-controlled trial. *Arch Gen Psychiatry* 2001;58:529-534.

Steiner M, Romano SJ, Babcock S, et al. The efficacy of fluoxetine in improving physical symptoms associated with premenstrual dysphoric disorder. *BJOG* 2001;108:462-468.

Studd JWW, Smith RNJ. Estrogens and depression in women. *Menopause* 1994;1:33-37.

Su TP, Schmidt PJ, Danaceau MA, et al. Fluoxetine in the treatment of premenstrual dysphoria. *Neuropsychopharmacology* 1997; 16:346-356.

Vogel W, Klaiber EL, Boverman DM. Roles of the gonadal steroid hormones in psychiatric depression in men and women. *Prog Neuropsychopharmacol* 1978;2:487-503.

Zweifel JE, O'Brien WH. A meta-analysis of the effect of hormone replacement therapy upon depressed mood. *Psychoneuroendocrinol* 1997;22:189-212.

J.05. Vulvovaginal changes

All women at midlife and beyond should have a thorough evaluation of vaginal health, regardless of whether they are symptomatic or sexually active.

Vulvovaginal changes, such as vaginal dryness and atrophic vaginitis, are common problems for postmenopausal women, but they usually do not become troublesome until several years after menopause. Clinical management depends on the pattern and severity of the symptoms, the woman's medical history, and her lifestyle. Often, the first noticeable change is reduced vaginal lubrication during sexual arousal.

Vulvovaginal changes should be investigated to determine the cause. Without treatment, the vaginal lining may deteriorate to a thickness of only a few cell layers, predisposing it to small vaginal ulcers. Vulvovaginal changes can result in vaginal pain and bleeding during sexual intercourse, which can intensify to the point where intercourse is no longer pleasurable or possible.

Vaginal lubricants and moisturizers available without a prescription may help maintain vaginal moisture in women with mild vaginal atrophy (see Section G.05). Water-soluble lubricants (rather than oil-based lubricants) are recommended. During sexual activity, they provide relief of vaginal dryness by decreasing the friction on atrophic vulvovaginal structures. A nonhormonal bioadhesive moisturizing gel may provide longer-lasting benefits. Improvements in vaginal dryness and dyspareunia may allow many postmenopausal women to resume premenopausal levels of sexual function. Regular sexual activity has also been shown to help maintain vaginal health.

Other nonprescription approaches that have been reported as helpful include soy foods and flaxseeds. However, inadequate data exist to evaluate the effect, if any, of foods high in phytoestrogens or isoflavones on vaginal dryness.

One therapeutic option is to develop an expanded view of sexual pleasure (eg, massage, extended caressing, and mutual masturbation, if penetration is difficult).

If nonprescription solutions are ineffective in treating vaginal dryness, estrogen is the treatment of choice. Estrogen has been proven to restore vaginal blood flow, decrease vaginal pH, and improve the thickness and elasticity of these tissues. Both oral and transdermal estrogen products are FDA-approved for treatment of vulvar and vaginal atrophy; vaginal estrogen products are FDA-approved for the treatment of atrophic vaginitis and kraurosis vulvae.

Improvements in vulvovaginal health usually occur within a few weeks of starting ERT; however, some atrophic changes require weeks or months before an improvement is seen. Severe atrophic changes will respond more quickly to vaginal estrogen (ie, cream, tablet, or ring) than systemic estrogen.

Localized therapy with an estrogen cream typically consists of a loading dose of 2 to 4 g/day for 2 weeks. After the initial therapeutic response is seen, the frequency and dosage can be reduced to maintain the response. A maintenance schedule of 1 to 3 doses per week is usually sufficient. There are anecdotal reports that a schedule of 0.5 to 1.0 g/day is another effective option. One small, uncontrolled study reported efficacy in treating urogenital atrophy with a dose of 10 μg estradiol cream (10% the strength of the marketed product: Estrace Vaginal Cream).

In one trial, the vaginal tablet (Vagifem) containing 25 μg estradiol had greater patient acceptance than estrogen cream and lower withdrawal rates (10% vs 32%). The vaginal tablet was as effective as 1.25 mg conjugated equine estrogens vaginal cream in relieving symptoms of atrophic vaginitis, without appreciable systemic estradiol increases or estrogenic side effects.

The vaginal ring (Estring) releases 5 to 10 μg/day of estradiol for up to 90 days. One study has shown that the ring provided therapeutic efficacy for vaginal atrophy but did not increase serum estradiol levels above the normal postmenopausal range.

Although vaginal ERT is not FDA-approved for systemic effects, concerns exist regarding the stimulatory effects the estrogen vaginal tablet and cream may have on the endometrium. Studies have shown that even low doses of these products can result in endometrial proliferation, hyperplasia, or carcinoma. Vaginal ERT that is unopposed by a progestogen, even for short courses of treatment, should not be prescribed without proper monitoring of the endometrium (see Section N.01).

Vaginal estrogen is not generally used in combination with oral or transdermal estrogen, as oral and transdermal routes result in estrogen effects on vaginal tissues. Yet, for women with atrophic vaginitis, some clinicians recommend a regimen of starting on vaginal ERT (unopposed, so as to avoid potential progestogen-related side effects and enhance well-being) for a few weeks for an immediate vaginal effect, then switching to oral or transdermal estrogen for systemic effects, if needed. At the switch (which should not be long after starting estrogen), women with an intact uterus should receive progestogen with systemic estrogen.

Bibliography

Ayton RA, Darling GM, Murkies AL, et al. A comparative study of safety and efficacy of continuous low dose oestradiol released from a vaginal ring compared with conjugated equine oestrogen vaginal cream in the treatment of postmenopausal urogenital atrophy. *Br J Obstet Gynaecol* 1996;103:351-358.

Bachmann GA, Ebert GA, Burd ID. Vulvovaginal complaints. *Treatment of the Postmenopausal Woman: Basic and Clinical Aspects.* 2nd ed. Philadelphia, PA: Lippincott Williams & Wilkins; 1999:195-201.

Nachtigall LE. Clinical trial of the estradiol vaginal ring in the US. *Maturitas* 1995;22:(suppl):S43-S47.

The North American Menopause Society. Clinical challenges of perimenopause: consensus opinion of The North American Menopause Society. *Menopause* 2000;7:5-13.

The North American Menopause Society. The role of isoflavones in menopausal health: consensus opinion of The North American Menopause Society. *Menopause* 2000;7:215-229.

Rioux JE, Devlin MC, Gelfand MM, Steinberg WM, Hepburn DS. 17ß-Estradiol vaginal tables versus conjugated equine estrogen vaginal cream to relieve menopausal atrophic vaginitis. *Menopause* 2000;7:156-161.

Santen RJ, Pinkerton JV, Conaway M, et al. Treatment of urogenital atrophy with low-dose estradiol: preliminary results. *Menopause* 2002;9:179-187.

J.06. Sexual dysfunction

Changes in sexual desire, decreased sexual frequency, and diminished responsiveness may occur during midlife, independent of physical vaginal changes. Data from the National Health and Social Life Survey indicate that nearly one-half of midlife women have a problem in one or more aspects of sexual functioning. A range of psychologic, sociocultural, interpersonal, and biologic factors can contribute to sexual dysfunction.

If sexual dysfunction is present, a physical exam is required to identify any physical causes. ERT should be considered for the treatment of urogenital symptoms. Options include systemic ERT and vaginal estrogen products (cream, tablet, ring). Treating the underlying cause of the dryness with local application of estrogen may ameliorate or prevent other sexual problems from developing. These include delayed or less robust orgasm and urogenital symptoms. Water-based vaginal lubricants and moisturizers are effective OTC alternative for the treatment of minor cases of vaginal dryness.

Complaints of decreased sexual desire require an evaluation of potential causes, such as depression, fatigue, or sexual dysfunction in the woman's sexual partner. Relationship issues can be key and often women need encouragement to reveal or even recognize them. Decreases in sexual arousal, ability to achieve orgasm, and perceived sexual satisfaction may be a result of diminished estrogenic effects on the vascular system, which impair arterial blood flow or decrease estrogenic effects on the central and peripheral nervous system. These effects can impair touch and vibration perception, which could cause a delay or absence of orgasm.

An assessment of all potential physical, psychological, or social factors amenable to intervention should be the primary therapeutic consideration for women with a specific complaint of loss of sexual desire. It is also important to evaluate the potential side effects of medications, herbal remedies, or other OTC supplements.

Various treatment strategies for decreases in sexual desire are listed in Table 3.

Table 3. Treatment strategies for decreases in libido

Nonmedical interventions

- Allow more time for manual or oral stimulation

- Experiment with erotic materials, sexual fantasies, vibrators, dildos

- Try a sensual massage or a warm bath

- Change the sexual routine, such as the location or the time of day

- Use vaginal lubricants (water-based)

- Explore noncoital sexual activity, such as oral sex or mutual masturbation

- Encourage communication about sexual and other concerns between the woman and her partner

Medical interventions

- Androgen therapy

- Offer alternatives to drugs that adversely affect sexual function

---

Although ERT improves vaginal health and may improve sexual function by restoring vaginal lubrication and reducing dyspareunia, its effect on libido is uncertain. No studies have confirmed a beneficial effect of ERT on sexual desire. There is some evidence that very high levels of ERT may decrease or impair libido due to increased levels of sex hormone-binding globulin, which binds to testosterone and interferes with its bioavailability.

Testosterone plays a role in women's sex drive, although published data have not conclusively confirmed how the change in testosterone levels affects perimenopausal women. In the United States, the only FDA-approved androgen product for women (Estratest, containing methyltestosterone plus estrogen) is approved for treating vasomotor symptoms that do not respond to estrogen alone. Estratest has demonstrated efficacy for improving libido, particularly after surgical menopause. No drug product containing testosterone or methyltestosterone is FDA-approved to increase libido in women. In Canada, two oral testosterone products are used in women: methyl testosterone (Metandren) and testosterone undecanoate (Andriol). An intramuscular product, testosterone enanthate (Climacteron, Delatestryl), is also available.

Some clinicians prescribe compounded methyltestosterone formulations (0.5 to 2.5 mg/day), either alone (in breast cancer patients) or in combination with other ERT formulations. Many clinicians believe that methyl-testosterone does not aromatize in the breast.

Custom-compounded unmethylated testosterone formulations are also prescribed by some clinicians, although trial data on efficacy and safety are lacking. These products have the problem of highly variable absorption and, thus, variable blood levels.

Testosterone products for women are in development. The research needed for FDA approval is hindered by the limitations of using male psychometric instruments for libido in female libido research and by using male endpoints, such as frequency of coitus, fantasy, or orgasm.

When loss of libido occurs in tandem with menopause, and in particular following bilateral oophorectomy, a trial of concomitant ERT and androgen is justified if the diagnosis of female androgen insufficiency is met (see Section H.03 for more on androgen therapy). Women with complaints of lifelong lack of libido likely need more extensive evaluation.

When using any testosterone preparation, liver function tests and fasting cholesterol panel should be monitored. Frequency recommendations vary. A baseline test with repeat tests at 3 months and then at 6 or 12 months could be appropriate, depending on the results. Synthetic testosterones are broken down in the liver, necessitating monitoring of liver function. Hirsutism, acne, lowering of the voice, and androgenic alopecia (thinning of the scalp hair) are all possible side effects, even at what is considered to be a female dose (1 to 2.5 mg/day methyltestosterone). No data are available for long-term (>2 years) use of androgen. Caution is advised.

Women should be advised regarding the adverse side effects that could occur with overdosage and to guard against self-medicating at a higher dose in an effort to achieve a greater libido-enhancing effect. In fact, any libido-enhancing effect may be lost at higher doses. Additionally, women may become addicted to testosterone because it raises central serotonergic activity leading to an elevated mood. Withdrawal from high doses of testosterone may lead to mild to moderate depression or depressive mood.

Some women use OTC products such as DHEA in an attempt to improve sexual function. This use is not recommended until more conclusive data are available (see Section G.03 for more).

Sildenafil (Viagra) at daily doses of 10, 50, and 100 mg did not improve sexual response in pre- or perimenopausal women with sexual dysfunction. Higher doses were associated with a significant increase in both headaches and flushing (a greater incidence than observed in other studies with men).

A couple's sexual problems are often exacerbated when the male partner is successfully treated for erectile dysfunction after the couple has not had intercourse for months or years. The woman may have extreme vaginal discomfort due to lack of lubrication and elasticity. On the other hand, women successfully treated for a lack of sexual drive may be frustrated if her partner is unable or unwilling to engage in sex after a long hiatus.

Counseling may help perimenopausal women and their partners prepare for the changes in sexual function that may occur with aging. A referral to a therapist should be considered for any woman with persistent sexual dysfunction or when no underlying cause for the dysfunction can be identified.

Bibliography

Basson R. Female sexual response: the role of drugs in the management of sexual dysfunction. *Obstet Gynecol* 2001; 98:350-353.

Brincat M, Magos A, Studd JW, et al. Subcutaneous hormone implants for the control of climacteric symptoms. A prospective study. *Lancet* 1984;1(8367):16-18.

Buster JE, Casson PR. Where androgens come from, what controls them, and whether to replace them. In: Lobo RA, ed. *Treatment of the Postmenopausal Woman: Basic and Clinical Aspects.* 2nd ed. Philadelphia, PA: Lippincott Williams & Wilkins; 1999:141-154.

Caruso S, Intelisano G, Lupo L, Agnello C. Premenopausal women affected by sexual arousal disorder treated with sildenafil: a double-blind, cross-over, placebo-controlled study. *BJOG* 2001;108:623-628

Ditkoff EC, Crary WG, Cristo M, Lobo RA. Estrogen improves psychological function in asymptomatic postmenopausal women. *Obstet Gynecol* 1991;78:991-995.

Gassman A, Santoro N. The influence of menopausal hormone changes on sexuality: current knowledge and recommendations for practice. *Menopause* 1994;1:91-98.

Gelfand MM, Witta B. Androgen and estrogen-androgen hormone replacement therapy: a review of the safety literature, 1941-1996. *Clin Therapeutics* 1997;19:383-404.

Graves G, Lea R, Bourgeois-Law G. Menopause and sexual function. *J SOGC* 2001;23:849-852.

Kolakowska T. The clinical course of primary recurrent depression in pharmacologically treated female patients. *Br J Psychiatry* 1975;126:336-345.

Montgomery JC, Appleby L, Brincat M, et al. Effect of oestrogen and testosterone implants on psychological disorders in the climacteric. *Lancet* 1987;1(8528):297-299.

The North American Menopause Society. Clinical challenges of perimenopause: consensus opinion of The North American Menopause Society. *Menopause* 2000;7:5-13.

Phillips NA, Rosen RC. Menopause and sexuality. In: Lobo RA, ed. *Treatment of the Postmenopausal Woman: Basic and Clinical Aspects.* 2nd ed. Philadelphia, PA: Lippincott Williams & Wilkins; 1999:437-443.

Schmidt PJ, Nieman L, Danaceau MA, et al. Estrogen replacement in perimenopause-related depression: a preliminary report. *Am J Obstet Gynecol* 2000;183:414-420.

Sherwin BB. Impact of the changing hormonal milieu on psychologic functioning. In: Lobo RA, ed. *Treatment of the Postmenopausal Woman: Basic and Clinical Aspects.* 2nd ed. Philadelphia, PA: Lippincott Williams & Wilkins; 1999:179-187.

Zweifel JE, O'Brien WH. A meta-analysis of the effect of hormone replacement therapy upon depressed mood [erratum in *Psychoneuroendocrinol* 1997;22:655]. *Psychoneuroendocrinol* 1997;22:189-212.

J.07. Incontinence

Although as many as 30% of women aged 45 to 64 have urinary incontinence, less than half seek evaluation and treatment. This is often because of embarrassment or because of the misconception that their condition is a normal part of aging and cannot be treated. It is not generally understood that effective nonsurgical treatments are available. Women often do not present for treatment until incontinence problems are severe. However, diagnosis and treatment can often completely cure the problem. If a cure is not possible, comfort can usually be improved. Incontinence should never be viewed as an inevitability of aging.

A large percentage of women with new-onset incontinence have a reversible cause, such as urinary tract infection, drug interaction, or cognition-related phenomena. However, pelvic floor muscle weakness and sphincter weakness are the major causes of urinary incontinence.

The types of incontinence are classified as follows:

- *Stress incontinence* is involuntary loss of urine that occurs with an activity that increases intra-abdominal pressure, such as coughing or sneezing. Leakage is usually in drops, at least at first. This is the most common type of incontinence. It may be due to displacement of the bladder base as well as bladder neck incompetence and urethral sphincter weakness.

- *Urge incontinence* is involuntary loss of urine that is provoked by uninhibited contraction of the detrusor muscle (smooth muscle of the bladder wall). This leakage is often preceded by an urgent sensation to urinate. Urge incontinence produces a large volume that may flood to the floor.

- *Mixed incontinence* is when both stress and urge incontinence occur simultaneously.

- *Overflow incontinence* occurs when the bladder fails to empty and remains partially full most of the time. Overflow leakage may occur while sleeping at night (nocturnal enuresis) or mimic stress or urge leakage. The bladder may become distended.

- *Extra urethral incontinence* is less common, occurring when there is an abnormal opening from the bladder, such as a vesico-vaginal fistula that might occur as a complication of hysterectomy.

Chronic dampness of underwear is sometimes mistaken for incontinence when the cause is an increase or change in vaginal secretions or perineal perspiration. A trial of phenazopyridine HCl (Pyridium), which will color the urine pink-orange, may help differentiate urine from watery vaginal secretions.

Diagnosis of the cause of a woman's incontinence requires a physical exam along with a medical and sexual history (see Section E.11). The examination includes a pelvic exam and analysis of a urine sample. In some cases, specialized studies of the bladder are required. Treatment of incontinence focuses on the root cause — and the type (eg, stress, urge).

Many women have more than one cause or contributing factor to urinary incontinence, necessitating more than one intervention to gain urinary control. The most troublesome symptoms should be addressed first. Treatment also depends on the significance of incontinence to the *individual* — not how often she leaks or if she needs to wear pads for protection. Significance is determined by the impact of incontinence on quality of life.

Modifiable contributors to incontinence, such as a chronic cough from smoking or undiagnosed asthma, should also be indicated. Treating asthma to eliminate persistent cough will simultaneously treat stress incontinence. Diuretic therapy could be a contributor to incontinence; taking the diuretic in divided doses may provide relief. Lack of mobility may contribute to not reaching the toilet with urge incontinence. Increasing mobility and/or moving the bed closer to the bathroom may help.

Drug therapy, behavior modification, biofeedback techniques, and electrical neurostimulation are some of the treatment options (see Table 4). The most effective approach teams the woman with a continence educator (typically a nurse) for coaching and personal support, as well as a physician.

Treating stress incontinence. Pelvic floor strengthening exercises improve stress incontinence. In a study comparing surgery with Kegel exercises, superior results were obtained with surgery. However, 42% of women performing Kegel exercises improved sufficiently so that surgery was no longer necessary. In another study, Kegel exercises helped 56% of women improve or cure their stress incontinence.

Table 4. Strategies for managing and treating urinary incontinence

Avoid bladder irritants — Certain foods and beverages high in caffeine or acid (eg, grapefruit juice, tomatoes, coffee, cola soft drinks) can contribute to incontinence by irritating the bladder.

Avoid fluid restriction — A common self-help strategy for urinary incontinence is fluid restriction. However, urine is more dilute and less irritating to the bladder when ample water is consumed.

Skin care tips — Women must be counseled as to good hygiene and care of the skin that may be exposed to urine for prolonged periods.

Pelvic floor exercises (Kegel exercises) — Contraction and relaxation to strengthen the muscles that control urine flow. When performed correctly, Kegel exercises can produce a cure in 50%-70% of women, but they must be performed regularly and indefinitely.

Functional electrical stimulation — Small devices inserted by the woman into the vagina that painlessly stimulate the muscles involved in urination (used in conjunction with Kegel exercises).

Vaginal cones — Small cones placed and held in the vagina to help a woman determine which muscles to contract and relax for Kegel exercises.

Biofeedback — A technique in which the senses are trained to affect bodily functions (usually with the help of a monitoring device).

Timed voiding — A technique for urge incontinence in which a woman urinates at regular, short intervals, then extends the intervals between voiding.

Medications — A variety of medications are available for different causes/types of incontinence, such as antibiotics to treat a UTI and anticholinergics (to control bladder contractions).

Surgery — Referral to a urologist or urogynecologist is appropriate for women with complex problems (such as neurologic conditions or anatomical defects) or when nonsurgical treatments are unsuccessful.

Kegel exercises consist of repeated contraction and relaxation of the urethral attempt the exercise while urinating to see if they can stop urine flow. When the correct muscles have been identified, the exercise should not be performed when urinating. The muscles are contracted to the count of 3 and then relaxed. Recommended frequency is 10 exercises 5 times each day. These exercises help maintain vaginal tone and increase circulation to the perineal area. Some women report an improvement in their sex life after a Kegel exercise program.

Overweight women who lose weight may find that pelvic relaxation is reduced and stress incontinence is improved.

Pharmacologic treatment for *stress* incontinence includes α-adrenergic agonists (eg, ephedrine, pseudoephedrine) for their potential to increase urethral closure.

Although estrogen is not FDA-approved for stress incontinence, ERT may help maintain muscle support to the urethra and pelvic floor. Studies on the effect of ERT on stress incontinence are inconsistent, although ERT in conjunction with pelvic strengthening exercises may benefit stress incontinence. Other treatments used in stress incontinence, although not FDA-approved for this indication, include the antihistamines pseudoephedrine (30 mg 1-3 times/day) and phenylpropanolamine (50 mg 1-3 times/day). Stress incontinence often requires surgery to correct the anatomic urinary tract structures.

Treating urge incontinence. With *urge* incontinence, the goal is to stop involuntary detrusor contractions. Drug therapy includes anticholinergic agents (eg, propantheline bromide), which suppress parasympathetic-mediated detrusor contractions. Musculotropic relaxants (eg, oxybutynin chloride and flavoxate HCl) suppress detrusor contractions through relaxation of the smooth muscles. Drug treatment can be enhanced with behavior modification. Tricyclic antidepressants have been used because of their relaxation effect on the smooth muscles of the bladder.

When bladder outlet dysfunction is the cause of incontinence, drug therapy can reduce the outlet resistance. Drugs such as α-adrenergic agonists (eg, methyldopa and clonidine) can stimulate the muscles of the bladder neck and proximal urethra to increase closure.

ERT does not have an established role in the treatment of urge incontinence, although the high concentration of estrogen receptors in the urethra suggests that ERT could have a benefit. Clinical trials using ERT to treat urge incontinence, however, have not produced clearly positive results. ERT is not FDA-approved to treat urge incontinence.

FDA-approved medications for treating urge urinary incontinence are found in Table 5. Other treatments that are sometimes used but are not FDA-approved for urge incontinence include imipramine HCl (10-25 mg 1-3 times/day) and propantheline bromide (15 mg 1-3 times/day).

If incontinence is not adequately controlled, the dosages of the selected drug can be increased every 3 to 5 days until clinical improvement is seen or until the woman experiences adverse side effects. Caution should be used when prescribing drugs to elderly women who have comorbidities and are being treated with other drugs.

Table 5. Medications in the United States and Canada for the treatment of urge urinary incontinence

Medication	Starting dosage
Oxybutynin chloride	
Ditropan	2.5-5 mg 1-3 times/day
Ditropan XL	5-15 mg daily
Tolterodine tartrate	1-2 mg 1-2 times/day
Detrol LA	2-4 mg daily
Detrol Unidet*	
Hyoscyamine sulfate	whole or half 0.375 mg tablet 1-2 times/day

* Available in Canada but not the United States.

Counseling. With any type of incontinence, counseling is appropriate regarding options to control urine. Many women are unaware of the options available. The use of containment pads may improve quality of life considerably.

Women with failed conservative management, extreme personal distress secondary to the incontinence, and with combined incontinence and recurrent bladder infections should be referred to a specialist.

Bibliography

Cardozo LD, Kelleher CJ. Sex hormones, the menopause and urinary problems. *Gynecol Endocrinol* 1995;9:75-84.

DeMarco EF. Urinary tract disorders in perimenopausal and postmenopausal women. In: Lobo RA, ed. *Treatment of the Postmenopausal Woman: Basic and Clinical Aspects.* 2nd ed. Philadelphia, PA: Lippincott Williams & Wilkins; 1999:213-227.

Elia G, Bergman A. Pelvic muscle exercises: when do they work? *Obstet Gynecol* 1993;81:283-286.

Fantl JA, Bump RC, Robinson D, McClish DK, Wyman JF. Efficacy of estrogen supplementation in the treatment of urinary incontinence: the Continence Program for Women Research Group. *Obstet Gynecol* 1996;88:745-749.

Griebling TL, Nygaard IE. The role of estrogen replacement therapy in the management of urinary incontinence and urinary tract infection in postmenopausal women. *Endocrinol Metab Clin North Am* 1997;26:347-360.

Henalla SM, Kirwan P, Castleden CM, Hutchins CJ, Breeson AJ. The effect of pelvic floor exercises in the treatment of genuine urinary stress incontinence in women at two hospitals. *Br J Obstet Gynaecol* 1988;95:602-606.

Johnson S. Canadian consensus on menopause and osteoporosis: urogenital health. *J SOGC* 2001;23:973-977.

Klarskov P, Belving D, Bischoff N, et al. Pelvic floor exercise versus surgery for female urinary stress incontinence. *Urol Int* 1986;41:129-132.

Wyman JF, Fantl JA, McClish DK, Bump RC. Comparative efficacy of behavioral interventions in the management of female urinary incontinence: Continence Program for Women Research Group. *Am J Obstet Gynecol* 1998;179:999-1007.

J.08. Urinary tract infection

To help prevent urinary tract infection (UTI), clinicians should first emphasize the importance of nonpharmacologic approaches. Although voiding, hygiene, and dietary measures have not been conclusively proven to prevent UTIs, they involve little risk or cost and may be beneficial to many women (see Table 6).

Table 6. Nonpharmacologic strategies for preventing urinary tract infection

- Void within 1 hour of the urge to urinate

- Wipe from front to back after a bowel movement to prevent spreading bacteria

- Change underwear daily

- Wear underwear with a cotton crotch to minimize moisture retention

- Avoid tight jeans and other pants (including pantyhose) that hold in heat and moisture

- Decrease use of hot tubs and highly chlorinated pools

- Avoid perfumed toilet paper, powders, and bubble baths

- Do not use feminine hygiene products that can irritate the urethra

- Abstain from food and beverage products believed to be bladder irritants

- Drink cranberry juice to decrease the pH of the urine in the bladder

After menopause, the vaginal pH increases and the vaginal flora changes. ERT may help reduce the risk of urinary tract infection by restoring the vagina to a healthier, more acidic environment. One randomized, placebo-controlled trial of 93 postmenopausal women found that vaginal ERT significantly reduced the risk of UTI.

However, a case-control trial of 3,616 women with first clinical UTI and 19,162 controls found that ERT use for 1 year significantly increased UTI risk, although this increase was observed only in women with an intact uterus. The investigators suggested that estrogen induced changes in bacterial attachment to urinary tract cells or antibody coating in the urinary tract. Another case-control study of 254 ERT users also did not support a reduced risk of UTIs with ERT.

Data from the Heart and Estrogen/Progestin Replacement Study (HERS) showed that HRT (conjugated equine estrogens plus medroxyprogesterone acetate) did not reduce the incidence of UTIs. The postmenopausal women receiving HRT actually had more UTIs than the placebo recipients, although the difference was not significant. No participants received ERT alone. The data also showed that the most significant risk factors for UTIs in these women were diabetes mellitus, vaginal dryness and/or itching, and urge incontinence.

In the postmenopausal woman presenting with recurrent lower UTI, therapy focuses on prophylactic antibiotic therapy.

Bibliography

Brown JS, Vittinghoff E, Kanaya AM, et al, for the Heart and Estrogen/Progestin Replacement Study Group. Urinary tract infections in postmenopausal women: effect of hormone therapy and risk factors. *Obstet Gynecol* 2001;9:1045-1052.

DeMarco EF. Urinary tract disorders in perimenopausal and postmenopausal women. In: Lobo RA, ed. *Treatment of the Postmenopausal Woman: Basic and Clinical Aspects*. 2nd ed. Philadelphia, PA: Lippincott Williams & Wilkins; 1999:213-227.

Griebling TL, Nygaard IE. The role of estrogen replacement therapy in the management of urinary incontinence and urinary tract infection in postmenopausal women. *Endocrinol Metab Clin North Am* 1997;26:347-360.

Oliveria SA, Klein RA, Reed JI, Cirillo PA, Christos PJ, Walker AM. Estrogen replacement therapy and urinary tract infections in postmenopausal women aged 45-89. *Menopause* 1998;5:4-8.

Orlander JD, Jick SS, Dean AD, Jick H. Urinary tract infections and estrogen use in older women. *J Am Geriatr Soc* 1992;40:817-820.

Privette M, Cade R, Peterson J, Mars D. Prevention of recurrent urinary tract infection in postmenopausal women. *Nephron* 1988;50:24-27.

Raz R, Stamm WE. A controlled trial of intravaginal estriol in postmenopausal women with recurrent urinary tract infections. *N Engl J Med* 1993;329:753-756.

J.09. Cognitive function

Memory and other cognitive abilities change throughout life, with a trend for declining performance with advancing age.

It is unclear whether ERT improves cognitive abilities. Most, but not all, studies of healthy, elderly postmenopausal women found that those taking ERT had higher scores on cognitive function tests than the controls, especially on verbal memory tests. Research findings in older women who began ERT some years after menopause generally fail to support the use of ERT solely to maintain or improve cognition.

Dementia — the loss of memory and other intellectual abilities, severe enough to interfere substantially with usual daily activities — is perhaps the most feared consequence of aging.

Observational studies suggest that ERT may delay brain aging and dementia. Short-term clinical trials of women undergoing surgical menopause suggest that ERT may help preserve memory, although any long-term benefit has not yet been demonstrated in randomized, controlled trials. Limited observational and clinical trial studies suggest that estrogen therapy has little, if any, effect on improving cognitive performance in postmenopausal women. There is a possibility that any beneficial effect of estrogen may be negated when combined with a progestogen.

The most common cause of dementia is Alzheimer's disease (AD), accounting for well over one-half of cases. Observational data indicate that higher education, maintaining an extensive social network, and remaining physically and mentally active may help protect against dementia. Few studies have focused on estrogen and vascular dementia. Estrogen may enhance cerebral blood flow, but limited clinical trial data do not indicate a substantial long-term effect of estrogen on cerebrovascular disease.

Diminished estrogen concentrations after menopause may also increase AD risk. Several pharmaceuticals have been investigated for use in preventing this disease, including ERT/HRT. A number of observational studies have associated the use of ERT/HRT with a reduced risk of developing AD, possibly by as much as one-third. One prospective, longitudinal study showed a protective effect on 1,124 postmenopausal women who were followed for 1 to 5 years. However, there are no data from randomized controlled trials to settle this important question. Several primary prevention trials are in progress.

Vitamin E was thought to have a protective effect against AD, based on its antioxidant properties, but this has not been confirmed in clinical trials. A report of lowered incidence of AD in individuals (both men and women) taking statins is a retrospective analysis and more study is required before statins can be considered for AD prevention.

Several therapies have been reported to decrease the risk for severe cognitive dysfunction, including ERT/HRT, nonsteroidal anti-inflammatory agents, and vitamin E. Moderate physical exercise also has been associated with less cognitive decline. These effects are not supported by well-controlled clinical trials.

For women with established AD, no therapies have yet been developed that persistently ameliorate the symptoms or retard the degenerative course of the disease. The FDA has approved several medications for treating patients with mild to moderate symptoms of Alzheimer's disease. These drugs, which include donepezil (Aricept), rivastigmine (Exelon), and tacrine (Cognex), act to increase brain levels of acetylcholine by blocking the breakdown of this key neurotransmitter. They are modestly effective but do not have a substantial clinical impact on the disease. There is limited evidence that the antioxidant vitamin E may slow disease progression in moderately impaired AD patients. Current evidence does not support an indication for ERT in the treatment of AD.

Bibliography

Asthana S, Baker LD, Craft S, et al. High-dose estradiol improves cognition for women with AD: results of a randomized study. *Neurology* 2001;57:605-612.

Baldereschi DM, DiCarlo A, Lepore V, et al. Estrogen-replacement therapy and Alzheimer's disease in the Italian Longitudinal Study on Aging. *Neurology* 1998;50:996-1002.

Binder EF, Schechtman KB, Birge SJ, Williams DB, Kohrt WM. Effects of hormone replacement therapy on cognitive performance in elderly women. *Maturitas* 2001;38:137-146.

Brenner DE, Kukull WA, Stergachis A, et al. Postmenopausal estrogen replacement therapy and the risk of Alzheimer's disease: a population-based case-control study. *Am J Epidemiol* 1994; 140:262-267.

Davis KL, Thal LJ, Gamzu ER, et al. Tacrine Collaborative Study Group: a double-blind, placebo-controlled multicenter study of tacrine for Alzheimer's disease. *N Engl J Med* 1992;327:1253-1259.

Funk JL, Mortel KF, Meyer JS. Effects of estrogen replacement therapy on cerebral perfusion and cognition among postmenopausal women. *Dementia* 1991;2:268-272.

Grodstein F, Chen J, Pollen DA, et al. Postmenopausal hormone therapy and cognitive function in healthy older women. *J Am Geriatr Soc* 2000;48:746-752.

Henderson VW. *Hormone Therapy and the Brain: A Clinical Perspective on the Role of Estrogen.* New York, NY: Parthenon Publishing Group; 2000.

Henderson VW. The role of sex steroids in Alzheimer's disease: prevention and treatment. In: Lobo RA, ed. *Treatment of the Postmenopausal Woman: Basic and Clinical Aspects.* 2nd ed. Philadelphia, PA; Lippincott Williams & Wilkins; 1999:269-276.

Henderson VW, Paganini-Hill A, Miller BL, et al. Estrogen for Alzheimer' disease in women: randomized, double-blind, placebo-controlled trial. *Neurology* 2000;54:295-301.

Henderson VW, Watt L, Buckwalter JG. Cognitive skills associated with estrogen replacement in women with Alzheimer's disease. *Psychoneuroendocrinol* 1996;21:421-430.

Hogervorst E, Williams J, Budge M, Riedel W, Jolles J. The nature of the effect of female gonadal hormone replacement therapy on cognitive function in post-menopausal women: a meta-analysis. *Neuroscience* 2000;101:485-512.

Kawas C, Resnick S, Morrison A, et al. A prospective study of estrogen replacement therapy and the risk of developing Alzheimer's disease: the Baltimore Longitudinal Study of Aging. *Neurology* 1997;48:1517-1521.

LeBlanc ES, Janowsky J, Chan BKS, Nelson HD. Hormone replacement therapy and cognition: systematic review and meta-analysis. *JAMA* 2001;285:1489-1499.

Maki P, Zonderman A, Resnick S. Enhanced verbal memory in nondemented elderly women receiving hormone-replacement therapy. *Am J Psychiatry* 2001;158:227-233.

Mulnard RA, Cotman CW, Kawas C, et al. Estrogen replacement therapy for treatment of mild to moderate Alzheimer disease: a randomized controlled trial. *JAMA* 2000;283:1007-1015.

Norberg A. Pharmacological treatment of cognitive dysfunction in dementia disorders. *Acta Neurol Scand* 1996;168:87-92.

Ohkura T, Isse K, Akazawa K, Hamamoto M, Yaoi Y, Hagino N. Long-term estrogen replacement therapy in female patients with dementia of the Alzheimer type: 7 case reports. *Dementia* 1995;6:99-107.

Paganini-Hill A, Henderson VW. Estrogen replacement therapy and risk of Alzheimer's disease. *Arch Intern Med* 1996;156:2213-2217.

Phillips SM, Sherwin BB. Effects of estrogen on memory function in surgically menopausal women. *Psychoneuroendocrinol* 1992; 17:485-495.

Polo-Kantola P, Portin R, Polo O, Helenuis H, Irjala K, Erkkola R. The effect of short-term estrogen replacement therapy on cognition: a randomized, double-blind, cross-over trial in postmenopausal women. *Obstet Gynecol* 1998;91:459-466.

Rice MM, Graves AB, McCurry SM, et al. Postmenopausal estrogen and estrogen-progestin use and 2-year rate of cognitive change in a cohort of older Japanese American women: The Kame Project. *Arch Intern Med* 2000;160:1641-1649.

Rogers SL, Farlow MR, Doody RS, et al. A 24-week, double-blind, placebo-controlled trial of donepezil in patients with Alzheimer's disease. *Neurology* 1998;50:136-145.

Rogers SL, Friedhoff LT. The efficacy and safety of donepezil in patients with Alzheimer's disease: results of a US multicentre, randomized, double-blind, placebo-controlled trial. *Dementia* 1996;7:293-303.

Rösler M, Anand R, Cicin-Sain A, et al. Efficacy and safety of rivastigmine in patients with Alzheimer' disease: international randomised controlled trial. *BMJ* 1999;318:633-640.

Sano M, Jacobs DM, Mayeux R. The epidemiology of Alzheimer's disease and the role of estrogen replacement therapy in the prevention and treatment of Alzheimer's disease and memory decline in older women. In: Lobo RA, ed. *Treatment of the Postmenopausal Woman: Basic and Clinical Aspects.* 2nd ed. Philadelphia, PA; Lippincott Williams & Wilkins; 1999;263-276.

Schneider LS, Farlow MR, Henderson VW, Pogoda JM. Effects of estrogen replacement therapy on response to tacrine in patients with Alzheimer's disease. *Neurology* 1996;46:1580-1584.

Shumaker SA, Reboussin BA, Espeland MA, et al. The Women's Health Initiative Memory Study (WHIMS): a trial of the effect of estrogen therapy in preventing and slowing the progression of dementia. *Controlled Clin Trials* 1998;19:604-621.

Silva I, Mor G, Naftolin F. Estrogen and the aging brain. *Maturitas* 2001;38:95-100.

Tang M-X, Jacobs D, Stern Y, et al. Effect of oestrogen during menopause on risk and age at onset of Alzheimer's disease. *Lancet* 1996;348:429-432.

Waring SC, Rocca WA, Petersen RC, O'Brien PC, Tangalos EG, Kokmen E. Postmenopausal estrogen replacement therapy and risk of AD: a population-based study. *Neurology* 1999;23:965-970.

Yaffe K, Barnes D, Nevitt M, et al. A prospective study of physical activity and cognitive decline in elderly women: women who walk. *Arch Intern Med* 2001;161:1703-1708.

Yaffe K, Sawaya G, Lieberburg I, Grady D. Estrogen therapy in postmenopausal women: effects on cognitive function and dementia. *JAMA* 1998;279:688-695.

J.10. Skin changes

Although skin collagen content and skin thickness decline significantly with aging, the skin ages relatively well. It is only with exposure to extrinsic factors, primarily sunlight and, to some extent, tobacco smoke, that aging of the skin occurs in a more marked fashion. While this problem is often medically insignificant, it is of profound cosmetic concern and will detract from the quality of life for many women at midlife and beyond.

It is important to keep skin hydrated by drinking adequate amounts of water. Most individuals consume far too little water; liquids like coffee, tea, and caffeinated soft drinks may quench thirst, but their diuretic action decreases hydration. Skin health is another reason to avoid excess alcohol consumption. Other skin-healthy habits include getting adequate exercise and sleep, and avoiding stress and smoking.

Xerosis (dry skin), the most common condition of aging skin, is a consequence of the skin's reduced oil production. Xerosis is usually more pronounced on the back and the ankles, and can cause significant itching and discomfort. It tends to be more marked in dry climates and during winter months.

Xerosis is best prevented by avoiding hot, soapy showers and baths, which overdry the skin. Women should be advised to use a bath oil or heavy lotion on wet skin immediately after showering or bathing. Products that have an oily feel, such as petroleum jelly and baby oil, are most effective, as common hand lotions often contain alcohol and little oil. Skin will become more resistant to physical and chemical insults if it is kept lubricated.

Use of a moisturizing sunscreen will have the greatest impact is protecting and improving the appearance of aging skin. Data support the importance of preventing ultraviolet A and B radiation. For optimal skin protection, women should use a sunscreen throughout the year. However, sunscreen use will block vitamin D absorption. Women using extensive sunscreen coverage should take a vitamin D supplement to obtain the recommended amount.

Antioxidants, alpha-hydroxy acids, and topical retinoids have been used to repair photoaged skin. Only topical retinoids have demonstrated well-documented ability to repair skin at the clinical, histological, and molecular level.

Many women today use exfoliant face creams to reduce wrinkling. These creams can be helpful but may cause stinging in women with sensitive skin. Retinoic acid (Retin-A) is an FDA-approved product for fine wrinkles, mottled pigmentation, and skin roughness. Any beneficial effects are seen only during product use. Retinoic acid can cause burning, itching, peeling, and increased sun sensitivity. Sunscreen protection should be used when sun exposure exceeds 20 min/day. Injections of collagen and botox are other wrinkle treatments.

Evidence indicates that ERT/HRT has at least some beneficial effects on skin. Clinical trial data on oral and transdermal ERT/HRT have shown it limits skin collagen loss and helps maintain skin thickness. In postmenopausal women treated with topical estrogen, 6 months of therapy markedly improved the elasticity and firmness of the skin and decreased wrinkle depth and pore size. Skin moisture increased and the measurement of wrinkles using skin profilometry revealed significant decreases in wrinkles. However, using only skin observations, it was not possible to distinguish ERT/HRT users from nonusers. ERT/HRT also appears to limit skin extensibility during perimenopause, exerting a preventive effect on skin slackness, although no effect on skin viscoelasticity has been noted. Although the data are not convincing enough to initiate ERT/HRT for skin benefits alone, the potential facial skin benefits may appeal to some women. ERT/HRT is not FDA-approved for any skin benefit.

ERT/HRT neither alters the effects of genetic aging or sun damage nor reduces or increases the risk of skin cancer. Some women taking high doses of estrogen may experience increased pigmentation (called melasma or cloasma) that may not be reversible.

Acne. Some women will develop acne in midlife, usually due to an increase in the ratio of androgen to estrogen. Circulating androgens are typically in the normal range, but levels have been shown to be significantly higher in women with acne than in women without acne. Women who had acne during their teen years will almost always have acne in midlife. The effects of androgens on acne are most evident in adult women.

The net effect of systemic hormonal treatment for acne is a reduction of sebum production from the sebaceous gland. Neither topical acne preparations nor oral antibiotics influence sebum production. In 1997, the FDA approved the first OC for the treatment of acne — norgestimate and ethinyl estradiol (Ortho Tri-Cyclen). Efficacy has been demonstrated in two multicenter, double-blind, placebo-controlled trials. At least one other OC (Estrostep) has also been approved for that indication.

DIANE-35 (cyproterone acetate and ethinyl estradiol) is approved in Canada for the treatment of severe acne in women who have associated symptoms of androgenization, including seborrhea and mild hirsutism. It also provides reliable contraception in this population.

Formication. Women presenting with formication (tactile sensation of insects crawling on the skin) may be treated with ERT/HRT and/or with psychopharmacologic therapies. There are no clinical studies addressing this problem and no known therapy has been identified as effective.

Skin cancer. Treatment of skin cancer is outside the scope of this guidebook.

Bibliography

Brincat MP. Hormone replacement therapy and the skin. *Maturitas* 2000;35:107-117.

Brincat M, Moniz CJ, Kabalan S, et al. Decline in skin collagen content and metacarpal index after the menopause and its prevention with sex hormone replacement. *Br J Obstet Gynaecol* 1987;94:126-129.

Castelo-Branco C, Duran M, Gonzalez-Merlo J. Skin collagen changes related to age and hormone replacement therapy. *Maturitas* 1992;15:113-119.

Creidi P, Faivre B, Agache P, Richard E, Hadiquet V, Sauvanet JP. Effect of a conjugated oestrogen (Premarin) cream on ageing facial skin: a comparative study with a placebo cream. *Maturitas* 1994; 19:211-223.

Dunn LB, Damesyn M, Moore AA, Reuben DB, Greendale GA. Does estrogen prevent skin aging? Results from the First National Health and Nutrition Examination Survey (NHANES I). *Arch Dermatol* 1997;133:339-342.

Griffiths CE. Drug treatment of photoaged skin. *Drugs Aging* 1999;14:289-301.

Griffiths CE, Kang S, Ellis CN, et al. Two concentrations of topical tretinoin (retinoic acid) cause similar improvement of photoaging but different degrees of irritation. A double-blind, vehicle-controlled comparison of 0.1% and 0.025% tretinoin creams. *Arch Dermatol* 1995;131:1037-1044.

Johnson SL, Graves GR, Kendler DL, Fluker MR. Medical and special conditions: Canadian consensus on menopause and osteoporosis. *J SOGC* 2001;23:1096-1101.

Lucky A, Henderson T, Olson W, Robish DM, Lebwohl M, Swinger LJ. Effectiveness of norgestimate and ethinyl estradiol in treating moderate acne vulgaris. *J Am Acad Dermatol* 1997;37: 746-754.

Maheux R, Naud F, Rioux M, et al. A randomized, double-blind, placebo-controlled study on the effect of conjugated estrogens on skin thickness. *Am J Obstet Gynecol* 1994;170:42-29.

Mercurio MG, Gogstetter DS. Androgen physiology and the cutaneous pilosebaceous unit. *J Gender-Specific Med* 2000;3:59-64.

Pierard GE, Letawe C, Dowlati A, Pierard-Franchimont C. Effect of hormone replacement therapy for menopause on the mechanical properties of skin. *J Am Geriatr Soc* 1995;43:662-665.

Pierard-Franchimont C, Cornil F, Dehavay J, et al. Climacteric skin ageing of the face: a prospective longitudinal comparative trial on the effect of oral hormone replacement therapy. *Maturitas* 1999;32:87-93.

Redmond G, Olson W, Lippman J, et al. Norgestimate and ethinyl estradiol in the treatment of acne vulgaris: a randomized, placebo-controlled trial. *Obstet Gynecol* 1997;89:615-622.

Schmidt JB, Binder M, Demschik G, Bieglmayer C, Reiner A. Treatment of skin aging with topical estrogens. *Int J Dermatol* 1996;35:669-674.

Thiboutot D, Gilliland K, Light J, Lookingbill D. Androgen metabolism in sebaceous glands from subjects with and without acne. *Arch Dermatol* 1999;135:1041-1045.

J.11. Ocular changes

Many ocular changes occur at midlife and beyond. Perhaps the most common change is dry eye.

Dry eye. Women presenting with symptoms of dry eye can be advised to use ocular lubricants such as drops, gels, and ointments. This treatment is palliative at best, resulting in temporary reduction of ocular surface-to-eyelid shear forces and transient symptomatic relief. Plugging of the lacrimal punctae, the openings through which tears drain from the surface of the eye into the nose, can increase the volume of tears on the ocular surface despite a decreased rate of tear production. This can be accomplished with temporary collagen plugs or with silicone plugs or cauterization; however, it may not relieve symptoms in all patients.

Although there are many causes of dry eye, an underlying cytokine/receptor-mediated inflammatory process is common to all ocular surface diseases. By treating this process, it may be possible to normalize the ocular surface/lacrimal neural reflex and facilitate ocular surface healing. Anti-inflammatory medications are now recognized as a more appropriate therapeutic strategy for dry eye than ocular drops. In women with moderate to severe dry eye, topical cyclosporine A has been shown to significantly increase tear production and significantly decrease ocular surface damage. Histopathologic evidence indicates that cyclosporine A treatment significantly reduces the numbers of activated T lymphocytes within the conjunctiva.

Similarly, there have been reports of symptomatic relief and reduction of signs of dry eye with the use of topical corticosteroids. Corticosteroids may have significant adverse effects, such as cataract formation and increased intraocular pressure, making them unsuitable for chronic use. A phase III clinical trial studying the effect of topical cyclosporine A in the treatment of moderate to severe dry eye in patients with Sjogren's syndrome and postmenopausal women is in progress.

Sex-hormone receptors have been identified in many ocular tissues, including the Meibomian glands, the lacrimal gland, the lens, the cornea, and conjunctiva, suggesting involvement of sex hormones in the maintenance of ocular surface homeostasis. Studies of topical androgen treatment in a dog model showed improvement in signs of dry eye with topical 19-nortestosterone treatment. The effects of topical application of estrogens or androgens in humans have not been completely identified, although studies are being conducted. A few studies have reported improvement in dry eye signs and symptoms with ERT, but these have involved relatively few patients. Recently, a review of data on 25,665 women from the Women's Health Study suggested that ERT is actually associated with an increased risk of either clinically diagnosed dry eye or severe symptoms of both ocular dryness and irritation. Treatment with HRT (estrogen plus a progestogen) was associated with an intermediate risk. Women who had never used estrogen had the lowest risk.

Oral pilocarpine (Salagen), a parasympathomimetic, and cevimeline HCl (Evoxac), a selective muscarinic cholinergic agonist, are indicated to treat dry mouth in Sjogren's syndrome. These drugs may also have beneficial effects in treating severe dry eye.

Cataract. There are no well-documented gender differences in cataract (lens opacities) formation, which rarely occurs during women's reproductive years. However, administration of estrogen was protective against cataract formation in several animal models. Two large cross-sectional studies, the Beaver Dam Eye Study and the Blue Mountain Study, reported a protective effect of current ERT/HRT on cataract formation. The Salisbury Eye Evaluation also showed a protective association between the use of HRT and both nuclear and posterior subcapsular cataract. In the Framingham Heart Study, 10 or more years of ERT use was inversely associated with nuclear cataract. Women who have undergone surgical menopause are more likely to develop posterior subcapsular cataract than women who enter menopause naturally. Women with breast cancer treated with tamoxifen have an increased risk of cataract, which is consistent with a protective role for estrogen in lens opacification.

Data from the Nurses' Health Study indicate that vitamin C supplements may diminish the risks for cortical cataracts in women younger than 60 and for posterior subcapsular cataracts in women who have never smoked.

Glaucoma. The relationship between gender and glaucoma remains controversial, with several large studies demonstrating conflicting results. However, in the population-based Rotterdam study, women who had reached natural menopause before age 45 had a higher risk of open-angle glaucoma after adjustment for age and ERT/HRT status. Nevertheless, intraocular pressure is higher in postmenopausal women than men of the same age or in premenopausal women.

Macular degeneration. Some researchers have suggested that ERT/HRT may help to prevent macular degeneration in postmenopausal women. The Women's Health Initiative: Sight Exam Study will assess possible protective effects of ERT/HRT against progression of macular degeneration.

Bibliography

Armaly MF. On the distribution of applanation pressure. I: Statistical features and the effect of age, sex, and family history of glaucoma. *Arch Ophthalmol* 1965;73:11-18.

Barrett-Connor E. Postmenopausal estrogen therapy and selected (less-often-considered) disease outcomes. *Menopause* 1999;6:14-20.

Benitez del Castillo JM, del Rio T, Garcia-Sanchez J. Effects of estrogen use on lens transmittance in postmenopausal women. *Ophthalmology* 1997;104:970-973.

Bigsby RM, Cardenas H, Caperell-Grant A, et al. Protective effects of estrogen in a rat model of age-related cataracts. *Proc Natl Acad Sci* 1999;96:9328-9332.

Cumming RG, Mitchell P. Hormone replacement therapy, reproductive factors, and cataract. The Blue Mountains Eye Study. *Am J Epidemiol* 1997;145:242-249.

Freeman EE, Munoz B, Schein OD, West SK. Hormone replacement therapy and lens opacities: the Salisbury Eye Evaluation Project. *Arch Ophthalmol* 2001;119:1687-1692.

Hulsman CA, Westendorp IC, Ramrattan R, et al. Is open-angle glaucoma associated with early menopause? The Rotterdam Study. *Am J Epidemiol* 2001;154:138-144.

Johnson SL, Graves GR, Kendler DL, Fluker MR. Canadian consensus on menopause and osteoporosis: medical and special conditions. *J SOGC* 2001;23:1096-1101.

The Eye Disease Case-Control Study Group. Risk factors for neovascular age-related macular degeneration. *Arch Ophthalmol* 1992;110:1701-1708.

Klein BE, Klein R, Ritter LL. Is there evidence of an estrogen effect on age-related lens opacities? The Beaver Dam Eye Study. *Arch Ophthalmol* 1994;112:85-91.

Kramer P, Lubkin V, Potter W, et al. Cyclic changes in conjunctival smears from menstruating females. *Ophthalmology* 1990;97:303-307.

Kunert KS, Tisdale AS, Stern ME, et al. Analysis of topical cyclosporine treatment of patients with dry eye syndrome: effect on conjunctival lymphocytes. *Arch Ophthalmol* 2000;118:1489-1496.

Metka M, Enzelsberger H, Knogler W, et al. Ophthalmic complaints as a climacteric symptom. *Maturitas* 1991;14:3-8.

Ogueta SB, Schwartz SD, Yamashita CK, Ferber DB. Estrogen receptor in the human eye: influence of gender and age on gene expression. *Invest Ophthalmol Vis Sci* 1999;40:1906-1911.

Paganini-Hill A, Clark LJ. Eye problems in breast cancer patients treated with tamoxifen. *Breast Cancer Res Treat* 2000;60:167-172.

Sall K, Stevenson OD, Mundorf TK, Reis BL. Two multicenter, randomized studies of the efficacy and safety of cyclosporine ophthalmic emulsion in moderate to severe dry eye diseases. *Ophthalmology* 2000;107:631-639.

Sator MO, Akramian J, Joura EA, et al. Reduction of intraocular pressure in a glaucoma patient undergoing hormone replacement therapy. *Maturitas* 1998;29:93-95.

Schaumberg DA, Buring JE, Sullivan DA, Dana MR. Hormone replacement therapy and dry eye syndrome. *JAMA* 2001;286:2114-2119.

Stern ME, Beuerman RW, Fox RI, Gao J, Mircheff AK, Pflugfelder SC. The pathology of dry eye: the interaction between the ocular surface and lacrimal glands. *Cornea* 1998;17:584-589.

Taylor A, Jacques PF, Chylack LT Jr, et al. Long-term intake of vitamins and carotenoids and odds of early age-related cortical and posterior subcapsular lens opacities. *Am J Clin Nutr* 2002;75:540-549.

Vecsei PV, Kircher K, Kaminski S, Nagel G, Breitenecker G, Kohlberger PD. Immunohistochemical detection of estrogen and progesterone receptor in human cornea. *Maturitas* 2000; 36:169-172.

Worzala K, Hiller R, Sperduto R, et al. Postmenopausal estrogen use, type of menopause, and lens opacities: the Framingham studies. *Arch Intern Med* 2001;161:1448-1454.

J.12. Hair changes

Hair growth aberrations can have significant psychological consequences that affect body image, self-esteem, and quality of life issues, underscoring the importance of effective medical management. Androgens have a significant impact on the modulation of hair growth. This is evidenced by the reduction in hair density that can be attained with antiandrogen treatments. The reason for the variable physiologic responses of hair follicles in different sites from the identical hormonal signal remains elusive.

Hirsutism. Excessive hair growth (hirsutism) typically occurs in areas of the body where the hair follicles are the most androgen-sensitive, including the chin, upper lip, and cheeks. Hirsutism is usually resulting from increased androgen production in the ovaries or adrenal glands. Most women with hirsutism have an exaggerated utilization of androgens as a result of enhanced local 5a-reductase activity.

Hirsutism usually does not signify major pathology, but it can be an early sign of a potentially serious underlying disorder. In rare cases, hirsutism accompanied by very obvious virilization may result from tumors of the adrenal gland or ovary, which produce extreme androgen excess. Especially important is the rapidity of development of symptoms. In the absence of androgen-producing tumors or classic adrenal hyperplasia, the symptoms of androgen excess develop slowly. Other women with hirsutism may have a functional disorder, such as polycystic ovary syndrome or late-onset congenital adrenal hyperplasia, resulting in mild to moderate serum androgen elevations.

Treatment for hirsutism focuses on a combination of mechanical depilation and hormonal therapies. A woman can remove hair by plucking, waxing, or shaving. Shaving is less traumatic than the other methods, but it may lead to folliculitis and ingrown hairs. Bleaching is also useful, particularly for mild conditions. Chemical depilatory agents may irritate the skin, particularly on the face. Electrolysis can usually destroy terminal hairs after 6 months of treatment.

Hormone therapy may sometimes delay the progression of hirsutism, but it will not change coarse terminal hairs into softer and less noticeable vellus hairs. Treatment options include combination oral contraceptives, antiandrogens (eg, spironolactone), and 5a-reductase inhibitors (eg, finasteride, either alone or in combination with cyproterone acetate).

To avoid progression of symptoms, treatment of androgen excess should begin as soon as the diagnosis is established. Response to hirsutism therapy may require 6 to 8 months. Hormonal suppression may need to be continued indefinitely. Androgen levels should be measured at regular intervals.

Hair loss. Androgenic (or sometimes called androgenetic) alopecia and hair thinning are typically genetically determined and respond to the shift in the androgen-to-estrogen ratio. Hair follicles in balding skin differ from those in nonbalding skin with respect to androgen metabolism.

After menopause, hyperandrogenic symptoms may worsen. Surgical menopause may result in an improvement of symptoms, since a significant amount of endogenous androgen is decreased.

Topical minoxidil solution (Rogaine) is the only drug available for promoting hair growth in women with androgenic alopecia. Trials with premenopausal women (aged 18-45 have demonstrated improved scalp coverage and slowed hair loss. No trials have been completed with menopausal women. Minoxidil therapy must be continued indefinitely because the condition may return to its pretreatment condition or worsen when the drug is stopped. It may take 3 to 4 months for hair growth to be noticed.

Finasteride (Propecia) is FDA-approved for treating androgenic alopecia in men, but a trial of finasteride (1 mg/day) in postmenopausal women with the same condition produced no significant difference in hair loss compared with placebo.

Numerous nutritional supplements (generally containing high doses of vitamin B complex, trace minerals, and amino acids) are available in pharmacies and health food stores. A shampoo containing hyaluronic acid has retarded hair loss in European clinical trials. None of these products are FDA-approved for treatment of hair loss, although some are recommended by pharmacists and dermatologists based on clinical experience. Some licensed acupuncturists use herbal therapies to stimulate hair growth with mixed success. These therapies, like pharmaceuticals, generally take 3 to 4 months before a change is noted.

When hormones (eg, ERT/HRT, contraceptives) are prescribed for a woman with androgenic alopecia, care should be taken to select a progestogen with little androgenic activity. Additionally, testosterone or androgen precursors, such as dehydroepiandrosterone (DHEA), may worsen androgenic alopecia. However, ERT/HRT has no recognized role in alopecia treatment. With all hair growth aberrations, photographs may be useful in monitoring therapeutic results.

Bibliography

Jacobs JP, Szpunar CA, Warner ML. Use of topical minoxidil therapy for androgenetic alopecia in women. *Int J Dermatol* 1993;32:758-762.

Price VH. Treatment of hair loss. *N Engl J Med* 1999;341:964-973.

Price VH, Roberts JL, Hordinsky M, et al. Lack of efficacy of finasteride in postmenopausal women with androgenetic alopecia. *J Am Acad Dermatol* 2000;43:768-776.

Redmond GP. Androgens and women's health. *Int J Fertil Womens Med* 1998;43:91-97.

J.13 Oral/dental changes

Hormone changes associated with menopause have been implicated in several oral and dental disorders including oral bone and tooth loss, temporomandibular disorders (TMDs), periodontal disease, and gingivitis.

Several studies have suggested that ERT/HRT may reduce tooth loss. The largest study of elderly women, the Leisure World Cohort, found that women using ERT/HRT had significantly less tooth loss and rates of endentia than nonusers, and the rates continued to improve with increasing duration of use. There may also be a reduction in gingival inflammation and bleeding associated with ERT/HRT.

The gender and age distribution of TMD suggests a potential link with the female hormonal axis. However, limited evidence suggests that ERT use does not place women at risk of developing TMDs.

Adequate intakes of calcium and vitamin D appear to have positive effects on oral health, although studies have been limited. Nevertheless, this may be an additional benefit to consuming the recommended levels of these two nutrients.

Bibliography

Campbell JH, Courey MS, Bourne P, Odziemiec C. Estrogen receptor analysis of human temporomandibular disc. *J Oral Maxillofac Surg* 1993;51:1101-1105.

Grodstein F, Colditz GA, Stampfer MJ. Post-menopausal hormone use and tooth loss: a prospective study. *J Am Dent Assoc* 1996; 127:370-377.

Grossi SG, Jeffcoat MK, Genco RJ. Osteopenia, osteoporosis, and oral disease. In: Rose LF, Genco RJ, Cohen DW, Mealey BL, eds. *Periodontal Medicine*. St Louis, MO: BC Decker, Inc; 2000:167-182.

Hatch JP, Rugh JD, Sakai S, Saunders MJ. Is use of exogenous estrogen associated with temporomandibular signs and symptoms? *J Am Dent Assoc* 2001;132:319-326.

Krall EA. The periodontal-systemic connection: implications for treatment of patients with osteoporosis and periodontal disease. *Ann Periodontol* 2001;6:209-213.

Krall EA, Dawson-Hughes B, Hannan MT, Wilson PW, Kiel DP. Postmenopausal estrogen replacement and tooth retention. *Am J Med* 1997;102:536-542.

Krall EA, Wehler C, Garcia RI, Harris SS, Dawson-Hughes B. Calcium and vitamin D supplements reduce tooth loss in the elderly. *Am J Med* 2001;111:452-456.

Paganini-Hill A. Benefits of estrogen replacement therapy on oral health. The Leisure World Cohort. *Arch Intern Med* 1995; 155:2325-2329.

Reinhardt RA, Payne JB, Maze CA, Patil KD, Gallagher SJ, Mattson JS. Influence of estrogen and osteopenia/osteoporosis on clinical periodontitis in postmenopausal women. *J Periodontol* 1999;70:823-828.

Postmenopausal osteoporosis is a major health problem in Western countries, especially among thin Caucasian women who are older than 70 years. Fractures of the spine and hip are the most important complications of osteoporosis, but fractures of the distal forearm, pelvis, ribs, and other limb bones are also consequences of osteoporosis.

In adults, the primary goal of osteoporosis management is to prevent fracture by slowing or preventing net bone loss, maintaining bone strength, and minimizing or eliminating factors that contribute to falls. Initiating preventive steps well into adulthood or old age can lessen a woman's risk of osteoporosis and fractures. With pharmacologic therapy, it is possible to reverse some loss of bone mass in adults.

K.01. Nutrition

A balanced diet is important for bone development as well as overall health. Many women, especially elderly women with reduced appetites or women who diet frequently or have eating disorders, may not consume adequate vitamins and minerals to maintain optimal bone mass. Very thin women also are at increased risk for osteoporosis and fracture. In addition, premenopausal women who over-diet or over-exercise can become so thin that their menstrual cycles stop temporarily, placing them at higher risk for osteoporosis later in life because of lowered estrogen levels and resultant bone loss.

All osteoporosis therapies should be used in conjunction with adequate calcium and vitamin D intake. Calcium is the most important nutrient for achieving peak bone mass and for preventing and treating osteoporosis. According to new guidelines from the National Academy of Sciences, women aged 19 to 50 should consume 1,000 mg/day of elemental calcium; women aged 51 and older should consume 1,200 mg/day. Older guidelines from the National Institutes of Health called for intakes of 1,500 mg/day for postmenopausal women. Clinicians need to help women develop strategies to ensure that they consume adequate calcium each day (see Table 1).

Table 1. Steps to ensure adequate calcium intake

- Estimate dietary calcium intake

- Provide counsel on increasing intake of calcium-rich foods

- If adequate intake cannot be achieved through diet, recommend an appropriate calcium supplement to make up the deficit

---

Because dairy products account for 75% to 80% of calcium intake in the typical North American diet, a good estimate of intake can be based on a woman's consumption of milk (~300 mg elemental calcium/8 oz), yogurt (~400 mg/8 oz), and cheese (~200 mg/oz), with 250 mg/day added for nondairy sources, such as grains and vegetables. Other ways to boost calcium intake include using milk instead of water when cooking hot cereals, and adding skim milk powder when preparing items such as soups, meatloaf, and mashed potatoes. Calcium can also be obtained from leafy, dark green vegetables, nuts, and dried beans.

Most people with lactase nonpersistence (ie, unable to metabolize lactose in dairy products) can consume yogurt and sometimes even milk in small (½-cup) servings, but they should avoid high-lactose foods (eg, condensed and evaporated milk, processed cheese) and focus on low-lactose products (eg, cottage cheese, cream cheese) and lactose-free products (ie, nondairy products) that are fortified with calcium. Other foods that may be fortified with calcium are soy milk and orange juice.

Women who are unable to consume adequate amounts of calcium in their diets should be encouraged to use calcium supplements. Any calcium supplement used in the United States should have the USP designation. In Canada, the DIN (drug identification number) and GP (general product) number indicate that products have met specific Canadian standards.

Calcium supplements include several different calcium salts; the most commonly used preparations are calcium carbonate and calcium citrate. Calcium carbonate provides 40% elemental calcium. These supplements should be taken with meals to aid absorption. Bedtime dosing may enhance calcium absorption. Calcium carbonate may cause constipation or gas, which can be managed by increasing fluid intake and physical activity. Calcium carbonate is inexpensive, is found in a wide range of generic formulations, and comes in flavored preparations that promote patient acceptance.

Calcium citrate does not need acid for solubilization and, thus, does not have to be taken with meals. Calcium citrate preparations typically cost more than calcium carbonate, however, and contain a lower percentage of elemental calcium (eg, 21% for the tetrahydrated form). Some women report less gastrointestinal upset with calcium citrate.

Table 2 provides recommendations regarding calcium supplements.

Table 2. Recommendations for calcium supplements

- Tailor the recommended dosage to the estimated dietary intake and calcium requirements.

- Base the total dosage of a calcium supplement on the amount of elemental calcium contained in a supplement. For example, 1,000 mg of calcium carbonate (40% elemental calcium) provides 400 mg of calcium.

- Recommend a divided dosage, taken throughout the day, and not with fiber or iron supplements. More than 500 mg at a time may not be absorbed.

- Advise taking calcium carbonate with meals and chewing the tablets to improve absorption and reduce the incidence of constipation.

- Caution against taking more than the recommended dose of a calcium supplement.

- Avoid bone meal and oyster shell calcium preparations that may contain dangerous levels of heavy metal contaminants.

- Review calcium intake at each visit and adjust the supplement dosage as necessary

---

Vitamin D figures prominently in osteoporosis prevention because it enhances intestinal absorption of calcium. Vitamin D is synthesized in the skin following sunlight exposure. Women at risk for inadequate vitamin D include elderly women, women who have reduced sun exposure because of being bedfast or institutionalized, those living in northern latitudes where sunlight hours are lacking during the winter, those using sun screens with a high sun-protective factor (SPF) or avoiding the sun because of the concern about skin aging and skin cancer, and women whose diets are deficient in vitamin D. Treating vitamin D deficiencies in older women reduces hip fracture risk.

The current RDA for vitamin D is 400 IU daily for women aged 51 to 70 years and 600 IU daily for women over 70. The National Osteoporosis Foundation recommends 400 to 800 IU/day for women at risk of suboptimal intake.

Milk fortified with vitamin D is the only dietary source providing a significant amount of vitamin D (400 IU per quart or 946 mL). When milk intake is low, vitamin D supplements are required. Vitamin supplements, which usually contain 400 IU of vitamin D, are generally recommended for all women over age 65 unless contraindicated.

Other substances consumed in the diet (eg, caffeine, high dietary protein, phosphorus, sodium) appear to have minimal detrimental effects on bone health in women with adequate calcium and vitamin D intakes. Minerals, including magnesium and boron, may be important for bone health and are available in the diet or through a multivitamin/mineral supplement.

Soy foods and isoflavones are being evaluated for their potential effect on bone health. Although some studies suggest that soy and isoflavones may favorably affect bone health, few human studies have been conducted and all involved small numbers of subjects in trials of short duration. Further clinical trials are needed.

K.02. Exercise

Regular exercise is clearly linked to reducing osteoporosis risk. Early in life, exercise promotes higher peak bone mass. During midlife, exercise provides many health benefits, although its effect on BMD has not been empirically established. For both pre- and postmenopausal women, a meta-analysis of controlled trials published from 1966 to 1996 showed that exercise training programs prevented or reversed almost 1% of bone loss per year in the lumbar spine and femoral neck. Later in life, exercise probably has a modest effect on slowing the decline in BMD, provided calcium and vitamin D intakes are adequate. Complete bed rest is highly detrimental to bone density.

The type of exercise is important. Most experts agree that there are two types of exercises that provide the most bone benefits: weight-bearing exercises and progressive strength training (resistance).

Weight-bearing exercises are those in which bones and muscles work against gravity. These include any exercise in which the feet and legs bear one's body weight, such as jogging/running, brisk walking/hiking, climbing stairs, dancing, and racquet sports.

Strength-training exercises are those activities that improve muscle mass through muscle resistance, such as free weights or weight machines.

At all ages, even in those over age 90, exercise can increase muscle mass and strength. Exercise programs for the elderly reduce their risk of falling by 10%, and programs that include training for balance reduce the risk nearly 20%. Exercise for women with established osteoporosis should not include heavy weight-bearing or vigorous activity that may trigger fracture. In the elderly, the importance of exercise in preserving independence and enhancing quality of life cannot be overemphasized.

Exercise is also important to early postmenopausal women. For bone benefits, muscle strength training should be a component of their exercise program. Strength training can be performed as little as twice a week and need not involve special equipment other than simple weights. Exercises that are not strength training or weight bearing have minimal effect on BMD, although they have beneficial effects on other aspects of health.

The recommended minimum for healthy midlife women is 30 minutes of moderate intensity physical activity performed on most, preferably all, days of the week. Some exercise, however, is better than none — and even minimal changes in routine that encourage physical activity can be an important beginning.

Because exercise has such wide-ranging benefits, clinicians should encourage all peri- and postmenopausal women to exercise regularly. Some women may need guidance regarding which type(s) and level of exercise are appropriate initially, and encouragement to incorporate physical activity into their daily routine.

K.03. Smoking cessation

Smoking can lead to lower bone mass and fractures, in addition to a wide range of health problems. Smoking cessation should be encouraged for all women who are smokers. A clinician's recommendation to quit smoking can have a powerful influence on a woman's decision to kick the habit. A wide array of smoking cessation aids are available, including prescription products (with and without nicotine) and behavior-modification smoking cessation programs.

K.04. Fall prevention

In the United States, about 30% of people over age 60 fall at least once a year. In Canada, between 23% to 39% of seniors fall at least once yearly. The prevalence of falls increases with age, rising to a 50% annual rate in people over 80 years of age. Older women have a significantly higher risk for falls than men of the same age. Prevention of falls should be an aspect of routine care for all older women.

After menopause, a woman's risk for falls should be assessed at least annually. Conditions that increase the risk for falls include a history of falls, fainting, or loss of consciousness; muscle weakness, dizziness, or balance problems; problems with muscle coordination; and impaired vision. Medications that affect balance and coordination (eg, sedatives, benzodiazepines, narcotic analgesics, anticholinergics, antihypertensives) should also be reviewed. Adjustments of dosages or a change of therapy may be necessary. Clinicians should also advise against overuse of alcohol, which leads to falls.

Safety hazards in the home and work environment, such as obstacles, scatter rugs, and poor lighting, also contribute to the risk of falls and injuries. These should be assessed by questioning the woman or through a visit to the home or workplace by an occupational therapist or other healthcare professional knowledgeable in fall prevention. Women and their caregivers need to be advised of hazards and preventive measures (see Table 3).

Table 3. Recommendations for fall prevention

Lighting
Provide ample lighting
Locate switches to light rooms and stairs before entry
Use night lights to illuminate path to bathroom

Obstructions
Remove clutter, low-lying objects
Remove raised door sills to ensure smooth transition

Floors and carpets
Provide nonskid rugs on slippery floors
Repair/replace worn, buckled, or curled carpet
Use nonskid floor wax

Furniture
Arrange to provide clear pathways
Remove or avoid low chairs and armless chairs
Adjust bed height if too high or low

Storage
Install shelves and cupboards at accessible height
Keep frequently used items at waist height

Bathroom
Install grab bars in tub, shower, near toilet
Use chair in shower and tub
Install nonskid strips/decals in tub/shower
Elevate low toilet seat or install safety frame

Stairways and halls
Install handrails on both sides of stairs
Remove or tape down throw/area rugs and runners
Repair loose and broken steps
Install nonskid treads on steps

Falls to the side are the most likely to result in hip fracture. For frail elderly adults at high risk for falling, hip protectors may reduce hip fracture risk. These are specialized undergarments with specially engineered cups that fit over the hip (trochanter) that shunt the energy of the fall into soft tissues. Finding an appropriate size and style for each woman, along with appropriate education about the value of the devices, is necessary to achieve compliance and efficacy. One randomized trial of hip protectors in a group of nursing home residents found that the only residents sustaining a hip fracture in the hip protector group were those who were not wearing the garment at the time of the fall. No drug has achieved this level of success. Some manufacturers of hip protectors can be found at www.hipsaver.com, www.safehip.com, and www.hipguard.com. (This mention does not imply that these brands are better than other brands.)

K.05. Pharmacologic interventions

Drugs approved for the prevention and treatment of osteoporosis include ERT/HRT, bisphosphonates, selective estrogen-receptor modulators (SERMs), and calcitonin (see Sections H.02 and H.04). Regardless of the medical therapy prescribed, clinicians should remind each woman that adequate intake of both calcium and vitamin D is essential.

The objective of therapy for osteoporosis is to reduce fracture risk. Fracture reduction has been documented with drug therapy in women with previous vertebral fractures or low BMD.

NAMS recommends considering pharmacologic therapy for osteoporosis in the following populations:

- All postmenopausal women with an osteoporotic vertebral fracture (no BMD is needed).

- All postmenopausal women with total hip or spine T scores worse than –2.5.

- All postmenopausal women with total hip or spine T scores –2.0 to –2.5 and at least one additional risk factor for fracture.

The indications for beginning therapy in women at lower risk are less clear. In women without osteoporosis, neither ERT nor bisphosphonate therapy had any effect on fracture rates in trials of up to 6 years.

K.06. Management of osteoporotic fractures

When osteoporotic fractures occur, pain management and rehabilitation are important clinical objectives. Healthcare providers should be alert to the need for pain management, especially in those elderly women who may attempt to "tough out" pain, and in those who may not exhibit usual pain behavior or are unable to express pain due to confusion or cognitive function decreased by dementia.

Chronic back pain, a common complication of osteoporotic vertebral fractures, can be reduced by improving muscle strength and posture. A back support is sometimes helpful. Because the pain frequently is related to strain on extensor muscles, exercises that improve extensor muscle strength and endurance can help. Some women achieve complete pain relief through an appropriately designed and monitored exercise program. Others achieve partial relief that enables them to resume many normal activities.

For women who have severe or intractable pain, drug therapy and site-specific analgesia are indicated. Multiple modalities, such as milder systemic pain medication in combination with site-specific analgesia, can help reduce the risk of side effects from any single pain therapy. They may provide alternatives to systemic narcotics and anticholinergics, which the elderly tolerate poorly. Trigger-point injections can decrease pain and improve the range of motion. If the woman's pain persists, referral to an anesthesiologist or pain management clinic may be warranted.

Open surgical management of vertebral fractures due to osteoporosis is rarely required. Vertebroplasty and kyphoplasty are invasive procedures in which bone cement is injected through a percutaneous needle into a fractured vertebra in an attempt to provide pain relief. Kyphoplasty may also partially reduce the height loss. More studies are needed to evaluate the long-term outcome of these procedures on both symptoms and subsequent fracture risk.

Hip fractures are nearly always treated surgically, either by internal fixation or hip replacement. Appropriate management of the comorbidities frequently found in these patients is essential, and adequate postoperative pain management is important. Physical medicine and rehabilitation can help many patients regain function after hip fracture. Despite therapy, the consequences of osteoporotic hip fracture for frail, elderly women are often devastating, frequently confining them to long-term care.

All patients with a hip fracture should receive calcium and vitamin D supplements. Oral nutritional supplements containing protein have been shown to reduce further bone loss in elderly women who have sustained hip fracture. These supplements may also shorten hospital stay after hip fracture and improve the clinical outcome. Patients with a hip fracture should have BMD testing and be considered for bisphosphonate treatment if osteoporosis is present.

Bibliography

Bone HG, Greenspan SL, McKeever C, et al for the Alendronate/Estrogen Study Group. Alendronate and estrogen effect in postmenopausal women with low bone mineral density. *J Clin Endocrinol Metab* 2000;85:720-726.

Chapuy MC, Arlot ME, Duboeuf F, et al. Vitamin D_3 and calcium to prevent hip fractures in elderly women. *N Engl J Med* 1992; 327:1637-1742.

Dawson-Hughes B, Dallal GE, Krall EA, et al. A controlled trial of the effect of calcium supplementation on bone density in postmenopausal women. *N Engl J Med* 1990;323:878-883.

Gallagher E, Hunter M, Scott V. The nature of falling among community dwelling seniors. *Can J Aging* 1999;18:348-362.

Greendale GA, Barrett-Connor E, Ingle S, et al. Late physical and functional effects of osteoporotic fractures in women: the Rancho Bernardo Study. *J Am Geriat Soc* 1995;43:955-961.

Harrison JE, Chow R, Dornan J, et al. Evaluation of a program for rehabilitation of osteoporotic patients (PRO): 4-year follow-up. *Osteoporosis Int* 1993;3:13-17.

Kannus P, Parkkari J, Niemi S, et al. Prevention of hip fractures in elderly people with use of a hip protector. *N Engl J Med* 2000; 343:1506-1513.

LeBoff MS, Kohlmeier L, Hurwitz S, et al. Occult vitamin D deficiency in postmenopausal US women with acute hip fracture. *JAMA* 1999;281:1505-1511.

Malmos B, Mortensen L, Jensen MB, et al. Positive effects of physiotherapy on pain and performance in osteoporosis. *Osteoporos Int* 1998;8:215-221.

Marshall D, Johnell O, Wedel H. Meta-analysis of how well measures of bone mineral density predict occurrence of osteoporotic fractures. *BMJ* 1996;312:1254-1259.

Meyer HJE, Tverdal A, Falch JA, et al. Factors associated with mortality after hip fracture. *Osteoporos Int* 2000;11:228-232.

National Academy of Sciences. Standing Committee on the Scientific Evaluation of Dietary Reference Intakes. *Dietary Reference Intakes: Calcium, Magnesium, Phosphorus, Vitamin D and Fluoride.* Washington, DC: National Academy Press; 1997.

National Institutes of Health Consensus Development Panel on Osteoporosis Prevention, Diagnosis, and Therapy. Osteoporosis prevention, diagnosis, and therapy. *JAMA* 2001;285:785-795.

National Osteoporosis Foundation. *Osteoporosis: Physician's Guide to Prevention and Treatment of Osteoporosis.* Belle Mead, NJ: Excerpta Medica; 1998.

Nelson ME, Fiatarone MA, Morganti CM, et al. Effects of high-intensity strength training on multiple risk factors for osteoporotic fractures: a randomized controlled trial. *JAMA* 1994;272:1909-1914.

The North American Menopause Society. Management of postmenopausal osteoporosis: position statement of The North American Menopause Society. *Menopause* 2002;9:84-101.

Province MA, Hadley EC, Hornbrook MC, et al, for the Frailty and Injuries: Cooperative Studies of Intervention Techniques (FICSIT) trials. The effects of exercise on falls in elderly patients: a preplanned meta-analysis of the FICSIT trials. *JAMA* 1995; 273:1341-1347.

Recker RR, Hinders S, Davies KM, et al. Correcting calcium nutritional deficiency prevents spine fractures in elderly women. *J Bone Miner Res* 1996;11:1961-1966.

Ross P. Risk factors for osteoporotic fracture. *Endocrinol Metab Clin North Am* 1998;27:289-301.

Schurch MA, Rizzoli R, Slosman D, et al. Protein supplements increase serum insulin-like growth factor-I levels and attenuate proximal femur bone loss in patients with recent hip fracture: a randomized, double-blind, placebo-controlled trial. *Ann Intern Med* 1998;128:801-809.

Taaffe DR, Duret C, Wheeler S, et al. Once-weekly resistance exercise improves muscle strength and neuromuscular performance in older adults. *J Am Geriatr Soc* 1999;47:1208-1214.

Tinetti ME, Baker DI, McAvay G, et al. A multifactorial intervention to reduce the risk of falling among elderly people living in the community. *N Engl J Med* 1994;331:821-827.

Wolff I, van Croonenborg JJ, Kemper HC, Kostense PJ, Twisk JW. The effect of exercise training programs on bone mass: a meta-analysis of published controlled trials in pre- and postmenopausal women. *Osteoporos Int* 1999;9:1-12.

Risk factors associated with cardiovascular disease (CVD) in women have been identified as cigarette smoking, sedentary lifestyle, hypertension, diabetes mellitus, abnormal plasma lipids, obesity, and stress. A decline in estrogen levels has been hypothesized to be a risk factor based on the association between increased risk of CVD and postmenopausal age. However, evidence of a direct relationship has yet to be established. The higher the risk of CVD, the more aggressive the prevention strategy should be.

L.01. Lifestyle modification

Women with any modifiable risk factors for CVD should be urged to initiate lifestyle changes that will decrease their overall risk. Counseling should focus on the following long-term benefits of lifestyle issues.

Smoking. Use of tobacco is the single most important preventable risk factor for CVD in women. A woman who smokes is 2 to 6 times more likely to have a heart attack than a woman who does not smoke. The effect of smoking on risk of fatal CVD is dose-related (ie, heavier smokers have a greater relative risk). However, if a woman stops smoking — no matter how long or how much she has smoked — her risk of heart disease drops rapidly. A number of effective programs and aids are available to help with smoking cessation.

Exercise. Physical inactivity is almost as great a risk factor as smoking. Studies have shown that middle-aged women who exercise regularly have lower weight, blood pressure, and plasma glucose levels, as well as more favorable lipid profiles than sedentary women. Regular physical activity, particularly aerobic exercise, promotes cardiovascular health. Adoption of a regular aerobic exercise program reduces the risk of coronary events in women. In the Nurses' Health Study, sedentary women who became active in middle adulthood or later had a lower risk of coronary events than their counterparts who remained sedentary, independent of obesity status. Physical activity need not be of high intensity to reduce CVD risk substantially, and lower intensity activity may result in better adherence over the long term; however, in the Nurses' Health Study, women who walked at a brisk pace were shown to have less CVD than slower walkers.

Weight management. Maintaining an ideal weight has been estimated to reduce the overall risk of CVD by 35% to 55%. Central obesity (ie, apple shape) is more dangerous for heart health. A combined approach of exercise and diet appears to be superior to diet only. For weight loss, three 10-minute exercise sessions have been shown to be more effective than one 30-minute session. A reasonable goal is losing 10% of body weight over a 6-month period.

Nutrition. Heart disease risk can be lowered by a diet that includes five or more servings of fruits and vegetables daily; little or no cholesterol and animal fat; little or no hydrogenated oil and trans-fatty acids; limiting salt to less than 2,400 mg/day; and limiting alcohol to one or two drinks per day but no more than seven drinks per week. There is some evidence that light-to-moderate use of alcohol lowers the cardiovascular mortality rate among women over age 50 who are at greater risk for coronary heart disease; however, higher levels (more than seven drinks per week) may increase risk of hypertension, stroke, and coronary disease. Data have shown that eating one egg daily is unlikely to affect the overall risk of CVD or stroke among healthy women.

As concluded in the NAMS consensus opinion, studies have associated consumption of soy/isoflavones with statistically significant reductions in low-density lipoproteins (LDL) and triglycerides, as well as increases in high-density lipoproteins (HDL). Women may consider adding soy foods (eg, soy milk, soy nuts, tofu) to their diet. More research is needed, however, to clarify the role that soy foods, isoflavones, and other phytoestrogens play in the management of CVD.

Antioxidants. To date, no large, randomized, controlled trials have established a benefit to taking supplemental antioxidants, such as vitamins C, vitamin E, beta-carotene, lycopene, and folic acid. The data on the role of vitamin E are inconclusive. Epidemiologic studies have shown a lower incidence of heart disease in those who eat more fruits and vegetables high in antioxidants and whole grains. Eating less meat and taking supplements of the B vitamins folate, B_6, and B_{12} will lower homocysteine levels, although no studies document that lowering homocysteine prevents CVD.

Stress management. Stress reduction can have a positive impact on cardiovascular health. The mechanisms by which stress affects CVD risks are unclear. Studies have shown a reduction in blood pressure when relaxation exercises are combined with lifestyle changes.

L.02. Pharmacologic therapy

Prevention is described as *primary* for women without diagnosed CVD and *secondary* for women with known CVD. A series of randomized clinical trials have dramatically altered the risk-benefit ratio between estrogen replacement therapy (ERT) or hormone replacement therapy (estrogen plus progestogen; HRT) and CVD, moving from a presumption of benefit to evidence of harm, at least for one regimen of continuous-combined HRT. This highlights the complexity of hormone therapy and underscores the value of randomized clinical trials to verify the safety and efficacy of therapeutic interventions. Despite the new data, there remain many questions regarding ERT/HRT and CVD risk.

L.02.a. Primary prevention

Increased serum levels of cholesterol can cause coronary artery atherosclerosis, limiting the blood flow to the heart. Severe atherosclerosis increases an individual's risk for myocardial infarction. More than one-third of women have abnormal cholesterol levels, which increases risk for heart disease. It is estimated that a 25% reduction in total blood cholesterol can reduce heart disease risk by 50%. Reducing cholesterol to a normal range is a therapeutic goal.

Optimal total cholesterol levels are less than 200 mg/dL (5.18 mmol/L). Elevated plasma levels of triglycerides are associated with an increased risk of CVD. The desirable range is less than 150 mg/dL (1.69 mmol/L).

Hypertension is defined as blood pressure greater than 140/90 mm Hg. Even mild elevations of blood pressure can double the risk for stroke. The risk for hypertension increases with age. Postmenopausal women are at greater risk — with more than 50% affected beyond age 55 — and black women are especially susceptible. Since hypertension rarely has symptoms, regular screening is important.

Peri- and postmenopausal women with abnormal lipids and/or hypertension should be encouraged to modify diet and exercise habits to improve their profile. When diet and exercise are not effective, therapy with lipid-lowering agents and/or antihypertensive agents should be considered. Lovastatin (20-40 mg/day), in addition to a low-saturated fat, low-cholesterol diet, has been shown to reduce the risk for the first acute major coronary event in women with average triglycerides and LDL levels and below-average levels of HDL. A wide variety of antihypertensive agents can be prescribed, including diuretics.

Diabetes mellitus is an independent risk factor for cardiovascular disease morbidity and mortality. Diabetes accelerates atherosclerosis and increases the risk of acute coronary ischemia in women. Diabetes is usually associated with obesity, hypertension, and unfavorable plasma lipid profiles, which can act synergistically to raise the woman's CVD risk. Programs aimed at reducing CVD risk in women with diabetes mellitus focus on controlling plasma glucose and insulin levels, reducing obesity, and promoting exercise. (For more information about diabetes, see Section P.01.)

Role of ERT/HRT in primary CVD prevention. The use of ERT/HRT as an option for the prevention of CVD in high-risk women is controversial. Data from observational studies had suggested that women who take oral ERT/HRT longer than 3 years may have a reduced incidence of cardiovascular events. However, recent data from the Women's Health Initiative (WHI), a large, randomized, placebo-controlled trial in mostly healthy postmenopausal women (N = 16,608), have changed the benefit-risk ratio. Initial reports from this trial indicated that a pattern of increased risk was emerging in both the ERT and HRT arms that resembled the pattern of early risk observed in the Heart and Estrogen/progestin Replacement Study (HERS). The WHI trial was allowed to continue because the risk was not statistically significant and because of the possibility that other noncoronary benefits might produce an overall net clinical benefit. However, the HRT arm of the trial, with continuous-combined conjugated equine estrogens (CEE) 0.625 mg/day plus medroxyprogesterone acetate (MPA) 2.5 mg/day, was stopped prematurely after a mean of 5.2 years of follow-up (original study design was for 8 years) owing to a significantly increased risk for CVD events, stroke, venous thromboembolic events, and breast cancer that outweighed the statistically significant beneficial effects of reduced hip fracture and colorectal cancer. Women taking unopposed ERT did not have the same results; thus, the ERT arm was allowed to continue. It is expected to be complete in 2005.

As a result, recommendations for the use of ERT/HRT for primary prevention are being revised. It appears that long-term use of the continuous-combined HRT regimen of CEE plus MPA, which is the most commonly used form in the United States, may not be appropriate for most healthy postmenopausal women, except for the short-term relief of menopause-related symptoms and unusual cases of severe osteoporosis not adequately treated with other therapies. Whether these findings extend to other regimens besides continuous-combined CEE/MPA or to other HRT hormones is unknown. The ongoing WHI arm of CEE alone will hopefully provide some answers about long-term ERT.

The mechanisms by which ERT might reduce the risk for CVD are believed to include beneficial effects on lipoprotein levels, endothelial function, and other metabolic effects. Oral estrogen alters the ratio of lipoproteins, raising HDL, lowering LDL, and slowing the progression of atherosclerosis. However, oral estrogens also tend to increase triglyceride levels. Serum levels of HDL have been suggested to be the best predictor of CVD risk in some women, although some experts now believe that homocysteine and C-reactive protein levels may be as predictive as HDL.

The observed effects differ markedly among regimens and vary according to the steroid administered, dosage, and route of administration. In the PEPI trial, CEE alone or in combination with either MPA or oral micronized progesterone significantly increased HDL and decreased LDL. The addition of MPA slightly reduced the lipid benefits of using estrogen alone; progesterone had less of an adverse effect.

Transdermal estrogen has been shown to increase HDL and to lower LDL to a lesser degree than the oral estrogens. Transdermal administration does not affect triglycerides. Nonoral estrogens avoid the first-pass hepatic metabolism, which is partially responsible for diminished lipid effects.

The beneficial effect of estrogen on endothelial function may occur via the promotion of nitric oxide release, which results in vasodilation, inhibition of adhesion molecule expression, and increased endothelial proliferation and migration to repair areas of injury. The improved lipid profile and endothelial cell function are thought to contribute to stabilization of atherosclerotic plaques. Estrogen increases the production of prostacyclin in the endothelium of blood vessels and decreases the production of thromboxane A_2 by platelets, thus reducing platelet adhesiveness. These effects may contribute to a lowered risk of myocardial infarction and stroke observed in some studies of women who receive ERT.

At least four observational studies have found that hormone therapy lowered the risk of stroke. However, the Women's Estrogen for Stroke Trial (WEST), a randomized, placebo-controlled study, found that estrogen therapy did not reduce mortality or the recurrence of stroke in postmenopausal women with cerebrovascular disease. The Framingham Study reported an increased risk, but confidence intervals were not calculated. Most studies have determined that ERT has no effect on the risk of stroke in healthy women.

An epidemiologic review of the literature published from 1989 through 1998 concluded that postmenopausal ERT doubles or triples the risk of deep vein thromboses and pulmonary embolism and may precipitate thromboses in the arterial circulation as well. This has been confirmed in the Heart and Estrogen/progestin Replacement Study (HERS) trial. Because these disorders are rare in healthy women, the increased absolute risk is small. However, caution should be exercised when administering any form of ERT to a woman with a personal or family history of thromboembolism. Neither should ERT be used during prolonged immobilization.

Most of the retrospective observational studies support the use of estrogen to prevent heart disease in postmenopausal women. A meta-analysis of these data suggests a 35% to 50% risk reduction in CVD risk. The effect appears to be independent of age, type of menopause (surgical or natural), or presence or absence of cardiovascular disease. In the Nurses' Health Study, a survival benefit was observed in women with one or more cardiovascular risk factors; among women with no risk factors, a 30% reduction in risk was observed. However, the Nurses' Health Study has also reported an increase in CVD events in the first few years of HRT use, similar to findings in the HERS data.

Guidelines from the American Heart Association (AHA), American College of Cardiology (ACC), and the National Cholesterol Education Program Second Report of the Expert Panel on Detection, Evaluation, and Treatment of High Blood Cholesterol in Adults— Adult Treatment Panel III (NCEP III) do not recommend hormone replacement (either ERT or HRT) to lower cardiovascular risk. A similar joint position statement from the Heart and Stroke Foundation of Canada, the Society of Obstetricians and Gynacologists of Canada (SOGC), and the Canadian Cardiovascular Society (CCS) was issued in December 2001. The WHI findings reinforce this position.

L.02.b. Secondary prevention

Postmenopausal women have an extremely high risk for recurrent myocardial infarction and CVD mortality. Thus, therapies that can reduce that risk, even a small reduction, would have a major impact on public health. In postmenopausal women with preexisting CVD, dietary and pharmacologic management of hypertension, hyperlipidemia, and diabetes mellitus should be initiated, where appropriate, according to established guidelines from the AHA, ACC, NCEP III, the American Diabetes Association, and the Sixth Report of the Joint National Committee on Prevention, Detection, Evaluation, and Treatment of High Blood Pressure (JNC VI).

A low dose (81 mg) of aspirin taken daily should be recommended for women with preexisting heart disease, who have no contraindications to aspirin. Vitamin E (400-800 IU/day) may also be of benefit. Both aspirin and vitamin E can aggravate bleeding, so caution is advised with concomitant use. Synergistic effects may result with other coagulants as well.

Role of ERT/HRT in secondary CVD prevention. Several observational, secondary prevention studies had suggested that ERT use could lower the risk of mortality and future cardiac events. However, there are a series of randomized clinical trials that have found no effect of ERT/HRT on clinical or anatomic progression of cardiovascular disease. Several of these trials used CEE combined with MPA while others used oral or transdermal 17β-estradiol (either alone or with a progestogen) or unopposed ERT regimens. In the recent HERS follow-up (HERS II), investigators noted a pattern of early increased risk for CVD events associated with HRT use, which appeared to be offset by an emerging pattern of benefit in the latter years of the trial. However, no long-term benefit was observed during the additional follow-up. Furthermore, there was a significant risk for venous thromboembolic events and need for gallbladder surgery in the women with established CVD. Based on these new data, the AHA, ACC, and CCS now recommend that ERT/HRT not be used for secondary prevention of cardiovascular disease. For women with CVD, it would be prudent to emphasize cardiovascular risk reduction with established evidence-based treatments.

Bibliography

Abramson B, Derzko C, Lalonde A, Reid R, Turek M, Wielgosz A. Hormone replacement therapy and cardiovascular disease: position statement of the Canadian Cardiovascular Society. Ottawa, ON, Canada: Canadian Cardiovascular Society; 2001. Accessible at http://www.ccs.ca/society/position/hormone.cfm.

Angerer P, Störk S, Kothny W, Schmitt P, van Schacky C. Effect of oral postmenopausal hormone replacement on progression of atherosclerosis: a randomized, controlled trial. *Arterioscler Thromb Vasc Biol* 2001;21:262-268.

Austin MA. Plasma triglycerides as a risk factor for coronary heart disease. *Am J Epidemiol* 1989;120:249-259.

Barnes RB, Levrant SG. Pharmacology of estrogens. In: Lobo RA, ed. *Treatment of the Postmenopausal Woman: Basic and Clinical Aspects.* 2nd ed. Philadelphia, PA: Lippincott Williams & Wilkins; 1999:95-104.

Barrett-Connor E. Postmenopausal estrogen therapy and selected (less-often-considered) disease outcomes. *Menopause* 1999;6:14-20.

Best PJM, Berger PB, Miller VM, Lerman A. The effects of estrogen replacement therapy on plasma nitric oxide and endothelin-1 levels in postmenopausal women. *Ann Intern Med* 1998;128:285-288.

Criqui MH, Suarez L, Barrett-Connor E, McPhillips J, Wingard DL, Garland C. Postmenopausal estrogen use and mortality. *Am J Epidemiol* 1988;128:606-614.

Crook D, Cust MP, Gangar KF, et al. Comparison of transdermal and oral estrogen-progestin replacement therapy: effects on serum lipids and lipoproteins. *Am J Obstet Gynecol* 1992;166:950-955.

Cummings SR, Eckert S, Krueger KA, et al. The effect of raloxifene on risk of breast cancer in postmenopausal women: results from the MORE randomized trial. Multiple Outcomes of Raloxifene Evaluation [published erratum appears in *JAMA* 1999;282:2124]. *JAMA* 1999;281:2189-2197.

Daly E, Vessey MP, Hawkins MM, Carson JL, Gough P, Marsh S. Risk of venous thromboembolism in users of hormone replacement therapy. *Lancet* 1996;348:977-980.

Despres JP, Lamarche B, Mauriege P, et al. Hyperinsulinemia as an independent risk factor for ischemic heart disease. *N Engl J Med* 1996;334:952-957.

Downs JR, Clearfield M, Weis S, et al. Primary prevention of acute coronary events with lovastatin in men and women with average cholesterol levels: results of AFCAPS/TexCAPS, Air Force/Texas Coronary Atherosclerosis Prevention Study. *JAMA* 1998;279:1615-1622.

Expert Panel on Detection, Evaluation, and Treatment of High Blood Cholesterol in Adults. Executive summary of the third report of the National Cholesterol Education Program (NCEP) Expert Panel on Detection, Evaluation, and Treatment of High Blood Cholesterol in Adults (Adult Treatment Panel III). *JAMA* 2001; 285:2486-2497.

Falkeborn M, Persson I, Terent A, Adami HO, Litchell H, Bergstrom R. Hormone replacement therapy and the risk of stroke: follow-up of a population-based cohort in Sweden. *Arch Intern Med* 1993;153:1201-1209.

Finucane FF, Madams JH, Bush TL, Wolf PH, Kleinman JC. Deceased risk of stroke among postmenopausal hormone users: results from a national cohort. *Arch Intern Med* 1993;153:73-79.

Folsom AR, Mink PJ, Sellers TA, Hong CP, Zheng W, Potter JD. Hormonal replacement therapy and morbidity and mortality in a prospective study of postmenopausal women. *Am J Public Health* 1995;85:1128-1132.

Gorodeski GI, Utian WH. Epidemiology and risk factors of cardiovascular disease in postmenopausal women. In: Lobo RA, ed. *Treatment of the Postmenopausal Woman: Basic and Clinical Aspects.* 2nd ed. Philadelphia, PA: Lippincott Williams & Wilkins; 1999:331-359.

Grady D, Herrington D, Bittner V, et al, for the HERS Research Group. Heart and estrogen/progestin replacement study follow-up (HERS II). Part 1: Cardiovascular outcomes during 6.8 years of hormone therapy. *JAMA* 2002;288:49-57.

Grady D, Rubin SM, Petitti DB, et al. Hormone therapy to prevent disease and prolong life in postmenopausal women. *Ann Intern Med* 1992;117:1016-1037.

Grodstein F, Stampfer MJ, Colditz GA, et al. Postmenopausal hormone therapy and mortality. *N Engl J Med* 1997;336:1769-1775.

Grodstein F, Stampfer MJ, Goldhaber SZ, et al. Prospective study of exogenous hormone and risk or pulmonary embolism in women. *Lancet* 1996;348:983-987.

Guetta V, Cannon RO III. Cardiovascular effects of estrogen and lipid-lowering therapies in postmenopausal women. *Circulation* 1996;93:1928-1937.

Henderson BE, Paganini-Hill A, Ross RK. Decreased mortality in users of estrogen replacement therapy. *Arch Intern Med* 1991; 151:75-78.

Herrington DM, Reboussin DM, Brosnihan KB, et al. Effects of estrogen replacement on the progression of coronary-artery atherosclerosis. *N Engl J Med* 2000;343:522-529.

Hodis HN, Mack WJ, Lobo RA, et al, for the Estrogen in Prevention of Atherosclerosis Trial (EPAT) research group. Estrogen in the prevention of atherosclerosis: a randomized, double-blind, placebo-controlled trial. *Ann Intern Med* 2001;135:939-953.

Hulley S, Furberg C, Barrett-Connor E, et al, for the HERS Research Group. Heart and estrogen/progestin replacement study follow-up (HERS II). Part 2: Non-cardiovascular outcomes during 6.8 years of hormone therapy. *JAMA* 2002;288:58-66.

Hulley S, Grady D, Bush T, et al, for the Heart and Estrogen/progestin Replacement Study (HERS) Research Group. Randomized trial of estrogen plus progestin for secondary prevention of coronary heart disease in postmenopausal women. *JAMA* 1998;280:605-613.

Manson JE, Colditz GA, Stampfer MJ, et al. A prospective study of obesity and risk of coronary heart disease in women. *N Engl J Med* 1990;322:882-889.

Manson JE, Tosteson H, Ridker PM, et al. The primary prevention of myocardial infarction. *N Engl J Med* 1992;326:1406-1416.

Mosca L, Collins P, Herrington DM, et al. Hormone replacement therapy and cardiovascular disease: a statement for healthcare professionals from the American Heart Association. *Circulation* 2001;104:499-503.

Mosca L, Grundy SM, Judelson D, et al. Guide to preventive cardiology for women. AHA/ACC scientific statement consensus panel statement. *Circulation* 1999;99:2480-2484.

National Institutes of Health, National Heart, Lung, and Blood Institute. Clinical guidelines on the identification, evaluation, and treatment of overweight and obesity in adults: the evidence report. *Obesity Res* 1998;6(suppl 2):51S-209S.

The North American Menopause Society. The role of isoflavones in menopausal health: consensus opinion of The North American Menopause Society. *Menopause* 2000;7:215-229.

The Sixth Report of the Joint National Committee on prevention, detection, evaluation, and treatment of high blood pressure. *Arch Intern Med* 1997;157:2413-2446.

Stampfer MJ, Willett WC, Colditz GA, Rosner B, Speizer FE, Hennekens CH. A prospective study of postmenopausal estrogen therapy and coronary heart disease. *N Engl J Med* 1985;313:1044-1049.

Stephens NG, Parsons A, Schofield PM, Kelly F, Cheeseman K, Mitchinson MJ. Randomised controlled trial of vitamin E in patients with coronary disease: Cambridge Heart Antioxidant Study. *Lancet* 1996;347:781-786.

Sullivan JM, VanderSwag R, Hughes JP, et al. Estrogen replacement and coronary artery disease: effect on survival in postmenopausal women. *Arch Intern Med* 1990;150:2557-2262.

Verhoef P, Stampfer MJ, Buring JE, et al. Homocysteine metabolism and risk of myocardial infarction: relation with vitamins B_6, B_{12}, and folate. *Am J Epidemiol* 1996;143:845-859.

Viscoli CM, Brass LM, Kernan WN, Sarrel PM, Suissa S, Horwitz RI. A clinical trial of estrogen-replacement therapy after ischemic stroke. *N Engl J Med* 2001;345:1243-1249.

The Writing Group for the PEPI Trial. Effects of estrogen/progestin regimens on heart disease risk factors in postmenopausal women. The Postmenopausal Estrogen/progestin Interventions (PEPI) Trial. *JAMA* 1995;273:199-208.

The Writing Group for the Women's Health Initiative Investigators. Risks and benefits of estrogen plus progestin in healthy postmenopausal women: principal results from the Women's Health Initiative randomized controlled trial. *JAMA* 2002;288:321-333.

For management of abnormal uterine bleeding (AUB) in peri- and postmenopausal women, clinicians have a number of effective options, both medical and surgical. The best option often depends on the woman's age and whether or not the bleeding is *organic* (ie, attributed to a systemic disease or reproductive tract lesion or disease).

Organic causes can be subdivided into *systemic disease* (eg, disorders of blood coagulation such as von Willebrand's disease and prothrombin deficiency; disorders that produce platelet deficiency such as leukemia, severe sepsis, idiopathic thrombocytopenic purpura; hypothyroidism; and cirrhosis) and *reproductive tract disease* (eg, accidents of pregnancy such as threatened, incomplete, or missed abortion and ectopic pregnancy; malignancies of the genital tract; uterine organic lesions such as submucous myomas, endometrial polyps, and adenomyosis; cervical lesions such as erosions, polyps, and cervicitis; traumatic vaginal lesions; and severe vaginal infections). Iatrogenic causes include uterine and vaginal foreign bodies, as well as use of certain drugs (eg, oral and injectable steroids, such as estrogen replacement therapy; hormones used for the management of dysmenorrhea, hirsutism, acne, or endometriosis; and tranquilizers that interfere with the neurotransmitters responsible for releasing and inhibiting hypothalamic hormones, thus causing anovulation and AUB).

After the above causes have been ruled out, the clinician must distinguish *ovulatory* from *anovulatory* AUB. (Some refer to both of these types of AUB as *dysfunctional uterine bleeding,* whereas others reserve that term only for anovulatory AUB).

Ovulatory AUB is not common, even in premenopausal women, and the exact mechanisms are unknown. It is generally demonstrated as regular menses every 24 to 35 days, but with excessive blood loss.

The predominant cause of AUB in perimenopausal women is anovulation secondary to alterations in neuroendocrine function. Anovulatory uterine bleeding presents as noncyclic menstrual blood flow ranging from spotting to heavy. It is usually caused by estrogen withdrawal (eg, midcycle spotting, bilateral oophorectomy, cessation of estrogen therapy), estrogen breakthrough (eg, polycystic ovarian syndrome, with chronic unopposed estrogen stimulation of the endometrium), or progesterone breakthrough (with a relatively high progesterone-to-estrogen ratio, as with progestin-only contraceptives). Without cyclic progesterone and regulated menstruation, the endometrium becomes hyperplastic and prone to localized bleeding. Timing of the bleeding episodes and the amount of blood loss are erratic.

Perimenopausal women experience an increase in anovulatory cycles due to depletion of ovarian oocytes. However, as polyps, submucosal fibroids, and endometrial hyperplasia and carcinoma become more prevalent with age, perimenopausal women with AUB should be examined for pathologic (ie, disease-altered) endometrial tissue. Chronic anovulation is associated with an increased risk for cancer in this population, although in younger perimenopausal women (under age 40), intracavity pathological conditions are the predominant cause of AUB.

After menopause, any unexpected uterine bleeding should be considered abnormal. The most common cause of AUB is endometrial atrophy. Up to 80% of postmenopausal women may have endometrial pathology, particularly if bleeding resumes after 1 year of amenorrhea. Pathology should also be suspected if uterine bleeding persists longer than 6 months with continuous-combined HRT.

M.01. Medical treatments

If there is no anatomic, organic, or systemic cause for the bleeding, medical treatment is the preferred treatment for perimenopausal women, especially those wishing to preserve fertility. The selection of a medical therapy is based on the woman's desire for conception or contraception, whether the AUB is ovulatory or anovulatory, and on any contraindications for the specific therapy. With anovulatory AUB, the cause should be identified and treated, allowing ovulation and regular menses to resume.

For perimenopausal women with AUB, the following therapies can be considered:

Combination estrogen-progestin contraceptives. Use of low-dose oral contraceptives (OCs) reduces blood loss by 50% (although no OC is FDA-approved for this use). However, OCs are not recommended for women over age 35 who smoke, those with a history of recurrent deep-vein thromboses, or those with other cardiovascular risk factors. Some clinicians may choose not to use these agents with obese perimenopausal women because of the thromboembolism risk. For women with vasomotor symptoms, OCs may offer additional benefits. Other contraceptive estrogen-progestogen options to regulate AUB include a monthly contraceptive injection containing medroxyprogesterone acetate and estradiol cypionate (Lunelle), a transdermal contraceptive patch delivering ethinyl estradiol and norelgestromin (Ortho Evra), and a contraceptive vaginal ring releasing ethinyl estradiol and etonogestrel (NuvaRing). (Lunelle and NuvaRing are not available in Canada.) Although use of these formulations should regulate perimenopausal periods, clinicians should be aware that no clinical trials have assessed the use of combination products other than OCs in the treatment of AUB.

Cyclic oral progestin. The standard medical therapy for anovulatory AUB in perimenopausal women has been cyclic oral progestin (continuous progestin therapy could result in breakthrough bleeding). Cyclic progestin therapy reverses hyperplastic changes and, in most studies, controls abnormal bleeding, although some studies have shown varying effects on bleeding, ranging from no change to increased bleeding. Cyclic progestin therapy is particularly useful for obese, well-estrogenized women. See Table 1 for suggested dosages of common oral progestins. Cyclic progestin should be administered for 12 to 14 days each month to result in predictable bleeding episodes. Prior to initiating therapy, an endometrial biopsy is recommended, which characteristically reveals proliferative or hyperplastic changes. Adding menopause doses of estrogen may be indicated if vasomotor symptoms occur or withdrawal bleeding ceases. Withdrawal bleeding may continue indefinitely in some obese perimenopause women treated with cyclic progestin-only therapy. If this occurs, it is appropriate to continue progestin therapy due to increased risk for endometrial hyperplasia and neoplasia in these women. For ovulatory AUB, continuous progestin is a better choice (cyclic progestin offers little advantage, as ovulatory women have regular menses). Continuous progestin (eg, intrauterine device) reduces blood loss by 80% to 90%.

Continuous progestin. For ovulatory perimenopausal women with AUB, continuous progestin therapy reduces blood loss by 80% to 90%. Use of cyclic progestin offers little advantage, as ovulatory women have regular menses. Continuous progestin is also an option for treatment of anovulatory AUB. In a 12-month study in symptomatic perimenopausal women, the intrauterine device (IUD) releasing levonorgestrel (Mirena) effectively prevented endometrial proliferation in women using oral estrogen replacement therapy. This IUD has also been demonstrated to profoundly reduce menstrual blood loss in women with menorrhagia. The Mirena IUD inserted during perimenopause may remain in place postmenopause. It can be combined with low-dose estrogen to relieve vasomotor symptoms, prevent vaginal atrophy, and positively affect bone while minimizing uterine bleeding and endometrial hyperplasia and cancer.

Low-dose continuous-combined hormone replacement therapy. For anovulatory perimenopausal women with AUB, menopause doses of estrogen plus progestogen (hormone replacement therapy; HRT) presents another useful approach. HRT delivers hormone levels much lower than the levels found in OCs. Moreover, those women with vasomotor symptoms may receive additional benefits. However, in ovulatory perimenopausal women with AUB, HRT is not a good choice, as HRT may not suppress ovulation and could consequently aggravate the problem of uterine bleeding.

Parenteral estrogen. For acute, excessive AUB — whether ovulatory or anovulatory — treatment with parenteral estrogen can be considered. In one controlled study, intravenous administration of conjugated equine estrogens stopped AUB in 71% of women compared with 38% who received placebo.

Tranexamic acid. If fertility is desired, an option to treat an ovulatory perimenopausal women with AUB is tranexamic acid (Cyklokapron), a synthetic derivative of the amino acid lysine. This drug exerts an antifibrinolytic effect by blocking plasminogen, but it has no effect on blood coagulation parameters or dysmenorrhea. Uterine bleeding is reduced by up to 40% with a dose of 1 g every 6 hours for the first 4 days of menses. One-third of women experience side effects, including nausea and leg cramps. Antifibrinolytics are not recommended to treat anovulatory AUB.

Table 1. Examples of cyclic progestin-only regimens for the treatment of anovulatory AUB in perimenopausal women

Progestin	Tablet strengths (mg)	Daily dosage (mg)*
Medroxyprogesterone acetate	2.5, 5.0, 10.0	5.0-10
Norethindrone acetate	5.0	2.5-5.0 (½ to 1 tablet/day)
Norethindrone	0.35	0.7-1.0 (2 to 3 tablets/day)

*Administered for 12-14 days each month

NSAIDs. Nonsteroidal anti-inflammatory drugs (NSAIDs) inhibit cyclooxygenase and reduce endometrial prostaglandin levels. In a review of randomized controlled trials, NSAIDs taken with menses decreased menstrual blood loss by 20% to 50% and improved dysmenorrhea in up to 70% of women. Therapy is usually started on the first day of menses and then continued for 5 days or until cessation of menstruation. However, NSAIDs are recommended only for ovulatory, not anovulatory, AUB.

GnRH agonists. Gonadotropin-releasing hormone (GnRH) agonists (eg, goserelin acetate) induce a reversible hypoestrogenic state, thus reducing total uterine volume. In the Leuprolide Study Group, treatment with 3.75 mg IM leuprolide acetate depot every 4 weeks for 24 weeks reduced uterine volume by 45%. A 25% reduction in volume was observed in 75% of the participants. The effect is temporary, as uterine volume expands to pretreatment levels within months of stopping therapy. GnRH agonists are effective in reducing menstrual blood loss (even after therapy) in perimenopausal women with either ovulatory or anovulatory AUB, but are limited by their side effects, including hot flashes and reduction of bone density.

Danazol. Danazol (Danocrine) is a synthetic steroid with mild androgenic properties. It has a profound effect on endometrial tissues, reducing menstrual blood loss by up to 80%. In one study, use of danazol (100-200 mg/day) resulted in amenorrhea in 20% of women and oligomenorrhea in another 70%. The side effect profile was mild, with approximately 70% of women reporting either minor or no side effects. Weight gain is the most common complaint. The recommended dosing for AUB is 100 to 200 mg/day for 3 months.

Iron. All women experiencing AUB should be evaluated for iron deficiency. Dietary sources provide adequate iron to replace that lost in menstrual blood volumes of up to 60 mL per month. Menstrual volumes above that amount may lead to iron-deficiency anemia. The primary symptom is fatigue. Anemia can be treated by adding a supplement providing 60 to 180 mg/day of iron.

If endometrial proliferation or hyperplasia without atypia is found, progestogen-based therapy is indicated. A follow-up endometrial biopsy should be performed after 3 to 4 months of treatment. If histological regression does not occur with progestogen therapy, dilation and curettage (D&C) may be appropriate prior to surgery to rule out underlying endometrial malignancy. There is nearly a 30% chance that complex endometrial hyperplasia with atypia will progress to cancer if untreated; therefore, hysterectomy represents appropriate surgical management in this setting.

M.02. Surgical management

Dilation and curettage is now considered obsolete for the treatment of AUB. D&C does not completely remove intracavity tissue.

Until the development of newer techniques, hysterectomy was the only definitive cure for benign AUB that failed to respond to medical treatment. Although surgical mortality is low, postoperative complications occur in approximately 30% of patients. In addition, hysterectomy is expensive and often medically unnecessary due to the absence of uterine pathology in many women.

Endometrial resection and ablation techniques have emerged as effective, safe, and cost-effective alternatives to hysterectomy for the treatment of AUB. Several issues should be considered when employing endometrial ablation in the treatment of AUB in perimenopausal women. First, endometrial histologic evaluation should take place prior to endometrial ablation. Second, thermal balloon ablation does not involve visualization of the endometrial cavity and will not effectively treat AUB caused by endometrial polyps or submucous fibroids. Clinicians should evaluate the endometrial cavity with sonohysterography or diagnostic hysteroscopy prior to thermal balloon ablation or any other endometrial destructive therapy. Clinicians planning hysteroscopic endometrial ablation should be prepared to resect any polypoid lesions encountered intraoperatively. Finally, endometrial ablation will not successfully treat AUB caused by anatomic lesions located in the uterine wall, either intramural fibroids or adenomyosis.

Bibliography

Andersch B, Milsom I, Rybo G. An objective evaluation of flurbiprofen and tranexamic acid in the treatment of idiopathic menorrhagia. *Acta Obstet Gynecol Scand* 1988;67:645-648.

Association of Professors of Gynecology and Obstetrics. *Clinical Management of Abnormal Uterine Bleeding: Educational Series on Women's Health Issues.* Crofton, MD: Association of Professors of Gynecology and Obstetrics; 2002.

Bayer SR, DeCherney AH. Clinical manifestations and treatment of dysfunctional uterine bleeding. *JAMA* 1993;269:1823-1828.

Bonduelle M, Walker JJ, Calder AA. A comparative study of danazol and norethisterone in dysfunctional uterine bleeding presenting as menorrhagia. *Postgrad Med J* 1991;67:833-836.

Chuong CJ, Brenner PF. Management of abnormal uterine bleeding. *Am J Obstet Gynecol* 1996;175(3 part 2):787-792.

Colacurci N, De Placido G, Mollo A, Perino A, Cittadini E. Short-term use of goserelin depot in the treatment of dysfunctional uterine bleeding. *Clin Exp Obstet Gynecol* 1995;22:212-219.

Crosignani PG, Vercellini P, Mosconi P, Oldani S, Cortesi I, De Giorgi O. Levonorgestrel-releasing intrauterine device versus hysteroscopic endometrial resection in the treatment of dysfunctional uterine bleeding. *Obstet Gynecol* 1997;90:257-263.

Davis A, Godwin A, Lippman J, Olson W, Kafrissen M. Triphasic norgestimate-ethinyl estradiol for treating dysfunctional uterine bleeding. *Obstet Gynecol* 2000;96:913-920.

Dockeray CJ, Sheppard BL, Bonnar J. Comparison between mefanamic acid and danazol in the treatment of established menorrhagia. *Br J Obstet Gynaecol* 1989;96:840-844.

Edlund M, Andersson K, Rybo G, Lindoff C, Astedt B, von Schoultz B. Reduction of menstrual blood loss in women suffering from idiopathic menorrhagia with a novel antifibrinolytic drug (Kabi 2161). *Br J Obstet Gynaeceol* 1995;102:913-917.

Farquhar CM, Lethaby A, Sowter M, et al. An evaluation of risk factors for endometrial hyperplasia in premenopausal women with abnormal menstrual bleeding. *Am J Obstet Gynecol* 1999; 181:525-529.

Frazer IS. Changes in the menstrual pattern during the perimenopause. In: Lobo RA, ed. *Treatment of the Postmenopausal Woman: Basic and Clinical Aspects*. 2nd ed. Philadelphia, PA: Lippincott Williams & Wilkins; 1999:69-74.

Fraser IS. Treatment of ovulatory and anovulatory dysfunctional uterine bleeding with oral progestogens. *Aust N Z J Obstet Gynaecol* 1990;30:353-356.

Fraser IS, McCarron G. Randomized trial of 2 hormonal and 2 prostaglandin-inhibiting agents in women with a complaint of menorrhagia. *Aust N Z J Obstet Gynaecol* 1991;31:66-70.

Friedman AJ, Hoffman DI, Comite F, Browneller RW, Miller JD. Treatment of leiomyomata uteri with leuprolide acetate depot: a double-blind, placebo-controlled, multicenter study. The Leuprolide Study Group. *Obstet Gynecol* 1991;77:720-725.

Gambrell RD Jr. Strategies to reduce the incidence of endometrial cancer in postmenopausal women. *Am J Obstet Gynecol* 1997; 177:1195-1204.

Gervaise A, Fernandez H, Capella-Allouc S, et al. Thermal balloon ablation versus endometrial resection for the treatment of abnormal uterine bleeding. *Hum Reprod* 2000;15:1424-1425.

Good AE. Diagnostic options for assessment of postmenopausal bleeding. *Mayo Clin Proc* 1997;72:345-349.

Higham JM, Shaw RW. A comparative study of danazol, a regimen of decreasing doses of danazol, and norethindrone in the treatment of objectively proven unexplained menorrhagia. *Am J Obstet Gynecol* 1993;169:1134-1139.

Hurskainen R, Teperi J, Rissanen P, et al. Quality of life and cost-effectiveness of levonorgestrel-releasing intrauterine system versus hysterectomy for treatment of menorrhagia: a randomised trial. *Lancet* 2001;357:273-277.

Irvine GA, Campbell-Brown MB, Lumsden MA, Heikkila A, Walker JJ, Cameron IT. Randomised comparative trial of the levo-norgestrel intrauterine system and norethisterone for treatment of idiopathic menorrhagia. *Br J Obstet Gynaecol* 1998;105:592-598.

Lamb MP. Danazol in menorrhagia: a double blind placebo controlled trial. *J Obstet Gynecol* 1987;7:212-216.

Munro MG. Abnormal uterine bleeding in the reproductive years. Part II: Medical management. *J Am Assoc Gynecol Laparosc* 2000; 7:17-35.

Munro MG. Abnormal uterine bleeding: surgical management. Part III. *J Am Assoc Gynecol Laparosc* 2001;8:18-44.

Munro MG. Medical management of abnormal uterine bleeding. *Obstet Gynecol Clin North Am* 2000;27:287-304.

The North American Menopause Society. Clinical challenges of perimenopause: consensus opinion of The North American Menopause Society. *Menopause* 2000;7:5-13.

Oriel KA, Schrager S. Abnormal uterine bleeding. *Am Fam Physician* 1999;60:1371-1380.

Preston JT, Cameron IT, Adams EJ, Smith SK. Comparative study of tranexamic acid and norethisterone in the treatment of ovulatory menorrhagia. *Br J Obstet Gynaecol* 1995;102:401-406.

Smith SK, Abel MH, Kelly RW, Baird DT. Prostaglandin synthesis in the endometrium of women with ovular dysfunctional uterine bleeding. *Br J Obstet Gynaecol* 1981;88:434-442.

Speroff L. Management of the perimenopausal transition. *Contemp OB/GYN* 2000;45:16-37.

Stabinsky SA, Einstein M, Breen JL. Modern treatments of menorrhagia attributable to dysfunctional uterine bleeding. *Obstet Gynecol Surv* 1999;54:61-72.

Thomas EJ. Add-back therapy for long-term use in dysfunctional uterine bleeding and uterine fibroids. *Br J Obstet Gynaecol* 1996; 14(suppl):S18-S21.

Townsend DE, Fields G, McCausland A, Kauffman K. Diagnostic and operative hysteroscopy in the management of persistent postmenopausal bleeding. *Obstet Gynecol* 1993;82:419-421.

Vilos GA, Lefebvre G, Graves GR. Guidelines for the management of abnormal uterine bleeding. *J SOCG* 2001;23:704-709.

The risk for most cancers increases with age, but menopause is not associated with increased cancer risk. However, some of the therapies used for menopause are associated with an increase or a decrease in certain types of cancers.

N.01. Endometrial cancer

A woman's lifetime risk of developing endometrial cancer is small and unrelated to menopause. Use of unopposed estrogen replacement therapy (ERT), however, is associated with increased risk related to the dosage and duration of the ERT. Studies have revealed that unopposed ERT, when used for more than 3 years, is associated with a 5-fold increased risk of endometrial cancer; if used for 10 years, the risk increases 10-fold. This increased risk persists for several years after discontinuation of estrogen. Studies have also found that most endometrial cancer that occurs while taking unopposed ERT does not reduce life expectancy.

Adding progestogen therapy to ERT reduces the risk of endometrial cancer induced by estrogen to the level found in women not taking hormones. Data from the Postmenopausal Estrogen/Progestin Interventions (PEPI) trial showed that women who took unopposed ERT during the 3-year trial had a significantly increased risk of hyperplasia (34%) while those taking ERT plus progestogen had a risk of only 1%. Progestogen does not eliminate endometrial cancer risk completely because there is a risk independent of hormone use.

Women with an intact uterus should use ERT plus progestogen (ie, hormone replacement therapy; HRT) to protect against endometrial hyperplasia. With some women and some dosage schedules of progestogen, the endometrial lining sheds and passes from the uterus as bleeding, similar to a menstrual period. This progestogen-induced bleeding is not associated with menstrual cramps. Ovulation does not occur.

Some women regard this progestogen-induced bleeding as an unacceptable nuisance. For many women, it is difficult to decide whether to tolerate the uterine bleeding in exchange for the ERT-reductions in short-term menopausal symptoms, such as hot flashes, and lowering the risk of other diseases later in life.

With an oral progestin used in a cyclic regimen, the minimum effective dosage for endometrial protection is 5 mg/day of medroxyprogesterone acetate (MPA) or the equivalent for 12 to 14 days each month. With oral micronized progesterone, the minimum effective dosage is 200 mg/day for 12 to 14 days each month.

The newer continuous-combined HRT dosage schedules, in which a smaller amount of progestogen is taken daily along with estrogen, usually result in amenorrhea over time. However, many women (particularly those who are recently postmenopausal) have vaginal spotting and bleeding during the first year or so of this regimen. With continuous-combined HRT, the minimum effective dose of oral progestin for endometrial protection is 2.5 mg/day of MPA (or the equivalent) or 100 mg/day of oral micronized progesterone. The continuous-combined regimen is the most popular regimen in the United States.

Other alternatives to reduce uterine bleeding include dosing progestogen every few months or not at all. However, ERT without a progestogen is rarely advisable for a woman with an intact uterus. If either of these options is chosen, an endometrial biopsy must be performed every year to monitor for endometrial cancer. Uterine bleeding can also occur when ERT is taken alone and may be associated with endometrial hyperplasia or carcinoma.

Women who use a cyclic progestogen regimen can expect uterine bleeding when the progestogen is withdrawn. These women should be encouraged to report any uterine bleeding that occurs at times other than usual. All postmenopausal women — whether or not they use hormones — should report any uterine bleeding, such as prolonged, excessive, or unexpected bleeding, as well as any bleeding or spotting after several months of no bleeding.

Management of endometrial cancer survivors
ERT/HRT has traditionally been withheld from women with a history of endometrial cancer, based on the belief that hormone therapy might increase the risk of recurrence. Despite epidemiologic studies linking prolonged use of unopposed ERT with the development of endometrial cancer, two recent retrospective studies in women who received ERT/HRT following their treatment for an endometrial cancer do not appear to have an excessive increased risk for recurrence. A prospective, placebo-controlled study is underway to further determine the impact of estrogen on endometrial cancer recurrence.

The American College of Obstetricians and Gynecologists (ACOG) has advised that, in the absence of well-designed studies, the decision to recommend estrogen therapy for women following endometrial cancer should be based on prognostic indicators, including depth of invasion, degree of differentiation, and cell type. The Society of Obstetricians and Gynaecologists of Canada (SOGC) similarly recommends that HRT may be used by women who have been treated for endometrial cancer and who fall in a low-risk group (ie, with stage I disease, grade 1 or 2 histology, and less than 50% depth of myometrial invasion). Careful counseling regarding perceived benefits and risks should be conducted to assist each woman in making an informed decision. The need for adding progestogen therapy is undetermined, although progestogen supplementation has not been found to affect the recurrence rate. Use of androgen therapy is not a substitute for progestogen, as some androgens may aromatize to estrogen.

Breast cancer survivors are often prescribed tamoxifen (Nolvadex), a selective estrogen-receptor modulator (SERM), to treat breast cancer. Tamoxifen is associated with increased risk of endometrial cancer. Although adding progestogen to ERT reduces the risk of endometrial cancer, the effect of adding progestogen to tamoxifen is undetermined. ACOG recommends that women using tamoxifen be educated about its risks on the endometrium and monitored closely. Tamoxifen use should be limited to 5 years. ACOG further advises that tamoxifen use may be considered following hysterectomy for endometrial cancer, provided that the women makes an informed decision.

Bibliography

The American College of Obstetricians and Gynecologists. Estrogen replacement therapy and endometrial cancer: ACOG Committee Opinion (no. 235). *Int J Gynaecol Obstet* 2001;73:283-284.

The American College of Obstetricians and Gynecologists. Tamoxifen and endometrial cancer. ACOG Committee Opinion (no. 232). *Int J Gynaecol Obstet* 2001;73:77-79.

Belisle S, Derzko C. Hormone replacement therapy and cancer: Canadian consensus on menopause and osteoporosis. *J SOGC* 2001;23:1198-1203.

Creasman WT, Henderson D, Hinshaw W, Clarke-Pearson DL. Estrogen replacement therapy in the patient treated for endometrial cancer. *Obstet Gynecol* 1986;67:326-330.

Gambrell RD Jr. Strategies to reduce the incidence of endometrial cancer in postmenopausal women. *Am J Obstet Gynecol* 1997; 177:1195-1204.

Grady D, Gebretsadik T, Kerlikowske K, Ernster V, Petitti D. Hormone replacement therapy and endometrial cancer risk: a meta-analysis. *Obstet Gynecol* 1995;85:304-313.

Kedar RP, Bourne TH, Powles TJ, et al. Effects of tamoxifen on uterus and ovaries of postmenopausal women in a randomised breast cancer prevention trial. *Lancet* 1994;343:1318-1321.

Lacey JV, Brinton LA, Barnes WA, et al. Use of hormone replacement therapy and adenocarcinomas and squamous cell carcinomas of the uterine cervix. *Gynecol Oncol* 2000;77:149-154.

Lee RB, Burke TW, Park RC. Estrogen replacement therapy following treatment of stage 1 endometrial carcinoma. *Gynecol Oncol* 1990; 36:189-191.

Persson I, Yuen J, Bergkvist L, Shairer C. Cancer incidence and mortality in women receiving estrogen and estrogen-progestin replacement therapy: long-term follow-up of a Swedish cohort. *Int J Cancer* 1996;67:327-221.

Schwartzbaum J, Hulka BS, Fowler WC Jr, Kaufman DG, Hoberman D. The influence of exogenous estrogen use on survival after diagnosis of endometrial cancer. *Am J Epidemiol* 1987;126: 851-860.

Suriano KA, McHale M, McLaren CE, Li KT, Re A, DiSaia PJ. Estrogen replacement therapy in endometrial cancer patients: a matched control study. *Obstet Gynecol* 2001;97:555-560.

The Writing Group for the PEPI Trial. Effects of hormone replacement therapy on endometrial biopsy in postmenopausal women. *JAMA* 1996;275:370-375.

N.02. Breast cancer

Breast cancer is a primary health concern for many women, particularly when deciding about menopause-related hormone therapy. Risk for breast cancer is not affected by menopause. There are some epidemiologic data, however, that suggest an association between timing of menopause and breast cancer risk, with early menopause associated with decreased risk, and delayed menopause associated with an increased risk.

The breast cancer risk associated with ERT/HRT use is controversial. Recent data from the Women's Health Initiative (WHI), a randomized, controlled trial, found that HRT (continuous-combined CEE plus MPA) significantly increased the risk of invasive breast cancer (relative risk, 1.26). The HRT-arm of the trial was discontinued prematurely after 5.2 years of a planned 8-year study, primarily because of the breast cancer findings. The increase in risk began during year 3; HRT-treated patients had lower risks during years 1 and 2. The unopposed ERT arm of the trial was allowed to continue, which suggests that combined HRT confers a greater breast cancer risk.

Similarly, data from the National Cancer Institute's Breast Cancer Detection Demonstration Project (BCDDP), a reanalysis of published data from 51 observational studies, and the Nurses' Health Study (published in abstract form only) found a positive association between both ERT and HRT use and increased breast cancer risk, especially in women using hormones for more than 5 to 15 years. Short-term or past users are not at significantly increased risk. The increased risk associated with hormone use disappeared within 5 years of its discontinuation.

Data on an association between progestogen use and breast cancer risk are inconsistent and controversial. The studies showing an association between progestogen use and increased breast cancer risk have not consistently associated any progestogen or HRT regimen with greater risk.

The woman's body mass index also may be a factor. The reports suggest an increased risk associated with use of ERT alone in long-term users who had lean body mass. This effect, however, may be no greater than the effect associated with increased estrogen production in overweight women. One case-control study from Sweden found a significantly increased risk of breast cancer associated with 10 or more years of current HRT use in women who were not overweight. This observational Swedish study also suggested, for the first time, that there is an increased risk for women who had discontinued HRT more than 10 years previously, and that a continuous-combined regimen is associated with a greater risk than was a cyclic-combined regimen. Some experts have pointed out that the data and the conclusions are not definitive.

Most of the studies that have examined the breast cancer mortality rates of women who have used postmenopausal ERT/HRT have documented improved survival rates. Even those studies that have found an increased risk of breast cancer in hormone users have found better outcomes, perhaps because of earlier diagnosis. In the reanalysis of the published data, among current or recent users of postmenopausal hormone therapy, the excess risk of breast cancer was confined to localized disease. There is also evidence to suggest that estrogen users develop smaller, lower-grade tumors.

In most of the studies that have examined the relationship between ERT/HRT and breast cancer, little attention was paid to the histologic type of breast cancer. In a recent case-control study of women aged 50 to 64, combined estrogen-progestin use for at least 6 months was found to increase the risk of lobular, but not ductal, breast cancer. Lobular tumors represent 5% to 10% of all breast cancer cases; ductal tumors

account for 80% to 85%. Lobular tumors are more difficult to palpate and are more likely to be missed by mammographic screening, but women with lobular cancer have a better prognosis than women with ductal cancer. The investigators concluded that, with respect to absolute risk, even if combined HRT use is associated with an increased risk of lobular breast cancer, only a small percentage of HRT users are likely to be affected.

Most women initiate ERT/HRT for relief of vasomotor symptoms. They usually experience prompt symptom relief and can taper off hormones long before breast cancer risk increases. The decision to continue ERT/HRT over the long term, is more complicated. It is especially important that each woman weigh known and probable risks and benefits. No simple rule will apply to every woman, as each has her own risk factor status and concerns.

Additional results from the WHI (expected in 2005) and other large clinical trials should provide more data to help women and their healthcare providers better understand the association between ERT/HRT and breast cancer.

Management of breast cancer survivors
The number of women surviving breast cancer has been increasing as a result of earlier detection due to widespread application of mammographic screening and the efficacy of adjuvant systemic therapies. While approximately 30% to 40% of US women and about 26% of Canadian women diagnosed with breast cancer will eventually succumb to their disease, the clinical course in any individual is difficult to predict. Thus, many women live with the constant threat of breast cancer recurrence. When such women reach menopause, they require special care.

Premenopausal women receiving ovary-damaging chemotherapy or radiation therapy have an increased risk of induced menopause. With chemotherapy, an increased risk of amenorrhea begins at approximately age 30, rising to more than 80% among women 45 years and older. Tamoxifen is likely to cause amenorrhea only among women approaching age 50. Induced menopause usually is associated with more severe menopausal symptoms, and early menopause may increase the risks of osteoporosis and cardiovascular disease.

A number of studies, mostly uncontrolled, have evaluated the effects of ERT/HRT in breast cancer survivors. Most have enrolled women 10 or more years after the initial breast cancer diagnosis. The weight of evidence is that initiating ERT/HRT at this point has no deleterious effects on tumor recurrence.

Having a history of or a high-risk profile for breast cancer is not considered to be an absolute contraindication for ERT/HRT use. No clinical trials have demonstrated that ERT/HRT increases the relapse rate. In certain situations, the clinician, in consultation with the woman's oncologist, may help the woman decide whether the benefits of such therapy outweigh its risks. The decision must be made with the full awareness that therapy might promote more rapid tumor growth, although observational studies have failed to show untoward effects of ERT/HRT even in estrogen receptor-positive breast cancer patients. A matched cohort analysis to evaluate the impact of ERT/HRT on mortality in breast cancer survivors matched 125 cases with 362 controls. Of those, 98% (n = 123) received systemic estrogen, with 72% (n = 90) also receiving a progestin. The median interval between the diagnosis of breast cancer and the initiation of ERT/HRT was 46 months. The median duration of ERT/HRT use was 22 months, and ERT/HRT users had a significantly reduced risk of breast cancer recurrence. This particular study suggested that ERT/HRT after the treatment of breast cancer is not associated with an adverse outcome.

ACOG and SOGC advise that the use of ERT/HRT may be considered in postmenopausal women with previously treated breast cancer. However, caution is recommended in all cases, since there are no specific data regarding particular stages or histologic types of the disease to provide guidance regarding patients at highest risk.

Nonetheless, breast cancer survivors and/or their healthcare providers generally do not choose ERT/HRT. The rationale is that avoiding hormones will reduce the risk of recurrence and of new contralateral tumors. In about one-third of women, stopping hormone therapy reduces mammographic density and, thereby, allows better surveillance for new breast cancer. However, women with debilitating menopause-related symptoms, primarily vasomotor and vaginal symptoms, often require the symptom relief that ERT/HRT offers, and abrupt withdrawal of therapy can exacerbate those symptoms. Fortunately, there are effective alternatives to ERT/HRT that can safely be used for symptom management in breast cancer survivors.

Vasomotor symptoms. Non-ERT/HRT therapies for the management of vasomotor symptoms vary in efficacy. Potentially effective therapies include transdermal clonidine, megestrol acetate, venlafaxine HCl, and various selective serotonin-reuptake inhibitors (SSRIs). The SSRIs are the most effective alternative and should be considered first line. Low doses of SSRIs can alleviate hot flashes, but high doses may make symptoms worse.

Soy protein isolate, 20 to 40 g/day, may reduce hot flashes 10% to 20% beyond reductions observed with placebo. Dietary supplementation with soy protein is FDA-approved for its potential benefit on cardiovascular disease risk. Its effect on breast cancer risk is uncertain.

Black cohosh did not reduce hot flashes better than placebo in breast cancer survivors receiving tamoxifen, but it has been shown to be effective in other populations with mild hot flashes. Vitamin E also has not been proven effective. In addition to drug and herbal remedies, a number of lifestyle options (eg, keeping rooms cool, avoiding hot flash triggers) may also provide relief.

Vaginal effects. Vaginal symptoms can be precipitated by discontinuation of ERT/HRT, onset of premature menopause, or administration of chemotherapy. Vaginal dryness and dyspareunia are common complaints among postmenopausal breast cancer survivors. Approximately 30% of women using tamoxifen may also experience vaginal discharge.

Vaginal moisturizers and vaginal lubricants are effective in relieving symptoms of vaginal dryness and dyspareunia. In the past, topical vaginal estrogen preparations have not been recommended for breast cancer survivors because of safety concerns related to systemic absorption of estrogen from these formulations. However, there are now several estrogen options that many oncologists consider safe. Use of one-quarter applicator of vaginal estrogen cream (various estrogen products available) once weekly can afford considerable relief of atrophic symptoms, producing only a very transient increase in serum estradiol level, if any. A silastic vaginal ring impregnated with estradiol (Estring) provides local estrogen release without significant systemic absorption; the ring remains active in the vagina for 3 months. The vaginal estradiol tablet (Vagifem), 25 µg tablet inserted daily for 2 weeks then twice weekly, also provides efficacy with minimal systemic absorption.

Sexual health and functioning. Several studies show that sexual interest and activity in breast cancer survivors are similar to age-matched postmenopausal women who are not taking ERT/HRT. Many of the factors affecting sexual health in postmenopausal breast cancer survivors are similar to those in postmenopausal women without cancer: vaginal dryness, emotional distress, body image, the quality of the partnered relationship, and sexual problems in the partner. These factors are potentially responsive to treatment.

Osteoporosis. In general, postmenopausal women with breast cancer have a lower risk of osteoporosis as a result of higher endogenous levels of estrogen throughout their lifetime. However, there have been studies linking lower bone mineral density (BMD) to younger women who have developed breast cancer. If uncertainty exists about a postmenopausal woman's risk for osteoporosis, clinical risk factors for osteoporosis should be assessed and BMD measured.

For women who cannot use ERT/HRT to prevent osteoporosis due to their risk profile for breast cancer, the SERM raloxifene (Evista) offers an attractive alternative. In the Multiple Outcomes of Raloxifene Evaluation (MORE), a multicenter, randomized, double-blind trial in which postmenopausal women with osteoporosis received raloxifene (60 mg or 120 mg daily) or placebo, raloxifene decreased the risk of estrogen receptor-positive breast cancer by 90%. No effect on estrogen receptor-negative breast cancer was found. During this 3-year trial, the risk of invasive breast cancer decreased by 76%. To determine the role of raloxifene in the primary prevention of breast cancer requires large, long-term studies. The ongoing Study of Tamoxifen and Raloxifene (STAR) will hopefully provide some answers. Raloxifene is FDA-approved only for osteoporosis therapy, not breast cancer prevention.

Another SERM, tamoxifen (Nolvadex), has been shown to decrease the incidence of breast cancer by 50% in high-risk women. It is FDA-approved for prevention as well as for treatment of breast cancer. Use for treatment is limited, however, to 5 years. In postmenopausal women, tamoxifen is likely to maintain BMD because it has some estrogen-agonist effects on bone. In premenopausal women, it is likely to induce bone loss because its major effect is blocking estrogen.

Tamoxifen is associated with increased risk of endometrial cancer, but this risk has not been seen with raloxifene. Both tamoxifen and raloxifene are associated with increased risk for venous thromboembolic events. In some clinical trials, tamoxifen has reduced the risk for and incidence of coronary heart disease. These data are not consistent, however, and were not supported by the Early Breast Cancer Trial or the Breast Cancer Prevention Trial.

Raloxifene is associated with an increase in hot flashes and leg cramps. It slightly lowers cholesterol and low-density lipoprotein (LDL) cholesterol. In a secondary analysis of the data from the MORE trial, raloxifene did not significantly affect overall risk for cardiovascular events in the total population, but it was associated with a significant 40% reduction in risk of cardiovascular events in high-risk women. The effect of raloxifene on the risk of cardiovascular events in postmenopausal women is being studied prospectively in the Raloxifene Use of The Heart (RUTH) trial.

Although low bone density and bone loss may eventually increase the risk of fracture, the primary short-term concern for breast cancer survivors should be prevention of breast cancer recurrence.

Cardiovascular disease. While the mortality risk from breast cancer varies substantially with the extent of the primary tumor, many women will survive their breast cancer and eventually reach the age when heart disease becomes common. It is not known to what extent breast cancer treatments and any subsequent induced menopause are associated with the risk of cardiovascular disease. This might also be complicated by the late effects of cardiotoxic drugs such as doxorubicin, which is widely used in the adjuvant therapy of breast cancer. Long-term observational studies to clarify these effects are underway.

Cognitive dysfunction. Complaints of difficulty with thinking and memory are often reported by women who reached menopause as a result of adjuvant therapy for breast cancer. These complaints could be the result of a direct neurotoxic effect of chemotherapy. Additional studies are needed to further define these effects. Similarly, little is known about the potential effects of tamoxifen on cognitive decline with aging.

Other conditions. Menopause appears to be a significant factor in the development of weight gain after breast cancer. This may be precipitated by adjuvant chemotherapy, decreased exercise during treatment, or to increased eating related to depression. Obesity is an important health concern for postmenopausal breast cancer survivors (as it is for all postmenopausal women) because it increases the risk for cardiovascular disease and diabetes. In some studies, weight gain has been associated with an increased risk of breast cancer recurrence, possibly due to higher levels of endogenous estrogen. Weight gain also affects body image and self-esteem, and it may be more of an issue for women than changes in the breast or mastectomy. Breast cancer survivors should be assisted in maintaining or achieving a healthy weight.

Managing women with benign breast disease

Women with premalignant breast disease are at increased risk for breast cancer. Compared with women with nonproliferative benign histology, those with proliferative, nonmalignant breast disease have an increased risk for developing breast cancer (relative risk of 3.6 and 1.8, respectively, with and without atypical hyperplasia). Hormone use has not been found to affect these risks.

Bibliography

The American College of Obstetricians and Gynecologists. Hormone replacement therapy in women with previously treated breast cancer: ACOG Committee Opinion (no. 226). Washington, DC: The American College of Obstetricians and Gynecologists; November 1999.

The American College of Obstetricians and Gynecologists. Risk of breast cancer with estrogen-progestin replacement therapy: ACOG Committee Opinion. *Obstet Gynecol* 2001;98:1181-1184.

Barrett-Connor E, Grady D, Sashegyi A, et al. Raloxifene and cardiovascular events in osteoporotic postmenopausal women: four-year results from the MORE (Multiple Outcomes of Raloxifene Evaluation) randomized trial. *JAMA* 2002;287:847-857.

Bentrem DJ, Jordan VC. Targeted antiestrogens for the prevention of breast cancer. *Oncol Res* 1999;11:401-409.

Belisle S, Derzko C. Hormone replacement therapy and cancer: Canadian consensus on menopause and osteoporosis. *J SOGC* 2001;23:1198-1203.

Brezden CB, Phillips KA, Abdolell M, Bunston T, Tannock IF. Cognitive function in breast cancer patients receiving adjuvant chemotherapy. *J Clin Oncol* 2000;18:2695-2701.

Byrne C, Connolly JL, Colditz GA, Schnitt SJ. Biopsy confirmed benign breast disease, postmenopausal use of exogenous female hormones, and breast carcinoma risk. *Cancer* 2000;89:2046-2052.

Burstein HJ, Winer EP. Primary care for survivors of breast cancer. *N Engl J Med* 2000;343:1086-1094.

Colditz GA, Hankinson SE, Hunter DJ, et al. Estrogen replacement therapy and progestins and the risk of breast cancer in postmenopausal women. *N Engl J Med* 1995;332:1589-1593.

Colditz GA, Rosner B. Cumulative risk of breast cancer to age 70 years according to risk factor status: data from the Nurses' Health Study. *Am J Epidemiol* 2000;152:950-964.

Colditz GA, Rosner B, for the Nurses' Health Study Research Group. Use of estrogen plus progestin is associated with greater increase in breast cancer risk than estrogen alone [abstract]. *Am J Epidemiol* 1998;147(suppl). Abstract 254.

Collaborative Group on Hormone Factors in Breast Cancer. Breast cancer and hormone replacement therapy: collaborative re-analysis of data from 51 epidemiological studies of 52,705 women with breast cancer and 108,411 women without breast cancer [erratum in: *Lancet* 1997;350:1484]. *Lancet* 1997;350:1047-1059.

Costantino JP, Kuller LH, Ives DG, et al. Coronary heart disease mortality and adjuvant tamoxifen therapy. *J Natl Cancer Inst* 1997;89:776-782.

Cummings SR, Eckert S, Krueger KA, et al. The effect of raloxifene on risk of breast cancer in postmenopausal women: results from the MORE randomized trial. Multiple Outcomes of Raloxifene Evaluation [erratum in: *JAMA* 1999;282:2124]. *JAMA* 1999; 281:2189-2197.

Day R, Ganz PA, Costantino JP, Cronin WM, Wickerham DL, Fisher B. Health-related quality of life and tamoxifen in breast cancer prevention: a report from the National Surgical Adjuvant Breast and Bowel Project P-1 study. *J Clin Oncol* 1999;17:2659-2669.

Delmas PD, Bjarnason NH, Mitlak BH, et al. Effects of raloxifene on bone mineral density, serum cholesterol concentrations, and uterine endometrium in postmenopausal women. *N Engl J Med* 1997;337:1641-1647.

DiSaia PJ, Brewster WR, Ziogas A, Anton-Culver H. Breast cancer survival and hormone replacement therapy: a cohort analysis. *Am J Clin Oncol* 2000;23:541-545.

Dupont WD, Page DL, Parl FF, et al. Estrogen replacement therapy in women with a history of proliferative breast disease. *Cancer* 1999;85:1279-1283.

Fisher B, Constantino J, Wickerham D, et al. Tamoxifen for the prevention of breast cancer: report of the NSABP Project P-1. *J Natl Cancer Inst* 1998;90:1371-1388.

Ganz PA, Desmond KA, Belin TR, Meyerowitz BE, Rowland JH. Predictors of sexual health in women after a breast cancer diagnosis. *J Clin Oncol* 1999;17:2371-2380.

Ganz PA, Greendale GA, Kahn B, et al. Are older breast carcinoma survivors willing to take hormone replacement therapy? *Cancer* 1999;86:814-820.

Ganz PA, Greendale GA, Petersen L, et al. Managing menopausal symptoms in breast cancer survivors: results of a randomized controlled trial. *J Natl Cancer Inst* 2000;92:1054-1064.

Ganz PA, Rowland JH, Desmond K, Meyerowitz BE, Wyatt GE. Life after breast cancer: understanding women's health-related quality of life and sexual functioning. *J Clin Oncol* 1998;16:501-514.

Gapster SM, Morrow M, Sellars TA. Hormone replacement therapy and risk of breast cancer with a favorable histology: results of the Iowa Women's Health Study. *JAMA* 1999;281:2091-2097.

Goldberg RM, Loprinzi CL, O'Fallon JR, et al. Transdermal clonidine for ameliorating tamoxifen-induced hot flashes [erratum in: *J Clin Oncol* 1996;14:2411]. *J Clin Oncol* 1994;12:155-158.

Goodwin PJ, Ennis M, Pritchard KI, et al. Adjuvant treatment and onset of menopause predict weight gain after breast cancer diagnosis. *J Clin Oncol* 1999;17:120-129.

Goodwin PJ, Ennis M, Pritchard KI, Trudeau M, Hood N. Risk of menopause during the first year after breast cancer diagnosis. *J Clin Oncol* 1999;17:2365-2370.

Holmgren PA, Lindskog M, von Schoultz B. Vaginal rings for continuous low-dose release of oestradiol in the treatment of urogenital atrophy. *Maturitas* 1989;11:55-63.

Kanis JA, McCloskey EV, Powles T, et al. A high incidence of vertebral fracture in women with breast cancer. *Br J Cancer* 1999;79:1179-1181.

Li CI, Weiss NS, Stanford JL, Daling JR. Hormone replacement therapy in relation to risk of lobular and ductal breast carcinoma in middle-aged women. *Cancer* 2000;88:2570-2577.

Lippman ME, Krueger KA, Eckert S, et al. Indicators of lifetime estrogen exposure: effect on breast cancer incidence and interaction with raloxifene therapy in the multiple outcomes of raloxifene evaluation study participants. *J Clin Oncol* 2001;19:3111-3116.

Loprinzi CL, Abu-Ghazaleh S, Sloan JA, et al. Phase III randomized double-blind study to evaluate the efficacy of a polycarbophil-based vaginal moisturizer in women with breast cancer. *J Clin Oncol* 1997;15:969-973.

Loprinzi CL, Kugler JW, Sloan JA, et al. Venlafaxine in management of hot flashes in survivors of breast cancer: a randomised controlled trial. *Lancet* 2000;356:2059-2063.

Loprinzi CL, Michalak JC, Quella SK, et al. Megestrol acetate for the prevention of hot flashes. *N Engl J Med* 1994;331:347-352.

Magnusson C, Baron JA, Correia N, Bergström R, Adami HO, Persson I. Breast cancer risk following long-term oestrogen- and oestrogen-progestin-replacement therapy. *Int J Cancer* 1999;81:339-344.

Meyerowitz BE, Desmond KA, Rowland JH, et al. Sexuality following breast cancer. *J Sex Marital Ther* 1999;25:237-250.

National Cancer Institute of Canada. *Canadian Cancer Statistics 2002.* Toronto, ON, Canada: National Cancer Institute of Canada; 2002.

Natrajan PK, Soumakis K, Gambrell RD Jr. Estrogen replacement therapy in women with previous breast cancer. *Obstet Gynecol* 1999;181:288-295.

Negri E, Tzonou A, Beral V, et al. Hormonal therapy for menopause and ovarian cancer in a collaborative re-analysis of European studies. *Int J Cancer* 1999;80:848-851.

Newcomb PA, Longnecker MP, Storer BE, et al. Long-term hormone replacement therapy and risk of breast cancer in postmenopausal women. *Am J Epidemiol* 1995;142:788-795.

Persson I, Yuen J, Bergkvist L, Shairer C. Cancer incidence and mortality in women receiving estrogen and estrogen-progestin replacement therapy: long-term follow-up of a Swedish cohort. *Int J Cancer* 1996;67:327-221.

Powles TJ, Hickish T, Kanis JA, et al. Effect of tamoxifen on bone mineral density measured by dual-energy x-ray absorptiometry in healthy premenopausal and postmenopausal women. *J Clin Oncol* 1996;14:78-84.

Ross RK, Paganini-Hill A, Wan PC, Pike MC. Effect of hormone replacement therapy on breast cancer risk: estrogen versus estrogen plus progestogen. *J Natl Cancer Inst* 2000;92:328-332.

Schagen SB, van Dam FS, Muller MJ, et al. Cognitive deficits after postoperative adjuvant chemotherapy for breast carcinoma. *Cancer* 1999;85:640-650.

Schairer C, Lubin J, Troisi R, Sturgeon S, Brinton L, Hoover R. Menopausal estrogen and estrogen-progestin replacement therapy and breast cancer risk. *JAMA* 2000;283:485-491.

Sellers TA, Mink PJ, Cerhan JR, et al. The role of hormone replacement therapy in the risk for breast cancer and total mortality in women with a family history of breast cancer. *Ann Intern Med* 1997;127:973-980.

Speroff L. Postmenopausal estrogen-progestin therapy and breast cancer: a clinical response to epidemiological reports. *Climacteric* 2000;3:3-12.

Stanford JL, Weiss NS, Voigt LF, Daling JR, Habel LA, Rossing MA. Combined estrogen and progestin hormone replacement therapy in relation to risk of breast cancer in middle-aged women. *JAMA* 1995;274:137-142.

van Dam FS, Schagen SB, Muller MJ, et al. Impairment of cognitive function in women receiving adjuvant treatment for high-risk breast cancer: high-dose versus standard-dose chemotherapy. *J Natl Cancer Inst* 1998;90:210-218.

Wagner TM, Moslinger RA, Muhr D, et al. BRCA1-related breast cancer in Austrian breast and ovarian cancer families: specific BRCA1 mutations and pathological characteristics. *Int J Cancer* 1998;77:354-360.

Walsh BW, Kuller LH, Wild RA, et al. Effects of raloxifene on serum lipids and coagulation factors in healthy postmenopausal women. *JAMA* 1998;279:1445-1451.

Wile AG, Opfell RW, Margileth DA. Hormone replacement therapy in previously treated breast cancer patients. *Am J Surg* 1993; 165:372-375.

The Writing Group for the PEPI Trial. Effects of hormone replacement therapy on endometrial biopsy in postmenopausal women. *JAMA* 1996;275:370-375.

The Writing Group for the Women's Health Initiative Investigators. Risks and benefits of estrogen plus progestin in healthy postmenopausal women: principal results from the Women's Health Initiative randomized controlled trial. *JAMA* 2002;288:321-333.

N.03. Cervical/ovarian cancer

Neither cervical nor ovarian cancer is linked with menopause. There is no convincing evidence that use of the postmenopausal hormone regimens available today is associated with either increasing or decreasing the risk of cervical or ovarian cancer.

Nevertheless, there is a relatively large volume of observational trial data that point to an association between ERT/HRT use and increased ovarian cancer risk. In a cohort of 44,241 postmenopausal women who had participated in the Breast Cancer Detection Demonstration Project (BCDDP), unopposed ERT use, especially use for more than 10 years, had an increased risk for ovarian cancer. Overall, ever-use of unopposed ERT was associated with a 60% greater risk of developing ovarian cancer compared with never-use. The risk increased with duration of use — those who used ERT for 10 to 19 years had a relative risk (RR) of 1.8 and those with 20 or more years had an RR of 3.2. Women who only used an estrogen-progestogen combination did not have a significantly increased risk of developing ovarian cancer.

Similar findings were reported previously. A large, prospective, epidemiologic observational study involving 211,581 postmenopausal women followed from 1982 through 1996 found that ever-users of hormone therapy (both ERT and HRT, but most were on ERT alone) had a significantly increased risk for death from ovarian cancer. Duration of use also was associated with a higher risk of ovarian cancer mortality. Women who used hormones for 10 or more years had a statistically increased risk for ovarian cancer mortality compared with never-users. Women using hormones for less than 10 years did not have an increased risk.

In this study, risk decreased with time since last use of hormones. Women who had not used hormones for at least 15 years did not have a significantly increased risk, whereas women who had stopped hormone use within 15 years did have a significantly increased risk. This series is limited by the relatively small number of ovarian cancer deaths in women who were hormone users at the time of study entry (n = 31) and those who were former users (n = 35). The impact of progestin therapy was unknown in this study.

A European study updated a collaborative reanalysis of European case-control ovarian cancer studies found a similar trend. Women who had stopped hormone therapy (both ERT and HRT) within the past 10 years had an increased risk for ovarian cancer that reached statistical significance. If the time since the last hormone use was 10 years or more, there was no increased risk for ovarian cancer.

Finally, a meta-analysis of 15 case-control studies of ERT/HRT and the risk of epithelial ovarian cancer failed to demonstrate that ERT/HRT has an important effect on risk of epithelial ovarian cancer.

These recent studies suggest that there may be a moderate, positive association of ERT/HRT use in postmenopausal women at risk for ovarian cancer, but additional epidemiologic studies are needed.

No epidemiological studies have linked ERT/HRT with squamous cell cancers of the cervix. One small epidemiologic study demonstrated a statistically increased risk for adenocarcinomas of the cervix among unopposed ERT users. It should be noted that in the same study, women using a progestogen had no statistical increased risk for the development of adenocarcinoma of the cervix. However, much larger epidemiologic studies are needed before these data should influence management of postmenopausal women considering ERT/HRT.

Bibliography

Coughlin SS, Giustozzi AG, Smith SJ, Lee NC. A meta-analysis of estrogen replacement therapy and risk of epithelial ovarian cancer. *J Clin Epidemiol* 2000;53:367-375.

Lacey JV Jr, Brinton LA, Barnes WA, et al. Use of hormone replacement therapy and adenocarcinomas and squamous cell carcinomas of the uterine cervix. *Gynecol Oncol* 2000;77:149-154.

Lacey JV Jr, Mink PJ, Lubin JH, et al. Menopausal hormone replacement therapy and risk of ovarian cancer. *JAMA* 2002;288:334-341.

Rodriguez C, Calle EE, Coates RJ, Miracle-McMahill HL, Thun MJ, Heath CW Jr. Hormone replacement therapy and fatal ovarian cancer. *Am J Epidemiol* 1995;141:828-825.

Rodriguez C, Patel AV, Calle EE, Jacob EJ, Thun MJ. Estrogen replacement therapy and ovarian cancer mortality in a large prospective study of US women. *JAMA* 2001;285:1460-1465.

Wagner TM, Moslinger RA, Muhr D, et al. BRCA1-related breast cancer in Austrian breast and ovarian cancer families: specific BRCA1 mutations and pathological characteristics. *Int J Cancer* 1998;77:354-360.

N.04. Colorectal cancer

Colorectal cancer risk is not associated with menopause. However, the risk increases with smoking, an inactive lifestyle, and age. The role of diet is controversial, although some evidence indicates that exercise and healthy eating habits (eg, low-fat, high-fiber diet) may have a protective effect. Aspirin and other nonsteroidal anti-inflammatory drugs also have been associated with some reduction in colorectal cancer risk. Evidence suggests that high calcium intake (1,200 mg/day) provides some chemoprotective properties against colorectal cancer. Further studies are needed before specific recommendations can be made.

Accumulating evidence indicates that postmenopausal ERT/HRT may reduce the risk of colorectal cancer. Studies have shown that oral estrogen decreases the production of certain bile acids that promote tumor growth.

In the WHI, a significantly decreased risk of colorectal cancer was found (overall RR, 0.63). The risk was lowest for longer use, with the year 5 RR at 0.47 and year 6 and later at 0.56.

The reductions are consistent with results found in observational studies. In a meta-analysis of 18 epidemiologic studies of postmenopausal hormone therapy and colorectal cancer, significant reductions in the risk of colon cancer (20%) and rectal cancer (19%) were found for women who had taken hormones compared with never-users. Current users had the greatest reduction in colorectal cancer risk (34% reduction).

A similar meta-analysis of 25 studies found that current ERT/HRT use significantly reduced the risk of colon cancer (by 33%) but not rectal cancer. Ever use of ERT/HRT did not substantially affect the risk for either colon or rectal cancer. Any conclusions are limited because none of the studies are randomized controlled trials.

This evidence suggests that women at risk for colorectal cancer could benefit from ERT/HRT. The optimal dose and duration are unknown. ERT/HRT is not FDA-approved for the prevention of colorectal cancer.

Bibliography

Baron JA, Beach M, Mandel JS, et al, for the Calcium Polyp Prevention Study Group. Calcium supplements for the prevention of colorectal adenomas. *N Engl J Med* 1999;340:101-107.

Jänne PA, Mayer RJ. Chemoprevention of colorectal cancer. *N Engl J Med* 2000;342:1960-1968.

Grodstein F, Newcomb PA, Stampfer MJ. Postmenopausal hormone therapy and the risk of colorectal cancer: a review and meta-analysis. *Am J Med* 1999;106:574-582.

Nanda K, Bastian LA, Hasselblad V, Simel DL. Hormone replacement therapy and the risk of colorectal cancer: a meta-analysis. *Obstet Gynecol* 1999;93:880-888.

Persson I, Yuen J, Bergkvist L, Shairer C. Cancer incidence and mortality in women receiving estrogen and estrogen-progestin replacement therapy: long-term follow-up of a Swedish cohort. *Int J Cancer* 1996;67:327-221.

The Writing Group for the Women's Health Initiative Investigators. Risks and benefits of estrogen plus progestin in healthy postmenopausal women: principal results from the Women's Health Initiative randomized controlled trial. *JAMA* 2002; 288:321-333.

Section O: Management strategies: Premature/induced menopause

Women who experience premature menopause (ie, before age 40) — whether induced or spontaneous — will spend more years without the protection of estrogen, increasing their lifetime risk for osteoporosis and, possibly, cardiovascular disease. The younger a woman is when she reaches menopause, the longer she is without high levels of endogenous estrogen. Women who experience premature menopause must be encouraged to change the modifiable risk factors related to lower estrogen levels.

Treatment options include psychological support (eg, for early loss of fertility, self-image and sexual function concerns) as well as pharmacologic therapy to treat acute menopause-related symptoms and to reduce the risk of osteoporosis and cardiovascular disease. Adoption of a more healthy lifestyle should be recommended for these women, regardless of their decision to initiate drug therapy.

Women experiencing premature menopause may consider estrogen replacement therapy (ERT) or, if their uterus is intact, hormone replacement therapy (HRT) to relieve acute symptoms of estrogen deficiency. Because of evidence from the Women's Health Initiative (WHI) showing greater risk than benefit for long-term therapy (>5 yrs) with continuous-combined conjugated equine estrogens (CEE) and medroxyprogesterone acetate, long-term HRT use is being re-evaluated. The WHI trial with CEE alone is still ongoing, with benefits presumably outweighing risks. More definitive data will be available after the trial ends in 2005.

Following premature menopause, some clinicians may manage the acute symptoms with ERT/HRT, and then choose a bone-specific agent (eg, bisphosphonate or SERM) for women who need long-term protection against bone loss. Cardiovascular risk can be lowered through other means as well. Some clinicians will be comfortable using HRT or estrogen alone long-term.

In some studies, 20% of women who experience premature menopause spontaneously ovulate within 4 months. If ERT/HRT is considered, women must be advised of this possibility. In some situations, the use of an oral contraceptive may be more appropriate than ERT/HRT. Assessment for associated endocrine and autoimmune disorders may also be indicated.

Women who experience induced menopause have additional needs because their ovarian levels fall dramatically, typically resulting in more sudden and severe menopausal symptoms. Higher starting doses of ERT are often used to manage these symptoms (ie, 1.25 mg or more of CEE or the equivalent). Many clinicians begin therapy the day of surgery, often using an estrogen patch since oral therapy is difficult to use immediately after surgery.

Androgen is reduced in women who experience induced menopause, and treatment with low-dose testosterone or methyltestosterone is often successful in restoring any loss of sexual desire that may result.

Bibliography

Anasti J. Premature ovarian failure: an update. *Fertil Steril* 1988;70:1-15.

Gorodeski GI, Utian WH. Epidemiology and risk factors of cardiovascular disease in postmenopausal women. In: Lobo RA, ed. *Treatment of the Postmenopausal Woman: Basic and Clinical Aspects.* 2nd ed. Philadelphia, PA: Lippincott Williams & Wilkins; 1999:331-359.

Kalantaridou SN, Davis SR, Nelson LM. Premature ovarian failure. *Endocrinol Metab Clin North Am* 1998;27:989-1006.

Nasir J, Walton C, Lindow, S, Masson E. Spontaneous recovery of chemotherapy-induced primary ovarian failure: implications for management. *Clin Endocrinol* 1997;46:217-219.

The North American Menopause Society. Clinical challenges of perimenopause: consensus opinion of The North American Menopause Society. *Menopause* 2000;7:5-13.

Pouilles JM, Tremollieres F, Bonneu M, Ribot C. Influence of early age at menopause on vertebral bone mass. *J Bone Miner Res* 1994;9:311-315.

Rebar RW, Cedars MI, Liu JH. Premature ovarian failure: a model for the menopause? In: Lobo RA, ed. *Perimenopause.* New York, NY: Springer-Verlag; 1997:7-11.

van Kasteren Y. Treatment concepts for premature ovarian failure. *J Soc Gynecol Invest* 2001;8(suppl 1):S58-S59.

Vega EM, Egea MA, Mautalen CA. Influence of the menopausal age on the severity of osteoporosis in women with vertebral fractures. *Maturitas* 1994;19:117-124.

The Writing Group for the Women's Health Initiative Investigators. Risks and benefits of estrogen plus progestin in healthy postmenopausal women: principal results from the Women's Health Initiative randomized controlled trial. *JAMA* 2002; 288:321-333.

This section will address clinical management of women reaching menopause who have concomitant health conditions. Included are conditions for which some data exist regarding their relationship to ovarian hormones, namely, diabetes, thyroid disease, arthritis, lupus, epilepsy, pancreatitis, gallbladder disease, asthma, and Raynaud's syndrome

P.01. Diabetes

As women age, they are more likely to develop non-insulin-dependent diabetes mellitus (type 2 DM). About 12.5% of women aged 50 to 59 have type 2 DM, with prevalence increasing to 17% to 18% at age 60 and older. The disease remains undiagnosed in about one-third of women with the disease. Type 2 DM is more prevalent in non-Caucasian women.

Some women reaching menopause have preexisting insulin-dependent diabetes mellitus (type 1 DM). Whether a woman has type 1 or type 2 DM, she has increased risks compared with women without DM.

A postmenopausal woman who has DM is three times more likely to develop cardiovascular disease (CVD) or stroke and is four times more likely to die from a myocardial infarction (MI) than a woman without DM.

Women who have DM are at increased risk for other diseases. Their risk for developing endometrial cancer or gallstones is doubled. The incidence of breast cancer does not appear to be affected by DM. The risk for osteoporosis may be lower, possibly because of the obesity associated with DM.

To address the difference between natural and induced menopause and the role that menopause plays in DM and its complications, NAMS developed a consensus opinion regarding type 2 DM. Some of the recommendations also apply to women with type 1 DM. Optimal glucose control (eg, glycated hemoglobin <7%) and controlling risk factors for cardiovascular events are primary goals of therapy for all women who have DM.

In 2000, NAMS published its recommendations for postmenopausal women who have or are at risk for developing type 2 DM. They include the following:

- Controlling CVD risk factors through pharmacologic and nonpharmacologic means can significantly decrease risk for cardiovascular events.

- A broad-based recommendation for estrogen replacement therapy (ERT; estrogen alone) or hormone replacement therapy (HRT; estrogen plus a progestogen) cannot be made; the benefits and risks must be weighed in the context of each woman's risk factors. Two large studies published in 2002 led to modification of NAMS recommendations. Given the results of the Heart and Estrogen/progestin Replacement Study (HERS) trial, ERT/HRT should not be initiated for the secondary prevention of CHD. Given the results of the Women's Health Initiative (WHI), HRT — at least continuous-combined conjugated equine estrogens (CEE) and medroxyprogesterone acetate (MPA) — cannot be recommended for primary prevention.

- If ERT/HRT is recommended, the greatest benefits may be obtained through the use of transdermal estrogen preparations and low doses of oral estrogens.

- If oral HRT is required, continuous-cyclic therapy is recommended, rather than continuous-combined therapy, to minimize exposure to progestogen. The use of low-dose, oral micronized progesterone is recommended, although vaginal or intrauterine progesterone formulations may also minimize the potential for negative metabolic events.

- Counseling can maximize the woman's adherence to multiple medication regimens and increase her understanding of the potential benefits and risks of ERT/HRT.

Peri- and postmenopausal women should undergo screening for DM, hyperlipidemia, and hypertension. Screening should be considered every 3 years for all women aged 45 years and older and for younger women who have other risk factors. DM is diagnosed when, on two or more occasions, the fasting plasma glucose is 126 mg/dL (6.99 mmol/L) or greater or the 2-hour postload glucose is 200 mg/dL (11.1 mmol/L) or greater.

In women who have DM, with or without CVD, the low-density lipoprotein (LDL) cholesterol target is below 100 mg/dL (2.59 mmol/L).

Target blood pressure in hypertensive women who have DM is below 130/85 mm Hg. Blood pressure control is especially important in the setting of DM, as higher blood pressure increases risks for renal dysfunction and CVD.

Women with DM should also be screened for the presence of microalbuminuria. If microalbuminuria and hypertension are both present, treatment with angiotensin-converting enzyme (ACE) inhibitors is recommended. This class of antihypertensive agents has been shown to delay the progression to nephropathy. The ACE inhibitors are also recommended for normotensive patients with type 1 DM who have microalbuminuria because a high proportion of them will develop overt nephropathy.

Because women with DM have an increased incidence of endometrial cancer, pelvic ultrasound or endometrial biopsy may be indicated before initiating ERT/HRT (especially if the woman is anovulatory). Particular vigilance is necessary for any unscheduled uterine bleeding in a postmenopausal woman with DM. The woman's medical history also should be reviewed for a predisposition to gallbladder disease.

Lifestyle modification is very important. Weight reduction has been shown to decrease insulin resistance. Because a weight-loss program limits fat intake, it also improves the lipid profile. Exercise has been shown to reduce insulin resistance and improve control of both glucose levels and lipids in individuals with DM. Excessive alcohol consumption is associated with hyper- and hypoglycemia and should be avoided, along with smoking.

Use of low-dose aspirin may be appropriate. A meta-analysis of 145 prospective, controlled trials of antiplatelet therapy estimated that 38 vascular events per 1,000 patients who have DM would be prevented if aspirin therapy were used for secondary prevention. This finding was further supported by the Early Treatment Diabetic Retinopathy Study.

In a study from The Netherlands, high serum levels of homocysteine were found to be related to 5-year mortality independent of other major risk factors. They appeared to be a stronger (1.9-fold) risk factor for mortality in men and women with type 2 DM than in those without DM. Homocysteine levels can be reduced by decreased consumption of animal protein and increasing intake of B vitamins, including folate.

Studies have consistently demonstrated that reductions in total cholesterol and LDL levels and increases in levels of high-density lipoprotein (HDL) cholesterol are associated with CVD risk reduction. Both pravastatin (Pravachol) and simvastatin (Zocor) have been shown to significantly reduce cardiovascular events in a subset of individuals who have DM to a greater extent than in those without DM. In a separate pravastatin study, although all treated individuals experienced a benefit, women older than age 65 had a greater benefit from therapy than did age-matched men. Women who have DM and elevated cholesterol levels should be treated as aggressively as men, because the presence of DM seems to inhibit the protective effect of female gender in cardiovascular risk.

Women with either type 1 or type 2 DM present a clinical challenge when hormone therapy is indicated (either as a contraceptive or menopause therapy). One comparative study in women with DM found that, compared with copper T 380A intrauterine device users, significantly higher triglycerides and HDL and lower LDL were observed in low-dose oral contraceptive (OC) users, while depot MPA users had significantly higher triglycerides and LDL and lower HDL. Partial thromboplastin time was prolonged in users of subdermal levonorgestrel (Norplant). The investigators concluded that, in women with DM, depot MPA has an unfavorable metabolic outcome and low-dose OCs produce some metabolic alterations, whereas Norplant has minimal metabolic alterations. In women aged 18 to 50 at high risk for DM, depot MPA was associated with a greater risk of diabetes compared with combination OCs.

In the Nurses' Health Study, after 12 years of follow-up, there was no evidence that the risk for DM was associated with the dose or duration of ERT/HRT or with the use of ERT versus HRT. In the Rancho Bernardo Study, a second prospective trial, the risk for DM was not significantly increased or decreased by ERT/HRT in postmenopausal women followed for 11 years. Another prospective study found no association between ERT/HRT use and risk of DM in more than 21,000 postmenopausal women. A 3-year randomized, double-blind clinical trial in women without DM found that oral CEE, either alone or in combination with a progestogen (MPA or oral micronized progesterone), slightly decreased fasting glucose levels compared with placebo while CEE in combination with MPA increased 2-hour glucose levels. Glucose levels are the strongest single predictor of risk for diabetes.

An epidemiologic review of the literature published from 1989 through 1998 found inconclusive evidence that postmenopausal ERT affects the risk of diabetes. However, the review did find that ERT increases the risk of gallbladder disease and cholecystectomy. Women who have DM and underlying gallbladder disease should be followed closely for the development of gallstones.

In women with DM, several short-term, randomized, placebo-controlled trials of ERT/HRT and glycemic control have been conducted. None included more than 60 women. In three trials that used oral estrogen, unopposed ERT (estradiol or CEE) improved glycemic control. Improved glycemic control was also observed in a trial that used oral CEE plus MPA. However, in other trials, no significant differences in glycemic control were observed for oral CEE plus cyclic medrogestone or transdermal estradiol plus oral norethisterone. In all these trials, only transdermal estradiol plus norethisterone did not worsen triglyceride levels.

The Wisconsin Epidemiologic Study of Diabetic Retinopathy concluded that use of OCs or ERT among women with either type 1 or type 2 DM does not appear to affect the severity of diabetic retinopathy or incidence of macular edema.

Women with type 2 DM have a high short-term risk for a coronary event and a particularly high mortality rate associated with those events. The most recent guidelines from the American Heart Association (AHA) have deemed that DM is a risk factor for CVD equivalent to that of having established CVD. For these women, the guidelines call for more aggressive treatment of high cholesterol as a means to reduce CVD risk, including lifestyle changes and drug intervention. The AHA and NAMS recommend cholesterol-lowering drugs as the preferred therapy, not ERT/HRT.

In women with DM who need ERT/HRT, transdermal ERT may offer advantages over the oral route. Serum triglyceride levels, often increased in women who have DM, are not increased further with transdermal ERT.

A daily dose equivalent to oral doses of 1 mg estradiol or 0.625 mg CEE or lower is recommended, even if vasomotor symptoms are still present at this dose. Higher doses have not been associated with increased benefit on the lipid profile, but they have been associated with decreased insulin sensitivity in a small study.

Observational studies have shown that ERT has beneficial effects on plasma lipids, insulin sensitivity, vasodilation, atherosclerosis, and arterial response to injury. While adding some progestogens may diminish these beneficial effects, in general, they do not eliminate them. Research suggests that the progestogen component of hormone therapy may attenuate the beneficial effects of estrogen on HDL, insulin sensitivity, and endothelial function. The NAMS consensus opinion concluded that, if HRT is required in a woman with DM, exposure to progestogen should be minimized. Selecting a metabolically neutral progestogen for HRT, such as micronized progesterone or norgestimate, is recommended to maintain higher plasma HDL. Progestins with a higher androgenic potency reduce more of the beneficial effects of estrogens on vasodilation; progesterone and 19-norpregnane derivatives have less of an adverse effect. For women with DM, continuous-cyclic HRT regimens are recommended to minimize progestogen exposure; low-dose oral micronized progesterone is also recommended.

Androgens should be used with caution in postmenopausal women who have DM. If androgen therapy is required, methyltestosterone should be avoided because it has been shown to decrease HDL levels and may also cause glucose intolerance.

Postmenopausal women who have DM are likely to be taking multiple medications to treat concomitant diseases, thereby increasing the likelihood of poor adherence to medication regimens. Counseling, therefore, is extremely important.

Bibliography

American Diabetes Association. Position statement: standards of medical care for patients with diabetes mellitus. *Diabetes Care* 2002;25(suppl 1):S33-S44.

Andersson B, Mattsson LA, Hahn L, et al. Estrogen replacement therapy decreases hyperandrogenicity and improves glucose homeostasis and plasma lipids in postmenopausal women with noninsulin-dependent diabetes mellitus. *J Clin Endocrinol Metab* 1997;82:638-643.

Antiplatelet Trialists' Collaboration. Collaborative overview of randomised trials of antiplatelet therapy. I: Prevention of death, myocardial infarction, and stroke by prolonged antiplatelet therapy in various categories of patients. *BMJ* 1994;308:81-106.

Barnard RJ, Jung T, Inkeles SB. Diet and exercise in the treatment of NIDDM: the need for early emphasis. *Diabetes Care* 1994; 17:1469-1472.

Barrett-Connor E. Postmenopausal estrogen therapy and selected (less-often-considered) disease outcomes. *Menopause* 1999;6:14-20.

Barrett-Connor E, Grady D. Hormone replacement therapy, heart disease, and other considerations. *Ann Rev Public Health* 1998; 19:55-72.

Brussaard HE, Gevers Leuven JA, Frolich M, Kluft C, Krans HM. Short-term oestrogen replacement therapy improves insulin resistance, lipids and fibrinolysis in postmenopausal women with NIDDM. *Diabetologia* 1997;40:843-849.

Diab KM, Zaki MM. Contraception in diabetic women: comparative metabolic study of Norplant, depot medroxyprogesterone acetate, low dose oral contraceptive pill and CuT380A. *J Obstet Gynaecol Res* 2000;26:17-26.

Expert Panel on Detection, Evaluation, and Treatment of High Blood Cholesterol in Adults. Executive summary of the Third Report of the National Cholesterol Education Program (NCEP) Expert Panel on Detection, Evaluation, and Treatment of High Blood Cholesterol in Adults (Adult Treatment Panel III). *JAMA* 2001; 285:2486-2497.

Friday KE, Dong C, Fontenot RU. Conjugated equine estrogen improves glycemic control and blood lipoproteins in postmenopausal women with type 2 diabetes. *J Clin Endocrinol Metab* 2001;86:48-52.

Gabal LL, Goodman-Gruen D, Barrett-Connor E. The effect of postmenopausal estrogen therapy on the risk of non-insulin-dependent diabetes mellitus. *Am J Public Health* 1997;87:443-445.

Goldberg RB, Mellies MJ, Sacks FM, et al. Cardiovascular events and their reduction with pravastatin in diabetic and glucose-intolerant and myocardial infarction survivors with average cholesterol levels: subgroup analyses in the cholesterol and recurrent events (CARE) trial. *Circulation* 1998;98:2513-2519.

Goldberg RJ, Larson M, Levy D. Factors associated with survival to 75 years of age in middle-aged men and women. The Framingham Study. *Arch Intern Med* 1996;156:505-509.

Grady D, Herrington D, Bittner V, et al, for the HERS Research Group. Heart and estrogen/progestin replacement study follow-up (HERS II). Part 1: Cardiovascular outcomes during 6.8 years of hormone therapy. *JAMA* 2002;288:49-57.

Haffner SM, Diehl AK, Mitchell DB, Stern MP, Hazuda HP. Increased prevalence of clinical gallbladder disease in subjects with non-insulin-dependent diabetes mellitus. *Am J Epidemiol* 1990; 132:327-335.

Harris MI, Flegal KM, Cowie CC, et al. Prevalence of diabetes, impaired fasting glucose, and impaired glucose tolerance in U.S. adults. The Third National Health and Nutrition Examination Survey, 1988-1994. *Diabetes Care* 1998;21:518-524.

Herrington DM, Reboussin DM, Brosnihan KB, et al. Effects of estrogen replacement on the progression of coronary-artery atherosclerosis. *N Engl J Med* 2000;343:522-529.

Hoogeveen EK, Kostense PJ, Jakobs C, et al. Hyperhomocysteinemia increases risk of death, especially in type 2 diabetes: 5-year follow-up of the Hoorn Study. *Circulation* 2000;101:1506-1511.

Kaplan RC, Heckbert SR, Weiss NS, et al. Postmenopausal estrogens and risk of myocardial infarction in diabetic women. *Diabetes Care* 1998;21:1117-1121.

Kim C, Seidel KW, Begier EA, Kwok YS. Diabetes and depot medroxyprogesterone contraception in Navajo women. *Arch Intern Med* 2001;161:1766-1771.

Klein BE, Klein R, Moss SE. Exogenous estrogen exposures and changes in diabetic retinopathy. The Wisconsin Epidemiologic Study of Diabetic Retinopathy. *Diabetes Care* 1999;22:1984-1987.

Lawrenson RA, Leydon GM, Newson RB, et al. Coronary heart disease in women with diabetes. Positive association with past hysterectomy and possible benefits of hormone replacement therapy. *Diabetes Care* 1999;22:856-857.

Manning PJ, Allum A, Jones S, Sutherland WH, Williams SM. The effect of hormone replacement therapy on cardiovascular risk factors in type 2 diabetes: a randomized controlled trial. *Arch Intern Med* 2001:161:1772-1776.

Manson JE, Colditz GA, Stampfer MJ, et al. A prospective study of maturity-onset diabetes mellitus and risk of coronary heart disease and stroke in women. *Arch Intern Med* 1991;151:1141-1147.

Manson JE, Rimm EB, Colditz GA, et al. A prospective study of postmenopausal estrogen therapy and subsequent incidence of non-insulin-dependent diabetes mellitus. *Ann Epidemiol* 1992; 2:665-673.

Mosca L, Collins P, Herrington DM, et al. Hormone replacement therapy and cardiovascular disease: a statement for healthcare professionals from the American Heart Association. *Circulation* 2001;104:499-503.

The North American Menopause Society. Effects of menopause and estrogen replacement therapy or hormone replacement therapy in women with diabetes mellitus: consensus opinion of The North American Menopause Society. *Menopause* 2000;7:87-95.

Perera M, Sattar N, Petrie JR, et al. The effects of transdermal estradiol in combination with oral norethisterone on lipoproteins, coagulation, and endothelial markers in postmenopausal women with type 2 diabetes: a randomized, placebo-controlled study. *J Clin Endocrinol Metab* 2001;86:1140-1114.

Sacks FM, Pfeffer MA, Moye LA, et al. The effects of pravastatin on coronary events after myocardial infarction in patients with average cholesterol levels. *N Engl J Med* 1996;335:1001-1009.

The Sixth Report of the Joint National Committee on prevention, detection, evaluation, and treatment of high blood pressure. *Arch Intern Med* 1997;157:2413-2446.

Sowers JR. Diabetes mellitus and cardiovascular disease in women. *Arch Intern Med* 1998;158:617-621.

van Daele PL, Stolk RP, Burger H, et al. Bone density in non-insulin-dependent diabetes mellitus. The Rotterdam Study. *Ann Intern Med* 1995;122:409-414.

Weiderpass E, Gridley G, Persson I, et al. Risk of endometrial and breast cancer in patients with diabetes mellitus. *Int J Cancer* 1997;71:360-363.

Wingard DL, Barrett-Connor E. Heart disease and diabetes. In Harris MI, Courie CC, Beiber G, Boyko E, Stern M, Bennet P, eds. *Diabetes in America*. 2nd ed. (NIH Publication No. 95-1468). Washington, DC: US Government Printing Office; 1995.

The Writing Group for the PEPI Trial. Effects of estrogen or estrogen/progestin regimens on heart disease risk factors in postmenopausal women. *JAMA* 1995;273:199-208.

The Writing Group for the Women's Health Initiative Investigators. Risks and benefits of estrogen plus progestin in healthy postmenopausal women: principal results from the Women's Health Initiative randomized controlled trial. *JAMA* 2002;288:321-333.

P.02. Thyroid Disease

Approximately one in eight women will develop thyroid disease during their lifetime. *Hypothyroidism* occurs when too little thyroid hormone is released and the metabolic rate slows. Fatigue is the most common symptom. Hypothyroidism in women is frequently underdiagnosed because its symptoms can easily be mistaken for other conditions. *Hyperthyroidism* results from an overactive thyroid gland, which increases metabolism. The most common symptoms are goiter and exophthalmos (bulging eyes).

The rate of hypothyroidism has been noted to rise exponentially after menopause. It is unclear whether this increase is related to decreased level of endogenous estrogen or whether the incidence is affected by use of estrogen replacement therapy (ERT).

Recent cross-sectional data suggest that menopause symptoms are more frequent and cholesterol levels are higher in women with subclinical hypothyroidism. Longitudinal data suggest a significant risk of cardiovascular morbidity if hypothyroidism is not treated. Also, data have suggested that higher doses of thyroxine may be required for women who are using ERT.

It is important to consider the effects of thyroxine on bone mineral density (BMD) and fracture risk. In addition to cross-sectional reports of lower BMD in women on thyroxine, recent data suggest the risk of fracture is also increased. In a large cohort of women over 65 years of age, hip fracture risk was also increased in women with previously diagnosed Graves' disease.

Women on thyroxine supplements should have their serum thyroid-stimulating hormone (TSH) levels monitored. Free thyroxine levels are less accurate for assessing the adequacy of thyroxine supplements. Serum total thyroxine levels are not reliable in women using oral ERT, since the elevation of serum levels of thyroid-binding globulin will lead to misleading elevations of total thyroxine levels but normal free thyroxine and normal TSH levels.

As association has been made between lower estrogen levels occurring after menopause and the presence of thyroid nodularity, which is greater in postmenopausal women than in men of the same age. There is not enough evidence to substantiate this connection.

Bibliography

Arafah BM. Increased need for thyroxine in women with hypothyroidism during estrogen therapy. *N Engl J Med* 2001;344:1743-1749.

Bauer DC, Nevitt MC, Ettinger B, Stone K. Low thyrotropin levels are not associated with bone loss in older women: a prospective study. *J Clin Endocrinol Metab* 1997;82:2931-2936.

Cooper DS. Clinical practice: subclinical hypothyroidism. *N Engl J Med* 2001;354:260-266.

Hak AE, Pols HA, Visser TJ, Drexhage HA, Hofman A, Witteman JC. Subclinical hypothyroidism is an independent risk factor for atherosclerosis and myocardial infarction in elderly women: the Rotterdam Study. *Ann Intern Med* 2000;132:270-278.

Johnston SL, Graves GR, Kendler DL, Flunker MR. Medical and special conditions: Canadian consensus on menopause and osteoporosis. *J SOGC* 2001;23:1096-1101.

Uzzan B, Campos J, Cucherat M, Nony P, Boissel JP, Perret GY. Effects on bone mass of long term treatment with thyroid hormones: a meta-analysis. *J Clin Endocrinol Metab* 1996; 81:4278-4289.

Vanderpump MP, Tunbridge WM, French JM, et al. The incidence of thyroid disorders in the community: a twenty-year follow-up of the Whickham Survey. *Clin Endocrinol* 1995;43:55-68.

P.03. Arthritis

Osteoarthritis (OA) and rheumatoid arthritis (RA) are joint diseases that affect women at midlife and beyond. OA can involve the fingers and the knees, and unlike RA, does not usually produce soft tissue swelling and does not involve the wrists, elbows, shoulders, and ankles. RA typically presents as a symmetrical disease, involving three or more joint groups, and involves stiffness, pain, and swelling of joints. Varying degrees of depression, sometimes related to pain, have been noted in RA patients. RA can also have ocular manifestations (secondary Sjögren's syndrome, with dryness or feelings of sand in the eyes). Other chronic inflammatory forms of arthritis, such as psoriatic arthritis, can have a similar presentation to that of RA, underscoring the importance of a thorough skin examination. Women who develop musculoskeletal complaints along with unexplained mood swings, energy loss, low-grade fevers, and facial flushing should be examined for late-onset systemic lupus erythematosus (see Section P.04.). An abrupt onset of joint pain may indicate infectious causes of arthritis (eg, viral arthritis, including hepatitis).

Osteoarthritis
The most common form of joint disease is osteoarthritis (OA), which increases in frequency with aging. Women suffer more from OA than men. Following menopause, there is an increase in its frequency and severity, leading researchers to associate estrogen with the disease. The role of ERT in reducing the risk for OA has not been established. An epidemiologic review of the literature from 1989-1998 found some suggestion that postmenopausal ERT decreases OA risk, but there is no consistent association by joint site or symptomatology.

Management of women with OA of the knee or hip should be individualized and tailored to the severity of the disease. In mildly symptomatic disease, therapy may be limited to education, physical and occupational therapy, other nonpharmacologic modalities, and pharmacologic therapy that includes nonopioid oral analgesics.

Body weight is associated with knee OA. Studies support a stronger contribution of mechanical as opposed to systemic factors to explain this association. Maintaining a healthy weight is an important strategy for individuals with OA.

OA of the knee may respond to treatment with topical analgesics. Nonsteroidal anti-inflammatory drugs (NSAIDs) are the most commonly prescribed FDA-approved treatment; however, these agents are associated with a high incidence of toxicity, particularly as related to gastrointestinal disorders.

The COX-2 selective inhibitors — celecoxib (Celebrex), rofecoxib (Vioxx) — have demonstrated efficacy equal to NSAIDs but are less toxic to the gastrointestinal tract.

The nutritional supplements glucosamine and chondroitin have appeared to be symptomatically effective in a number of studies, although definitive trials have not been completed. These agents appear to be safe, based on 10 years of use in Europe.

In women with knee OA who have symptomatic effusions, judicious use of intraarticular steroid injections (either as monotherapy or as an adjunct to systemic therapy) is another option. Severe OA of the knee or hip requires a more aggressive approach. Referral for consultation with an orthopedic physician or rheumatologist may be advised.

Rheumatoid arthritis
Rheumatoid arthritis (RA) also has an increased incidence in women compared with men. Approximately 10% of patients with RA have a first-degree relative with the disease. Rheumatoid factor is an important prognostic marker, as those who test positive are more likely to have greater joint destruction and disability; however, the test is not reliable, as those with a negative rheumatoid factor test can still have RA and those with a positive test may not have the disease. During pregnancy, symptoms may improve, suggesting a connection to estrogen.

A matched-population study in Norway published in 2000 found that women who have RA and are older than age 50 have a significantly increased risk for low bone mineral density of the neck and spine compared with women without RA. Further study is required to determine if RA is a risk factor for the development and/or severity of osteoporosis or whether the diagnosis of RA simply provides a selection bias for the known risk factors for osteoporosis. Nevertheless, women with RA are at risk for osteoporosis because of use of corticosteroids and immobility.

An epidemiologic review of the literature from 1989-1998 found that studies of postmenopausal ERT/HRT use for RA are conflicting. Neither RA nor the agents used to treat it are contraindications to the use of ERT/HRT; however, no double-blind, randomized trials have shown that ERT/HRT has a significant effect on the clinical course or disease markers of RA.

Anemia is very common during the active phase of RA, usually attributable to active inflammation, but can also be caused by blood loss in patients taking OTC or prescription NSAIDs. When appropriate, iron therapy can be prescribed.

RA is a potentially debilitating condition that can profoundly affect quality of life. New drug treatments, along with physical and occupational therapy, are promising with respect to slowing or even stopping the progression of disease. Because much of the irreversible joint damage caused by RA occurs within the first 2 years of symptom onset, early recognition and referral to a rheumatologist are essential for achieving the best possible outcomes.

Bibliography

American College of Rheumatology. Guidelines for the management of rheumatoid arthritis. *Arthritis Rheum* 2002;46:328-346.

American College of Rheumatology. Recommendations for the medical management of osteoarthritis of the hip and knee. *Arthritis Rheum* 2000;43:1905-1915.

Barrett-Connor E. Postmenopausal estrogen therapy and selected (less-often-considered) disease outcomes. *Menopause* 1999;6:14-20.

Bijlsma JW, Van den Brink HR. Estrogen and rheumatoid arthritis. *Am J Reprod Immunol* 1992;28:231-234.

Deal C, Moskowitz RW. Nutraceuticals as therapeutic agents in osteoarthritis: the role of glucosamine, chondroitin sulfate, and collagen hydrolystate. *Rheum Dis Clin North Am* 1999;25:379-395.

Gabriel SE, Jaakkimainen L, Bombardier C. Risk for serious gastrointestinal complications related to use of nonsteroidal anti-inflammatory drugs: a meta-analysis. *Ann Intern Med* 1991; 115:787-796.

Hall GM, Spector TD, Delmas PD. Markers of bone metabolism in postmenopausal women with rheumatoid arthritis: effects of corticosteroids and hormone replacement therapy. *Arthritis Rheum* 1995;38:902-906.

Hannan MT, Felson DT, Anderson JJ, Naimark A, Kannel WB. Estrogen use and radiographic osteoarthritis of the knee in women: the Framingham Osteoarthritis Study. *Arthritis Rheum* 1990; 33:525-532.

Haugeberg G, Uhlig T, Falch JA, Halse JI, Kvein TK. Bone mineral density and frequency of osteoporosis in female patients with rheumatoid arthritis: results from 394 patients in the Oslo County Rheumatoid Arthritis register. *Arthritis Rheum* 2000;43:522-530.

Hernandez-Avila M, Liang MH, Willett WC, et al. Exogenous sex hormones and the risk of rheumatoid arthritis. *Arthritis Rheum* 1990;33:947-953.

Hochberg MC, Lethbridge-Cejku M, Scott WW, Reichle R, Plato CC, Tobin JD. The association of body weight, body fatness and body fat distribution with osteoarthritis of the knee: data from the Baltimore Longitudinal Study of Aging. *J Rheumatol* 1995;22:488-493.

MacDonald AG, Murphy EA, Capell HA, Bankowska UZ, Ralston SH. Effects of hormone replacement therapy in rheumatoid arthritis: a double-blind placebo-controlled study. *Ann Rheum Dis* 1994; 53:54-57.

McAlindon TE, La Valley MP, Gulin JP, Felson DT. Glucosamine and chondroitin for treatment of osteoarthritis: a systematic quality assessment and meta-analysis. *JAMA* 2000;283:1469-1475.

Nevitt MC, Cummings SR, Lane NE, et al, for the Study of Osteoporotic Fractures Research Group. Association of estrogen replacement therapy with the risk of osteoarthritis of the hip in elderly white women. *Arch Intern Med* 1996;156:2073-2080.

Oliveria SA, Felson DT, Klein RA, Reed JI, Walker AM. Estrogen replacement therapy and the development of osteoarthritis. *Epidemiology* 1996;7:415-419.

Silman AJ. Rheumatoid arthritis. In: Silman AJ, Hochberg MC, eds. *Epidemiology of the Rheumatic Diseases*. Oxford, Eng: Oxford University Press; 2001:31-71.

Sowers M. Osteoporosis and menopause. In: Lobo RA, Kelsey J, Marcus R, eds. *Menopause: Biology and Pathobiology*. San Diego, CA: Academic Press; 2000:535-542.

Spector TD, Nandra D, Hart DJ, Doyle DV. Is hormone replacement therapy protective for hand and knee osteoarthritis in women? The Chingford study. *Ann Rheum Dis* 1997;56:432-434.

Van Vollenhoven RF, McGuire JL. Estrogen, progesterone, and testosterone: can they be used to treat autoimmune disease? *Cleve Clin J Med* 1994;61:276-284.

Wolfe F, Pincus T. The level of inflammation in rheumatoid arthritis is determined early and remains stable over the longterm course of the illness. *J Rheumatol* 2001;28:1817-1824.

P.04. Lupus

Systemic lupus erythematosus (SLE) is much more common in women than men. SLE is more prevalent in African Americans and those of Hispanic or Asian descent. Outcomes and response to therapy may be affected by race, with African Americans being predisposed to aggressive and treatment-resistant nephritis.

SLE is an autoimmune system rheumatic disease of unknown etiology. SLE mimics many other diseases and often begins with vague flu-like symptoms. Women who develop musculoskeletal complaints along with unexplained mood swings, energy loss, low-grade fevers, and facial rash ("butterfly" rash) should be examined for late-onset systemic lupus erythematosus. It is the most common condition with a presentation similar to that of rheumatoid arthritis; however, SLE is a multisystem disease in which joint involvement is only one feature. Patients with SLE typically have skin involvement, and the lungs and kidneys can be affected as well. Anemia is common.

SLE typically begins in the reproductive years. Symptoms can vary with menses and pregnancy, although a modest decrease in disease activity, especially maximum activity, is seen after menopause. In addition, some women with SLE seem to have abnormal estrogen metabolism and a hypoestrogenic state. A small study conducted in Brazil found that premature menopause is common in women with SLE.

There are numerous reports suggesting an association between oral contraceptive use and lupus flares.

An epidemiologic review of the literature from 1989 to1998 found two studies that suggest a nearly 3-fold increased risk of lupus in women using ERT for 2 or more years. In the Nurses' Health Study, the only prospective study of ERT and SLE, ERT increased the risk of SLE from 1.8-fold to 2.5-fold, and the risk increased with duration of use. These results are similar to those observed in a case-control study in the UK. More studies are needed to confirm this effect.

Some experts believe that postmenopausal hormone use by women with preexisting, stable SLE is well-tolerated and safe. A retrospective study in the UK of postmenopausal women with SLE found, after 12 months of treatment with HRT or placebo, that HRT users experienced significant improvement in general well-being, libido, and depression. Also, in this study, there was no increase in the number of thromboembolic events in the user group, despite 7 of the 30 users having a positive thrombophilia screen associated with lupus. Other trials have also found no adverse impact of ERT/HRT on SLE.

The potential long-term benefits of ERT/HRT assume importance in women with SLE. Risk of osteoporosis is increased with corticosteroid use, which is a common therapy for SLE. In addition, CVD risk is approximately 10 times greater in individuals with SLE than in the general age- and sex-matched population; the prevalence of nonfatal coronary artery disease for those with SLE approaches 5% to 8%.

In 1997, the NIH-sponsored Safety in Lupus Erythematosus National Assessment (SELENA) was begun. In this multi-center, randomized, double-blind, placebo-controlled study inclusive of many ethnic groups, younger women (aged 18-40) with SLE are being treated with an estrogen-progestin contraceptive, whereas postmenopausal women are receiving CEE and MPA. An interim analysis failed to identify a trend regarding hormone use and its effect on disease activity. It is hoped that this trial can provide the basis for definitive recommendations.

SLE is a potentially life-threatening disease, yet advances in drug treatments, along with physical therapy, can help decrease morbidity and mortality. Referral to a rheumatologist is essential.

Bibliography

Arden NK, Lloyd ME, Spector TD, Hughes GR. Safety of hormone replacement therapy (HRT) in systemic lupus erythematosus. *Lupus* 1994;3:11-13.

Barrett-Connor E. Postmenopausal estrogen therapy and selected (less-often-considered) disease outcomes. *Menopause* 1999;6:14-20.

Buyon JP. Hormone replacement therapy in postmenopausal women with systemic lupus erythematosus. *J Am Med Womens Assoc* 1998;53:13-17.

Kreidstein S, Urowitz MB, Gladman DD, Gough J. Hormone replacement therapy in systemic lupus erythematosus. *J Rheumatol* 1997;24:2149-2152.

Medeiros MM, Silveira VA, Menezes AP, Carvalho RC. Risk factors for ovarian failure in patients with systemic lupus erythematosus. *Braz J Med Biol Res* 2001;34:1561-1568.

Meier CR, Sturkenboom MC, Cohen AS, Jick H. Postmenopausal estrogen replacement therapy and the risk of developing systemic lupus erythematosus or discord lupus. *J Rheumatol* 1998;25: 1515-1519.

Mok CC, Lau CS, Ho CT, Lee KW, Mok MY, Wong RW. Safety of hormonal replacement therapy in postmenopausal patients with systemic lupus erythematosus. *Scand J Rheumatol* 1998;27:342-346.

Petri M. Exogenous estrogen in systemic lupus erythematosus: oral contraceptives and hormone replacement therapy. *Lupus* 2001;10:222-226.

Petri M, Perez-Gutthann S, Spence D, Hochberg MC. Risk factors for coronary artery disease in patients with systemic lupus erythematosus. *Am J Med* 1992;93:513-519.

Sanchez-Guerrero J, Liang MH, Karlson EW, Hunter DJ, Colditz GA. Postmenopausal estrogen therapy and the risk for developing systemic lupus erythematosus. *Ann Intern Med* 1995;122:430-433.

Sanchez-Guerrero J, Villegas A, Mendoza-Fuentes A, Romero-Diaz J, Moreno-Coutino G, Cravioto MC. Disease activity during the premenopausal and postmenopausal periods in women with systemic lupus erythematosus. *Am J Med* 2001;111:464-468.

P.05. Epilepsy

Epilepsy is a chronic neurological disease characterized by recurrent seizures. Seizures do not occur randomly in most women and men with epilepsy. They tend to cluster in more than 50% of cases. Seizure clusters, in turn, may occur with temporal rhythmicity in a significant proportion of women (35%) and men (29%) with epilepsy.

In women, seizures may cluster in relation to the menstrual cycle, commonly known as catamenial epilepsy. This is attributable to the neuroactive properties of reproductive hormones and the cyclic variation of their serum levels. Statistical evidence supports the concept of catamenial epilepsy and the existence of at least three distinct patterns of seizure exacerbation in relation to the menstrual cycle: (1) perimenstrual or (2) preovulatory patterns in women with ovulatory cycles and (3) the entire luteal and perimenstrual phase exacerbation.

Natural progesterone therapy may benefit some women with catamenial epilepsy. Two open-label trials showed cyclic progesterone supplements at physiological dosages in the luteal phase of each cycle to be associated with substantially and significantly lower seizure frequencies than optimal antiepileptic drug therapy alone. In contrast, oral synthetic progestins, administered cyclically or continuously, have not proven to be effective therapy. An NIH-sponsored multicenter investigation is under way to evaluate the efficacy of progesterone as a supplemental treatment for epilepsy.

Some evidence suggests that menopause may occur earlier in women with epilepsy than in the general population, especially in women with a high lifetime seizure frequency. Perimenopause is sometimes associated with increased seizure frequency, especially in women who have shown previous evidence of hormonal sensitivity in the form of catamenial seizure exacerbation. This may result from the loss of ovulation and adequate endogenous progesterone production. The effects of HRT with CEE and MPA, the most commonly used HRT, have not been rigorously assessed and are the focus of a current NIH-sponsored multicenter investigation. Unopposed ERT in women with epilepsy who have had a hysterectomy is of theoretical concern because of the previously demonstrated epileptogenic effect of estrogen administration to women with epilepsy, albeit in much higher than the standard dosage.

Perimenopausal women with epilepsy should be counseled that certain antiepileptic drugs (eg, carbamazepine, oxcarbazepine, phenobarbital, phenytoin, primidone, topiramate) can make hormonal contraceptives ineffective, reducing their concentrations by up to 50%, and increasing a woman's risk for an unplanned pregnancy. Antiepileptic medications that do not appear to interfere with the effectiveness of hormonal birth control include felbamate, gabapentin, lamotrigine, levetiracetam, tiagabine, and zonisamide. Effects of antiepileptic medications on ERT/HRT efficacy have not been established.

Bibliography

Abbasi F, Krumholz A, Kittner SJ, Langenberg P. Effects of menopause on seizures in women with epilepsy. *Epilepsia* 1999;40:205-210.

Bäckström T. Epileptic seizures in women related to plasma estrogen and progesterone during the menstrual cycle. *Acta Neurol Scand* 1976;54:321-347.

Epilepsy Foundation. Epilepsy Answer Place. Accessible at http://www.efa.org/answerplace.

Foldvary N. Treatment issues for women with epilepsy. *Neurol Clin* 2001;19:409-425.

Harden CL, Pulver MC, Ravdin L, Jacobs AR. The effect of menopause and perimenopause on the course of epilepsy. *Epilepsia* 1999;40:1402-1407.

Harden CL, Nikolov BG, Koppel BS, et al. Seizure frequency and age of menopause in women with epilepsy. *Epilepsia* 2001; 42(suppl 7):S291.

Herzog AG. Progesterone therapy in women with complex partial and secondary generalized seizures. *Neurology* 1995;45:1660-1662.

Herzog AG. Progesterone therapy in women with epilepsy: a 3-year follow up. *Neurology* 1999;52:1917-1918.

Herzog AG, Klein P, Ransil BJ. Three patterns of catamenial epilepsy. *Epilepsia* 1997;38:1082-1088.

Klein P, Serje A, Pezzullo JC. Premature ovarian failure in women with epilepsy. *Epilepsia* 2001;42:1584-1589.

Mattson RH, Cramer JA, Caldwell BV, Siconolfi BC. Treatment of seizures with medroxyprogesterone acetate: preliminary report. *Neurology* 1984;34:1255-1258.

Shorvon SD, Tallis RC, Wallace HK. Antiepileptic drugs: coprescription of proconvulsant drugs and oral contraceptives: a national study of antiepileptic drug prescribing practice. *J Neurol Neurosurg Psychiatry* 2001;72:114-115.

P.06. Pancreatitis

Menopause does not change the risk of pancreatitis. However, ERT has been associated with pancreatitis in case reports, usually in the setting of severe hypertriglyceridemia (triglyceride level >750 mg/dL or 8.47 mmol/L). Oral ERT increases triglycerides by 15% to 30%; the effect occurs early in therapy and should be monitored. Women with elevated triglycerides at baseline, such as those with type 2 diabetes mellitus or familial hypertriglyceridemia, are at the greatest risk for severe hypertriglyceridemia on ERT.

An epidemiologic review of the literature from 1989 to 1998 concluded that pancreatitis caused by oral ERT/HRT appears to be rare and probably occurs only in women with severe underlying hypertriglyceridemia. The PEPI trial (which excluded women with high triglycerides at baseline) found similar elevated triglycerides in all arms of the study (ie, users of unopposed oral CEE, users of oral CEE plus oral MPA, and users of oral CEE plus oral progesterone).

Transdermal ERT has a neutral or beneficial effect on triglyceride levels, but whether the risk of pancreatitis is lower than with oral ERT has not been studied. Oral and transdermal ERT both increase the risk of gallstones, another mechanism by which the risk of pancreatitis may be increased. Progestins have not been associated with pancreatitis, and may mitigate the triglyceride-elevating effects of oral ERT.

In a study of women with triglyceride levels greater than 750 mg/dL (8.47 mmol/L), oral ERT was found to be contraindicated. Women with baseline triglyceride level greater than 250 mg/dL (2.82 mmol/L) should consider transdermal rather than oral ERT, or have triglycerides monitored while taking oral ERT, to avoid triglyceride-induced pancreatitis.

Bibliography

Barrett-Connor E. Postmenopausal estrogen therapy and selected (less-often considered) disease outcomes. *Menopause* 1999;6:14-20.

Glueck CJ, Lang J, Hamer T, Tracy T. Severe hypertriglyceridemia and pancreatitis when estrogen replacement therapy is given to hypertriglyceridemic women. *J Lab Clin Med* 1994;123:59-64.

Stone, NJ. Estrogen-induced pancreatitis: a caveat worth remembering [editorial]. *J Lab Clin Med* 1994;123:18-19.

Wilmink T, Frick T. Drug-induced pancreatitis. *Drug Saf* 1996;14:406-423.

The Writing Group for the PEPI Trial. Effects of estrogen or estrogen/progestin regimens on heart disease risk factors in postmenopausal women. *JAMA* 1995;273:199-208.

P.07. Gallbladder disease

The prevalence of gallstones in the US population has been estimated at 8% to 10%. Women are more likely to have gallstones than are men. A woman's risk of gallstones increases with obesity, parity, OC use. Both OCs and ERT increase biliary cholesterol saturation, and supersaturated bile is a prerequisite for cholesterol gallstone formation.

An epidemiologic review of the literature from 1989 to 1998 found that ERT increases risk for gallbladder disease and cholecystectomy. This was confirmed in epidemiologic studies, including the Nurses' Health Study and two clinical trials, PEPI and HERS. The HERS trial further found that estrogen plus progestin therapy among postmenopausal women with known coronary disease resulted in a marginally significant increase in the risk for biliary tract surgery.

The only randomized study that compared the impact of transdermal estrogens on biliary markers of gallstone formation found that both oral and nonoral administration of estrogen altered bile comparably in ways that would be expected to form gallstones.

ERT/HRT should be administered with caution to postmenopausal women who have gallstones or a history of gallbladder disease.

The HERS trial found that use of ascorbic acid supplements was associated with a decreased prevalence of gallbladder disease among postmenopausal women who consumed alcohol, but not among nondrinkers. Further study is necessary to confirm these findings.

Bibliography

Barrett-Connor E. Postmenopausal estrogen therapy and selected (less-often-considered) disease outcomes. *Menopause* 1999; 6:14-20.

Hulley S, Grady D, Bush T, et al, for the Heart and Estrogen/progestin Replacement Study (HERS) Research Group. Randomized trial of estrogen plus progestin for secondary prevention of coronary heart disease in postmenopausal women. *JAMA* 1998;280:605-613.

Manson JE, Rimm EB, Colditz GA, et al. A prospective study of postmenopausal estrogen therapy and subsequent incidence of non-insulin-dependent diabetes mellitus. *Ann Epidemiol* 1992; 2:665-673.

Simon JA, Grady D, Snabes MC, Fong J, Hunninghake DB. Ascorbic acid supplement use and prevalence of gallbladder disease. Heart & Estrogen-Progestin Replacement Study (HERS) Research Group. *J Clin Epidemiol* 1998;51:257-265.

Simon JA, Hunninghake DB, Agarwal SK, et al. Effect of estrogen plus progestin on risk for biliary tract surgery in postmenopausal women with coronary artery disease. The Heart and Estrogen/ progestin Replacement Study. *Ann Intern Med* 2001;135:493-501.

Uhler ML, Marks JW, Judd HL. Estrogen replacement therapy and gallbladder disease in postmenopausal women. *Menopause* 2000;7:162-167.

Uhler ML, Marks JW, Voigt BJ, Judd HL. Comparison of the impact of transdermal versus oral estrogen on biliary markers of gallstone formation in postmenopausal women. *J Clin Endocrinol Metab* 1998;83:410-414.

The Writing Group for the PEPI Trial. Effects of estrogen or estrogen/progestin regimens on heart disease risk factors in postmenopausal women. *JAMA* 1995;273:199-208.

P.08. Asthma

The relationship between sex hormones and asthma is complex. Compared with men, women have more hospital admissions due to the disease. Studies are not consistent regarding which phase of the menstrual cycle (premenstrual or preovulatory) is more associated with asthma flares. The relationship between estrogen therapy (either in oral contraceptives or estrogen replacement therapy for menopause) and asthma is also inadequately characterized.

During the reproductive years, women experience an increased incidence and severity of asthma. Some clinicians have postulated that ERT may increase susceptibility to this disease in midlife.

An epidemiologic review of the literature from 1989 to 1998 reported that limited data suggest ERT may increase the risk of new onset asthma. The Nurses' Health Study, the only epidemiologic study of ERT and asthma, found that current use of ERT was associated with increased asthma severity, and that longer use of ERT was associated with increased incidence of asthma. Women who used ERT for 10 or more years had twice the age-adjusted risk of asthma versus never-users. Previous use of oral contraceptives did not affect the results.

A more recent prospective, crossover study of asthmatic women (N = 20) who were at least 2 years postmenopausal found that neither discontinuation nor reinitiation of ERT had any effect on objective measures of airway function. However, women with corticosteroid-dependent asthma, those older than 70 years, and smokers were not studied. The authors concluded that, until data to the contrary are available, ERT should not be withheld from postmenopausal women due to concerns about its effects on asthma.

In a study of 55 asthmatic and 20 healthy postmenopausal women (aged 48-60), measurement of endocrine and spirometric parameters before and after 6 months of transdermal 17β-estradiol and cyclic oral MPA treatment led to the conclusion that HRT in postmenopausal asthmatic women has a favorable influence on the course of asthma. HRT was found to reduce daily use of glucocorticoids and frequency of asthma exacerbations, and normalize serum concentrations of estradiol, cortisol, and dehydroepiandrosterone sulfate (DHEA-S), which were decreased before HRT.

Bibliography

Barrett-Connor E. Postmenopausal estrogen therapy and selected (less-often-considered) disease outcomes. *Menopause* 1999;6:14-20.

Troisi RJ, Speizer FE, Willett WC, Trichopoulos D, Rosner B. Menopause, postmenopausal estrogen preparations, and the risk of adult-onset asthma: a prospective cohort study. *Am J Respir Crit Care Med* 1995;152:1183-1188.

Hepburn MJ, Dooley DP, Morris MJ. The effects of estrogen replacement therapy on airway function in postmenopausal, asthmatic women. *Arch Intern Med* 2001;161:2717-2721.

Los-Kudla B, Ostrowska Z, Marek B, et al. Effects of hormone replacement therapy on endocrine and spirometric parameters in asthmatic postmenopausal women. *Gynecol Endocrinol* 2001;15:304-311.

P.09. Raynaud's syndrome

Raynaud's syndrome is a vascular disorder characterized by intermittent bilateral attacks of ischemia of the fingers or toes (sometimes the ears and nose). It is marked by severe pallor, and is often accompanied by paresthesia and pain.

Reproductive-aged women exhibit the highest prevalence of Raynaud's syndrome. Some clinicians have postulated that hormonal factors may play an important role. Experimental studies have shown an increased vasoconstrictor response to estrogen, a response that can be prevented by the addition of progestogen.

An epidemiologic review of the literature from 1989 to 1998 found only one study on hormone therapy and Raynaud's syndrome. This study suggested an increased risk for Raynaud's syndrome with unopposed estrogen (ERT) but not estrogen plus progestogen (HRT).

In the Framingham Offspring Study of 497 postmenopausal women, 9.9% demonstrated Raynaud's syndrome. The prevalence of this phenomenon was 8.4% among women who did not receive hormone therapy, 19.1% among those receiving estrogen alone, and 9.8% among those receiving estrogen plus progestogen. More research is needed to clarify the association of postmenopausal hormones and Raynaud's syndrome.

Bibliography

Barrett-Connor E. Postmenopausal estrogen therapy and selected (less-often-considered) disease outcomes. *Menopause* 1999;6:14-20.

Fraenkel L, Zhang Y, Chaisson CE, Evans SR, Wilson PW, Felson DT. The association of estrogen replacement therapy and the Raynaud phenomenon in postmenopausal women. *Ann Intern Med* 1998; 129:208-211.

Menopause is a milestone in a woman's life and signals an opportunity to start, or continue, an individualized, appropriate lifestyle program. Women of this millennium can expect to live extended and healthy lives beyond menopause.

The following issues should be included when counseling women about menopause.

Q.01. View of menopause/aging

Menopause is a multidimensional change, which has different meanings and experiences for each woman. It is a major transition in a woman's life, not only because of biological changes but also because of the social and psychological challenges that take place during midlife. For some women, menopause initiates a period of independence, relief from menstrual difficulties, and freedom from contraceptive choices or threat of pregnancy. For others, it is a time associated with the loss of reproductive abilities.

While menopause is a universal fact of life, the physiological and psychological effects for women are not the same within or across all cultures. There is no typical menopause transition.

Various studies have found lifestyle, demographic factors, and attitudes toward menopause all influence a woman's perception of menopause. One study reported that 80% of women experiencing menopause reported no decrease in quality of life (QOL), and 75% of the women denied experiencing any loss of their attractiveness. The majority (62%) of women reported positive attributions to menopause itself. Another study found that most women view menopause as inconsequential, and that other events of midlife are more important or stressful for them. A cohort of well-educated, midlife women participating in the Seattle Midlife Women's Health Study described menopause as a normal developmental event. Only about 10% of peri- and postmenopausal women participating in community-based studies have reported feelings of despair, irritability, and fatigue during menopause. However, no direct connection between mental health issues and menopause-related estrogen decreases has been validated by research studies.

The majority (51%) of US postmenopausal women surveyed in a 1998 NAMS-sponsored Gallup poll reported being happiest and most fulfilled between the ages of 50 to 65 years compared with when they were in their 20s (10%), 30s (17%), or 40s (16%). Many women reported improvement in various areas of their lives since menopause. They reported a sense of personal fulfillment, ability to focus on hobbies or other interests, and improved relationship with spouse/partner, and with other friendships. Most (51%) said their sexual relationships had remained unchanged. Lifestyle behaviors were often initiated by women during this midlife period.

The QOL and health status of a generally low-income and poorly educated population of menopausal-aged women were examined in a cross-sectional design study. Women who were employed, had higher levels of education, or higher levels of income reported better overall health and fewer menopausal symptoms. There were no significant differences between ethnic groups with respect to either menopausal QOL or health status.

The surgical intervention of hysterectomy (with bilateral oophorectomy) did not appear to be a factor in decreasing QOL. Compared with women with an intact uterus, hysterectomized women expressed more improvement, especially in the areas of sexual relationships, spouse/partner relationships, personal fulfillment, and physical health; this improvement did not appear to be the result of hormone replacement therapy.

Survey research does not verify the concept of a "midlife crisis" as universal or even widely present in the general population. However, women in midlife may fear aging for a variety of reasons, some of which are universal, some peculiar to their culture, and the rest reflect their personal and family circumstances. Women may react to a multitude of midlife changes that could elicit fear and anxiety.

Healthcare professionals can be an integral part of the resources women use to make the lifestyle adjustments that enable them to thrive. Collaboration between the clinician and woman, characterized by mutual respect and trust, is the goal of menopause counseling, with discussions based on the woman's health, social history, and family history. The importance of individualized screening and management approaches for each woman is important.

Women need accurate information about physiological changes, and the prevention and treatment of typical midlife conditions. Although menopause is perhaps the most prominent physical event, general knowledge about the aging process is also needed. Additionally, psychological support, both through counseling and pharmacological intervention, may be required for the many psychosocial issues facing women in midlife.

Recognizing and reacting to women's emotional concerns, such as financial, relationship, and caregiving burdens, is a major preventive measure for the development of stress-related disorders. Considering the woman's preferences, values, and key concerns, the clinician should provide education and facilitate informed decision making. Additionally, validating the woman's confidence in the decision made and in her ability to carry it out or modify it over time should also be a focus of menopause counseling.

Bibliography

Administration on Aging. *A Profile of Older Americans: 2000.* Washington, DC: US Department of Health and Human Services/Administration on Aging; 2000.

Avis NE, Stellato R, Crawford S, et al. Is there a menopausal syndrome? Menopausal status and symptoms across racial/ethnic groups. *Soc Sci Med* 2001;52:345-356.

Brzyski RG, Medrano MA, Hyatt-Santos JM, Ross JS. Quality of life in low-income menopausal women attending primary care clinics. *Fertil Steril* 2001;76:44-50.

Gold EB, Sternfeld B, Kelsey JL, et al. Relation of demographic and lifestyle factors to symptoms in a multi-racial/ethnic population of women 40-55 years of age. *Am J Epidemiol* 2000;152:463-473.

Jacobs Institute of Women's Health, Expert Panel on Menopause Counseling. *Guidelines for Counseling Women on the Management of Menopause.* Washington, DC: Jacobs Institute of Women's Health; 2000.

Lock M, Kaufert P. Menopause, local biologies, and cultures of aging. *Am J Human Biol* 2001;3:494-504.

The North American Menopause Society. Clinical challenges of perimenopause: consensus opinion of The North American Menopause Society. *Menopause* 2000;7:5-13.

Obermeyer CM. Menopause across cultures: a review of the evidence. *Menopause* 2000;7:184-192.

Schneider HP, Schultz-Zehden B, Rosemeier H, Behre H. Assessing well-being in menopausal women. In: Studd J, ed. *The Management of the Menopause: The Millennium Review 2000.* Pearl River, NY: The Parthenon Publishing Group; 2000:11-19.

Sommer B, Avis N, Meyer P, et al. Attitudes toward menopause and aging across ethnic/racial groups. *Psychosom Med* 1999;61:868-875.

Utian WH, Boggs P. The North American Menopause Society 1998 menopause survey. Part I: Postmenopausal women's perceptions about menopause and midlife. *Menopause* 1999;6:122-128.

Winterich JA, Umberson D. How women experience menopause: the importance of social context. *J Women Aging* 1999;11:57-73.

Woods NF, Mitchell ES. Anticipating menopause: observations from the Seattle Midlife Women's Health Study. *Menopause* 1999;6:167-173.

Q.02. Social and cultural aspects of care

Social and cultural differences between middle-class Caucasian women and African American, Native American, Latino, and Asian American women have implications both for the way in which they experience menopause and for their future health and well-being. Risk factors, morbidity and mortality patterns, and access to health care all differ among these groups. However, there are few data on these differences as they relate to menopause and to estrogen replacement therapy (ERT) and hormone replacement therapy (estrogen plus progestogen; HRT).

Nearly 10% of the US population is foreign born. Nearly 15% speaks a foreign language at home. Hispanic Americans are the largest minority population in the United States. In 2000, there will be an estimated 30 million Hispanic Americans. Millions of American-born residents follow the traditions and beliefs of other cultures.

In 2000, there were approximately 40 million postmenopausal women in the United States. Within that number, an increasing percentage will be racially and ethnically diverse. This is estimated to include over 3.5 million African American women, 1 to 2 million Hispanic women, and 1 million Asian women. Thus, it is likely that most practitioners in the United States will care for women from other cultures.

Canadian healthcare professionals face similar social and cultural challenges in meeting the needs of an increasingly diverse population. In the 1996 census, 17.5% of the population were immigrants. This represented a 14.5% increase from 1991, three times the growth rate of the Canadian-born population. Sources of immigration to Canada have also changed. Throughout much of the 20th century, the United Kingdom, the United States, and Europe were the major sources. In more recent years, this trend has changed, with increasing number of immigrants from Asia, Central and South America, the Middle East, and Africa.

Also to be considered are the concerns of Native Canadian women. Although they represent less than one-third of the total Canadian population, an increasing disproportionate incidence and prevalence of chronic illnesses have been documented (eg, diabetes, cardiovascular disease, cancer, end-stage renal disease).

Unfortunately, the current body of health information is based on Caucasian, relatively healthy, middle-class women. Nevertheless, significant differences exist between racial and ethnic groups.

Morbidity and mortality from chronic diseases are significantly different among different races. In the United States, the rates of diabetes, hypertension, and obesity are much higher among African American, Latino, and Native American women than among Caucasian women. The lifetime probability of developing coronary heart disease is similar for African American and Caucasian women (46.5% and 46.1%, respectively) not receiving ERT/HRT. One major risk factors for developing heart disease is the presence of hypertension. African American women are reported to have a 50% higher prevalence of hypertension, and it is noted to develop at an earlier age. However, compared with Caucasian women treated for hypertension, African American women had significantly greater risk reductions in fatal and nonfatal cardiovascular events and all-cause mortality.

Rates of osteoporosis are higher among Caucasian women. This is most likely due to higher bone mineral densities in African American women than in Caucasian women. African American women also have lower rates of hip fracture (5.6% vs 15.3%, respectively). African American women also have lower rates of endometrial cancer (1.5% vs 2.6%) and breast cancer (7.3% vs 10.2%), although the cancer is more likely to be fatal.

With respect to menopause, there are great variations across racial and ethnic groups in the frequency and severity of menopause-related symptoms, attitudes toward menopause, attitudes toward ERT/HRT use, and healthcare utilization. The Study of Women's Health Across the Nation (SWAN) is a 10-year longitudinal trial with several ethnic groups of women — including African Americans, Caucasians, Chinese Americans, Japanese Americans, and Hispanic Americans — designed to examine the differences among them with respect to the transition to menopause. Results showed that, in general, women's attitudes toward menopause were neutral to positive. Among the groups, African American women were significantly more positive in attitude than other groups. The least positive groups were the less acculturated Chinese American and Japanese American women. The results also suggest that factors other than those directly associated with menopause status, including socioeconomics, smoking, and other demographic factors, had a substantial effect on attitudes.

Other US surveys have also found similar attitudinal differences regarding menopause. These studies have also shown that African American, Japanese American, and Chinese American women report significantly fewer symptoms associated with menopause than Caucasian women. However, African American women report more vasomotor symptoms than Caucasian women, although they do not find them as bothersome. Both Japanese and Chinese American women have shown more negative attitudes toward menopause than Caucasian women, despite their report of fewer symptoms.

While such variability can be partly attributed to differences in definitions, measurements, and analysis, some key comparative studies provide strong evidence that this variability is real, and it is possible to delineate the factors that account for it.

Some of these factors are biological. For example, in populations where many women experience surgical menopause, symptom frequency is higher than among those who experience spontaneous menopause. Similarly, where more women smoke or the incidence of obesity is high, symptoms frequently will be higher than in populations where these characteristics are rare.

It is also clear, however, that social factors play a significant role in explaining both the experience of particular symptoms and the meaning that are attached to menopause as a phase of life. Such factors include socioeconomic status, definitions of women's position across the life cycle, prevalent ideas about body functioning, and norms related to femininity and aging.

In addition, the healthcare industry has an important influence on the attitudes of both women and clinicians. Whether menopause is accepted as a natural phase of life or considered as a medical condition to be treated will depend on the extent to which therapies are available and accessible to the population and on clinicians' enthusiasm in recommending them.

The risk and benefits of ERT/HRT have mainly been evaluated in multicenter clinical trials using Caucasian women. A literature review found that less than 1% of the participants in these studies have been non-Caucasian. Treatment regimens differ among sociocultural groups. In one study, African American women predominately treated menopausal symptoms with nonprescription treatments (55% prefer diet, vitamins, exercise, or herbal remedies over ERT/HRT). Only 25% believed that the benefits of ERT/HRT outweigh the risks (compared with 44% of Caucasian women). However, knowledge deficits among African American women, especially among low-income women, were identified regarding menopause and ERT/HRT. The Commonwealth Fund Study found that hormone use is most prevalent among well-educated, white, non-Hispanic women living in the midwestern United States and having partners and middle- to upper-range incomes.

The sources of information for African American women suggest that practitioners are not providing adequate information regarding menopause. Only 14% identified their healthcare provider as the primary source of information on menopause; 60% identified their family and friends as the primary source, with literature second at 20%. In contrast, most Caucasian women (67%) rely on literature as their primary source, with their healthcare provider second at 17%.

The 1993 National Institutes of Health Act dramatically redirected the context of medical research in the United States by requiring that trials involving human subjects should include women and members of minority groups as research subjects. Two large, ongoing trials — the Women's Health Initiative (WHI) and SWAN — were designed with a significant commitment to recruiting minority group women. They promise to have a major impact on menopause research in general, but particularly on understanding the menopausal experiences of African American, Hispanic American, Asian American, and Native American women.

The research on menopause experiences of women in other cultures illustrates the need to learn about women's cultural beliefs and the variety of complementary and alternative therapies that women use. Educational material that addresses those issues should be made available.

Effective counseling requires that the clinician be aware of any cultural beliefs that can have an impact on a woman's view of menopause and various treatment options. However, it is a mistake to stereotype women of foreign descent — they do not all observe the same traditions or exhibit the same cultural traits. As always, delivery of health care must respect each woman as a unique individual (see Table 1).

One option when there is a language barrier is using medical translators, which is the optimal situation. Using a telephone-interpreter service is another option.

Be aware that some individuals who are able to converse quite well in English or another language are unable to read educational material either in English or their native language. One in five US adults is functionally illiterate. If illiteracy is suspected, then have visual instructions that illustrate when to take the medication, such as a clock face or depictions of sunrise.

There are multiple factors that increase diseases during menopause but there are also barriers that lead to disparities in the disease prevalence, such as income level, health insurance status, cultural values, transportation, and race or ethnicity. Many of these barriers can be overcome with more patient and clinician education.

Table 1. Suggestions for cross-cultural counseling

- Encourage the woman to explain her medical problems. Ask why she thinks she has the symptoms, what her family and friends say about the symptoms, and her concerns about it.

- Ask the woman if she is using alternative or folk remedies or if she is consulting with others, such as healers. It is important to know what other medications or treatments the woman is using before a treatment plan can be prescribed.

- Do not disparage her current practices. Be willing to compromise to devise a plan acceptable to the woman.

- In some cultures, healing and religion are inextricably linked. A medical treatment plan may need to be designed to complement her other treatments to ensure adherence. Consider a plan that will treat the woman both medically and traditionally.

- Have social workers experienced with a particular culture and interpreters available for consultation. Avoid using family members as interpreters.

- Consider the role of the woman's family. They can help the woman follow instructions as well as monitor therapy and keep records.

- If the woman does not speak English or is unfamiliar with Western medicine, set aside more time for counseling. Be aware that conversing in English does not necessarily mean that the woman can read English — or her native language.

- Clarify the limitations of Western medicine. If the woman has symptoms that may not respond to therapy, make it clear to her.

- Explain in advance what you are going to be doing during a physical examination. Some women may not understand why you are examining parts of their body other than those affected.

- Keep in mind differences between populations and the differences within populations. Major differences in social class, economic status, and background exist within all ethnic groups.

Bibliography

Berg JA, Taylor DL. Symptom experience of Filipino American midlife women. *Menopause* 1999;6:105-114.

Bohannon AD. Osteoporosis and African American women. *J Womens Health* 1999;8:609-615.

Boulet M, Oddens B, Lehert P, Verner HM, Visser A. Climacteric and menopause in seven South-east Asian countries. *Maturitas* 1994; 19:157-176.

Grady D, Rubin SM, Petitti DB, et al. Hormone therapy to prevent disease and prolong life in postmenopausal women. *Ann Intern Med* 1992;117:1016-1036.

Grisso JA, Freeman EW, Maurin E, et al. Racial differences in menopause information and the experience of hot flashes. *J Gen Intern Med* 1999;14:98-103.

Holmes-Rovner M, Padonu G, Kroll J, et al. African American women's attitudes and expectations of menopause. *Am J Prev Med* 1996;12:420-423.

Kaufert P. The social and cultural context of menopause. *Maturitas* 1996;23:169-180.

Lillie-Blanton M, Bowie J, Ro M. African-American women: continuing disparities in health. *Int J Health Serv* 1993;23:555-584.

Lock M. Menopause in cultural context. *Exp Gerontol* 1994; 29:307-317.

MacDougall LA, Brazilay JI, Helmick CG. Hormone replacement therapy awareness in a biracial cohort of women aged 50-54 years. *Menopause* 1999;6:251-256.

National Population Health Survey 1994-1995. Ottawa, ON, Canada: Statistics Canada, 1995. Catalogue no. 82-F0001XCB.

Nicholson WK, Brown AF, Gathe J, Grumbach K, Washington AE, Pérez-Stable EJ. Hormone replacement therapy for African American women: missed opportunities for effective intervention. *Menopause* 1999;6:147-155.

Obermeyer CM. Cross-cultural perspectives on menopause [abstract]. *Menopause* 1999;6:320. Abstract 11.

Oddens BJ. The climacteric cross-culturally: the International Health Foundation South-East Asia study. *Maturitas* 1994; 19:155-156.

Pham K, Freeman E, Grisso J. Menopause and hormone replacement therapy: focus groups of African American and Caucasian women. *Menopause* 1997;4:71-79.

Postl B. Native health: it's time for action [editorial]. *Can Med Assoc J* 1997;157:1655-1656.

Ramirez de Arellano A. Latino women: health status and access to health care. In: Falik M, Scott Collins K, eds. *Women's Health: The Commonwealth Fund Survey.* Baltimore, MD: Johns Hopkins University Press; 1996:123-144.

Rossouw JE, Hurd S. The women's health initiative: recruitment complete — looking back and looking forward. *J Womens Health* 1999;8:3-5.

Statistics Canada. 1996 *Census: Immigration and Citizenship.* Ottawa, ON, Canada: Statistics Canada, 1997. Accessible at http://www.statcan.ca/Daily/English/971104/d971104.htm.

US Department of Health and Human Services (US DHHS), National Institutes of Health (NIH). *Outreach Notebook for the NIH Guidelines on Inclusion of Women and Minorities as Subjects in Clinical Research.* Bethesda, MD: National Institutes of Health; 1994.

Woods NF. Midlife women: health care patterns and choices. In: Falik M, Scott Collins K, eds. *Women's Health: The Commonwealth Fund Survey.* Baltimore, MD: Johns Hopkins University Press; 1996:145-174.

Woods NF. Symptoms among midlife women: cultural lenses, research, and health care [editorial]. *Menopause* 1999;6:90-91.

Q.03. Behavior modification

Despite the proven heath benefits of lifestyle changes, many individuals choose not to alter undesirable lifestyle habits or they find making changes and maintaining compliance difficult. Often, the healthcare professional has no training or skills in behavior modification.

Various motivational factors have an impact on acceptance and continuance of therapy, including enjoyment of a habit, situational factors, costs, and family pressures. A woman's decision can also be influenced by her religion, the media, the advice of others, or many other factors. A women's perception of how the recommendation will affect her health often determines the effort that she puts forth.

Strategies to improve health behaviors need to consider three types of factors: motivational factors, factors that promote adherence to the health regimen, and reinforcement factors that help continuance of behavioral changes in the long run.

Motivational factors include perspectives on the health issue in question, health beliefs, preferences, and knowledge. Adherence and reinforcement factors include those related to the intervention or treatment in the context of the personal environment. The pros must outweigh the cons. Delivering instructions verbally and in writing has been shown to improve adherence with the instructions. Interactive approaches are more effective than simply handing over a pamphlet. A trusting relationship between a woman and her healthcare provider is also important, as is the support the woman receives from her family and friends.

It is important to determine each woman's preferences and beliefs regarding health care. This should be scheduled after the examination, when the woman may feel less vulnerable. She should be asked about her opinion regarding the treatment options. Although some women may have opinions based on unsound scientific evidence, practitioners must be sensitive to those beliefs. Health professionals should provide unbiased, comprehensive, and up-to-date information regarding the treatment options.

The Transtheoretical Model (TTM) assumes that individuals are at different stages of readiness for change, and that effectiveness is optimized by matching the intervention to the person's current stage of readiness. Identification of the stage of change is only the beginning. This approach focuses on improving motivation, effecting change, and maintaining the changed behavior.

Table 2 presents some strategies for changing behavior patterns.

Table 2. Strategies for changing behavior patterns

- Ask open-ended questions. These may elicit more responses regarding knowledge of the therapy and ability to adhere to regimens. It also provides the opportunity to share concerns and reservations about the treatment.

- Emphasize the most important information at the beginning and end of a discussion; first and last instructions are often remembered best.

- Keep the message simple. The fewer instructions that are given, the better. Clarify the goal(s). Ask the woman to repeat the key points.

- Have the woman generate a list of benefits for herself and her loved ones from the proposed change. Discuss the potential problems of continuing her current behavior.

- Provide the recommendations in writing as a follow-up to oral instructions.

- Modify the treatment regimens based on the woman's preferences and match the therapeutic plan to the woman's lifestyle. Try to make the plan fit her schedule. Have her generate a list of benefits from the proposed change. Some women may wish to change several areas of their lifestyle to enhance their health. It is difficult to sustain multiple changes in behavior over time. Support her intention to be healthy while encouraging her to incorporate one new health behavior at a time, thereby ensuring success that will be in her own incentive for other successes.

- Develop a contingency contract with the woman. This contract specifies her treatment goal and notes the obligations of both the woman and her provider. The goal is to create a sense of shared partnership to enhance adherence to the therapy plan.

- Simplify the medications. Individuals adhere better to regimens requiring infrequent dosing and few medications. Convenient, inexpensive plans usually work the best.

- Establish a health education clinic or menopause discussion group. Intensive education can enhance continuance with regimens, especially with long-term medications that do not produce readily apparent results. Individuals are more receptive to clinics that emphasize education rather than promoting specific products. (NAMS offers a booklet on how to develop a menopause discussion group.)

- Schedule frequent visits early in the regimen (at least every few months) to provide a communication link with the woman and to detect any concerns or problems and to enhance the continuance of the therapeutic program. Conduct periodic telephone contacts between office visits to offer support and encouragement.

Bibliography

Cramer JA. Optimizing long-term patient compliance. *Neurology* 1995;45(suppl 1):S25-S28.

Cramer JA. Partial medical compliance: the enigma in poor medical outcomes. *Am J Manag Care* 1995;1:45-52.

The North American Menopause Society. *How to Develop a Menopause Discussion Group.* Cleveland, OH: The North American Menopause Society; 2002.

Steele DJ, Jackson TC, Gutmann MC. The adherence-monitoring sequence in the medical interview. *J Fam Pract* 1990;30:294-290.

Q.04. Lifestyle modification

Menopause is an appropriate time for a complete review of and counseling about risk factor reduction. Lifestyle modification (altering the types of behaviors women can change) includes smoking cessation, exercise, weight control, stress reduction, and diet management. (Types of interventions and the benefits that can be achieved have been detailed elsewhere in this study guide.) In most instances, lifestyle modification should be the first "course of therapy."

Many postmenopausal women are active participants in their health. According to one survey, approximately 75% of postmenopausal women report making some type of health-related lifestyle change at menopause/midlife. These include eating a more healthy diet, maintaining a healthy weight, exercising regularly, taking vitamins, taking calcium supplements, stopping smoking, and using relaxation methods.

The annual physical examination provides an important opportunity for healthcare providers to counsel women regarding preventive care through lifestyle changes. Although smoking may be the single greatest preventable cause of illness and premature death, clinicians also need to stress the importance of other factors to overall health (see Table 3).

Bibliography

US Preventive Services Task Force. *Guide to Clinical Preventive Services.* 2nd ed. Washington, DC: US Department of Health and Human Services; 1996.

Warren MP, Artacho CA. Role of exercise and nutrition. In: Lobo RA, ed. *Treatment of the Postmenopausal Woman: Basic and Clinical Aspects.* 2nd ed. Philadelphia, PA: Lippincott Williams & Wilkins; 1999:417-436.

Table 3. Lifestyle counseling issues for peri- and postmenopausal women

Substance use
Tobacco cessation
Alcohol/drug safety (eg, avoid use while driving, swimming, boating, etc)
Alcohol/drug abuse

Diet and exercise
Limit fat and cholesterol intake
Maintain caloric balance
Consume a diet based on whole grains, fruits, vegetables, water
Ensure adequate vitamin and mineral intake, especially calcium
Emphasize importance of regular physical activity

Injury prevention
Wear lap/shoulder belts in the car
Institute fall prevention methods
Wear appropriate helmet and other safety equipment when riding motorcycle, bicycle, or all-terrain vehicle
Have adequate number of smoke detectors
Ensure safe storage or removal of firearms
Set water heater thermostat between 120-130° F or lower
Household members should be trained to deliver CPR

Sexual behavior
Institute prevention of sexually transmitted infections:
    Avoid high-risk sexual behavior
    Use condoms and/or female barrier
Prevent unintended pregnancies with appropriate contraceptives

Dental health
Stress importance of regular dental visits
Floss and brush with fluoride toothpaste daily

Source: US Preventive Services Task Force, 1996.

Q.05. Treatment counseling

When counseling a woman regarding menopause, a clinician should recognize that she needs to be fully informed and encouraged to take an active part in the decision-making process. Midlife women who have more confidence in their ability to participate and experience fewer barriers to participating are more likely to take an active role in the healthcare encounter and, in turn, are more satisfied with the decisions made.

The clinician should ask the woman about her priorities for treatment and concerns. The clinician can provide accurate and current information about the treatment options and help her examine the options and tradeoffs in light of the outcome that is most important to her.

The clinician should also reinforce the fact that menopause is a natural event, not a disease. Women who have no bothersome symptoms still need to understand the changes in risk profile at the time of menopause, and the options that are available for risk reduction.

Some women may experience menopause-associated symptoms that interfere with their daily life. These women may be uncertain about what is happening to their bodies and need to understand the hormonal changes involved in menopause. Clinicians must be sensitive to individual concerns, recognizing that each woman is distinctively different in her response to menopause. Culture may influence communication style. Skills and sensitivity in communicating with women from different cultural backgrounds are essential.

Many women use alternative therapies, including herbal preparations, for symptom relief or for disease prevention. Because they are understood to be "natural," women may not think of these preparations as medicines. It is important for the clinician to assess all therapeutic strategies, including herbal preparations, when taking the history and physical. Clinicians should have current information on alternative therapies and alert women to those that have been shown to be effective or not effective through clinical trials and those for which there are no data. Women should be informed about the lack of standardization among products, and they should know that side effects and interactions must be a consideration with so-called natural preparations as well as other medications.

Many women want an answer to the question, "Should I take hormones?" There will never be a universal answer because each woman is unique — not only in her biologic and psychologic response to menopause/aging, but also in her tolerance for various symptoms, her risk profile for disease in later years, contraindications to therapy, and her feelings about medications. Clinicians can reinforce the concept of uniqueness and help women to become informed about the options available to them to achieve the outcomes they desire.

Of the midlife women who use ERT/HRT, many do so for relief of symptoms rather than to protect against disease in later years. In the 1997 NAMS/Gallup survey (N = 749), a woman's decision to commence ERT/HRT was more often made on the basis of physical symptom relief rather than to prevent disease. In a study of a nationally representative sample of women in the Commonwealth Fund 1998 Survey of Women's Health (N = 884), the two most common reasons for initiating hormone therapy were following a doctor's or other provider's recommendation (57%) and seeking relief of menopause symptoms (36%).

Clinicians have a responsibility to provide counsel to ensure that women's decisions are informed and based on current information, including the risks and benefits of hormones. In the year 2000, menopause counseling became a HEDIS measure, designed to determine whether health plans and/or their clinicians have provided at least an adequate level of counseling (see Section Q.05.a). Improved counseling has been cited as a possible solution to the low rates of initiating and continuing ERT/HRT. A simple question asking women to rate their level of knowledge about menopause and hormone therapy appears to be a good estimation of their educational needs. In a telephone survey of 156 women in a managed care population, it was found that a global question about level of knowledge was an effective clinical tool for identifying women who need additional education about hormones and menopause. Race, income, and discussion with a provider were related to knowledge about hormones but not educational status.

A study of 421 women looked at HRT awareness among black and white women aged 50 to 54. HRT awareness among women is strongly influenced by race, educational level, and perception of being in or having completed menopause. Increased HRT use among educated women may partly result from increased awareness of HRT. Black race was associated with a lower likelihood of HRT awareness, even when adjusted for educational level. Black women may view menopause and menopause symptoms differently than white women, considering it a natural process that does not require treatment.

Few studies have addressed the prevalence of HRT counseling among US women. A report on counseling prevalence based on the 1994 National Health Interview Survey showed that among women aged 50 to 54, about 62% reported having received counseling regarding HRT. The 1998 NAMS/Gallup survey (Part II) showed that 75.4% of 749 US women aged 50 to 65 reported they had received counseling from healthcare providers. Women of low socioeconomic status and those who did not have a primary care physician were least likely to have received counseling. No differences were observed in prevalence of counseling between women in managed care settings and those with other types of health insurance.

In a survey of 1,800 Canadian women in 2000, 96% aged 45 to 64 felt comfortable discussing menopause with their physician and 70% felt that their physicians provided adequate information about HRT. However, 25% of women aged 50 to 54 had not discussed HRT for the main reason that they did not have menopause symptoms and a discussion was not necessary.

Q.05.a. HEDIS requirements

The Health Plan Employer Data and Information Set — called HEDIS 2000 — is a set of standards designed to enable purchasers to compare the performance of managed care plans in the United States. HEDIS is sponsored by the National Committee for Quality Assurance (NCQA). In HEDIS 2000, the NCQA introduced its management of menopause measures. These measures provide counseling requirements for women aged 47 to 55 about managing symptoms associated with perimenopausal and postmenopausal hormone changes.

The HEDIS survey measure was designed to determine whether some type of counseling occurred and to assess what components were included. Women are asked whether they received any information regarding the potential benefits and risks of HRT and alternative therapies or approaches to disease prevention and menopausal symptom relief. The survey also asks whether the counseling took into account the woman's medical history, family history, values, preferences, and concerns. Respondents are also queried about whether they had a chance to ask all of their questions.

The objectives of counseling, as stated by the NCQA, include addressing women's questions and concerns, providing education, facilitating informed decision making, and enhancing confidence in her decision and in her ability to carry it out or modify it over time. It further states that a partnership between the woman and her provider characterized by mutual respect and trust enhances counseling.

In HEDIS 2000, counseling refers to communication of information to help a woman make informed decisions about her health. As defined by the measure, counseling includes face-to-face contact and patient information, such as classes or support groups, print materials, audio and videotapes, telephone resource lines, and Internet tools.

The measure is scored as a composite of three components:

- exposure (whether and when counseling occurred),

- breadth (whether the counseling included information on risks, benefits, and alternatives to ERT/HRT), and

- personalization (whether the counseling involved consideration of the woman's personal and family medical histories and her own concerns).

To achieve the maximum score, plans must demonstrate that this level of counseling was provided within the last two years. The measure does not assess the results of the decisions the woman makes.

If a therapy was chosen, the woman and her provider should agree on the goals, whether they are short-term (menopause symptom relief), long-term (primary or secondary prevention of diseases associated with aging), or both. The clinician should revisit decisions about menopause management with the woman at subsequent visits, as new research is published and the woman's health status and preferences may change over time.

Continuance of therapy is another issue to evaluate. The clinician should determine if the woman changed or discontinued her treatment plan because she experienced troublesome side effects from pharmacologic agents or because the treatment failed to provide the expected or desired results.

Suggestions for meeting HEDIS requirements are found in Table 4.

Bibliography

Anderson LA, Caplan LS, Buist DS, et al. Perceived barriers and recommendations concerning hormone replacement therapy counseling among primary care providers. *Menopause* 1999; 6:161-166.

Angus Reid Group. Attitudes towards menopause and hormone replacement therapy [press release]. Toronto, ON, Canada: Angus Reid Group, September 7, 2000. Accessible at http://www.angusreid.com/pdf/media/mr000907.pdf.

Connelly MT, Rusinak D, Livingston W, Raeke L, Inui T. Patient knowledge about hormone replacement therapy: implications for treatment. *Menopause* 2000;7:266-272.

Ettinger B, Woods NF, Barrett-Connor E, Pressman A. The North American Menopause Society 1998 Menopause Survey: Part II. Counseling about hormone replacement therapy: association with socioeconomic status and access to medical care. *Menopause* 2000;7:143-148.

HEDIS 2000 Technical Specifications, vol 3. Washington, DC: National Committee for Quality Assurance; 1999.

Holmes-Rovner M, Padonu G, Kroll J, Breer L. African American women's attitudes and expectations of menopause. *Am J Prev Med* 1996:12:420-423.

Jacobs Institute of Women's Health Expert Panel on Menopause Counseling. *Guidelines for Counseling Women on the Management of Menopause.* Washington, DC: Jacobs Institute of Women's Health; 2000.

Kaufert P, Boggs PP, Ettinger B, Woods NF, Utian WH. Women and menopause: beliefs, attitudes, and behaviors: The North American Menopause Society 1997 Menopause Survey. *Menopause* 1998;5: 197-202.

Table 4. Suggestions to clinicians for meeting HEDIS 2000 requirements for counseling menopausal women

- Make an effort to address all of the woman's questions, including those about therapies you would not recommend. Treat the woman's questions respectfully, even if her facts or sources are not ones you endorse.

- Ensure that the scientific information presented to the patient is objective. Achieve balance in presenting options — be aware of any biases you may have.

- Educate the woman about relevant health conditions (such as heart disease and osteoporosis) so she appreciates how these diseases could affect her quality of life in the future.

- Discuss the known risks and benefits associated with each option, and present, in lay terminology, information about the strength of the existing evidence and what remains unknown.

- Personalize the discussions based on the woman's health, social history, and family history.

- Consider the woman's preferences, values, and key concerns (eg, family members' experiences, concerns about breast cancer).

- Tailor the use of materials to the needs and wants of the woman. For example, some women may want to read key scientific studies while others may prefer concise booklets that briefly summarize relevant information. Consider using educational materials and programs to enhance the office visit counseling session.

- Consider the woman's practical issues that she may face if medication will be part of her management plan, such as cost, convenience, and side effects that might affect her desire to continue therapy.

- Ensure that follow-up is routinely done with all women who start a treatment regimen. The interval for follow-up depends on the woman's needs and concerns.

- Menopause is an appropriate time for a complete review of osteoporosis risk status and counseling on risk status reduction. Because a woman may decide to take ERT (or HRT) only if she knows that she is at risk for osteoporotic fractures, her clinician must be able to assess her individual risk and involve her in the decision-making process.

- Constraints on time for office visits has been cited by primary care physicians as an important barrier to providing comprehensive counseling to women at the time of menopause. Although longer physician office visits might be an ideal approach, offering visits with nonphysician clinicians, as well as providing educational programs and materials in conjunction with visits, may be a more realistic one.

Source: NCQA; adapted with permission.

Kroll J, Rothert M, Davidson WS, et al. Predictors of participation in health care at menopause. *Health Communication* 2000;12:339-360.

MacDougall LA, Barzilay JI, Helmick CG. Hormone replacement therapy awareness in a biracial cohort of women aged 50-54 years. *Menopause* 1999;6:251-256.

MacLaren A, Woods NF. Midlife women making hormone therapy decisions. *Womens Health Issues* 2001;11:216-230.

Mort EA. HEDIS and menopause counseling: the management of menopause measure. *Menopause Management* 2001;10(5):8-12.

Padonu G, Holmes-Rovner M, Rothert M, et al. African-American women's perception of menopause. *Am J Health Behav* 1996; 20:242-251.

Utian WH, Boggs PP. The North American Menopause Society 1998 Menopause Survey. Part I: Postmenopausal women's perceptions about menopause and midlife. *Menopause* 1999;6:122-128.

Zhang P, Tho G, Anderson LA. Prevalence of and factors associated with hormone replacement therapy counseling: results from the 1994 National Health Interview Survey. *Am J Public Health* 1999; 89:1575-1577.

Q.06. Improving medication continuance

Continuance is defined as taking a medication regimen over the period of time and at the dosage needed to achieve the desired effect. It defines behavior. The word *adherence* can be used as a substitute. The words *compliance, comply,* and *compliant* are paternalistic words referring to yielding or obedience rather than following a mutual decision, and they should be avoided.

Most of the discussion about medication continuance centers around ERT/HRT. In the Massachusetts Women's Health Study, among 2,500 women aged 45 to 55 years given prescriptions for ERT/HRT, 30% never filled the prescription, 20% stopped within 9 months, and 10% used ERT/HRT only intermittently. Records from the Kaiser Health Plan for 1991-1995 revealed that, regardless of whether estrogen and progestogen were given cyclically or continuously, less than 50% of women were using estrogen 1 year after beginning therapy and less than 20% were still using estrogen 3 years later. Nonetheless, continuation rates with ERT/HRT are similar to those of other long-term therapies.

In a survey of Canadian women, 73% of women aged 45 to 64 believed that HRT can improve quality of life, but only 24% of women aged 45 to 64 were current users of HRT.

There is some evidence that continuance is greater with transdermal than with oral ERT. Continuance is also greater with oral ERT than with oral estrogen plus progestogen,

taken separately. In one study, 30% of women stopped using progestogen and continued taking estrogen alone. Experiencing side effects appears to be the most common reason given for discontinuance (42%), followed by recommendation of a healthcare professional (22%) and concerns about breast or endometrial cancer (10%). Cost of therapy has not been linked conclusively to continuance.

Continuance is correlated not with the number of drugs prescribed but with the number of dosing times per day of all therapies taken. The fewer the number of doses, the greater the rate of continuance.

A study of 449 women in a Massachusetts HMO found women who report therapeutic benefits from hormone therapy are more likely to continue using hormones long-term. The experience of certain side effects, such as irregular uterine bleeding, edema, and abdominal cramps/pelvic pain, were significantly associated with hormone therapy discontinuation, especially during the first few months of use. In this study, women who adjusted their own progestogen dosages without consulting their physician were approximately four times more likely to discontinue. Women whose symptoms were reduced after using hormone therapy were more likely than other women to continue using hormone therapy. Women who used alternative therapies or made lifestyle changes around menopause were not more likely to discontinue hormone therapy.

Many women are intolerant of uterine bleeding, especially older women. In one study, 52% of those older than 65 years discontinued HRT because of bleeding, compared with 29% of those 55 year old and younger for that reason.

Hysterectomy plays a significant role in both initiation and continuation of hormone therapy. The absence of a uterus enhances continuance, as uterine bleeding is eliminated. Following bilateral oophorectomy, women typically have severe symptoms, leading to improved HRT continuance.

Most studies show that older women are more likely to discontinue ERT/HRT than younger women. In one study, a relative risk of discontinuation was determined to be 1.1 for every 5 years of age.

Women who feel better using ERT/HRT are more likely to continue the regimen. When the woman is asymptomatic, continuation is more problematic. In a study of HRT for osteoporosis prevention, about 30% of new HRT users discontinued therapy during the first 6 months. It was determined that continuation could be improved 10% to 20% by switching to another regimen.

With the conflicting data in the literature, many women feel inadequately informed about the risks and benefits of ERT/HRT and this can lead to inaccurate expectations and uncertainty. It is useful to supplement discussions with written information. Women can be helped to address these issues by assisting them to become informed about the side effects of ERT/HRT and building realistic expectations of the therapy. The clinician should thoroughly discuss options and assess what is important to each woman. Women must be fully informed in order to participate in the decision. Women often have concerns about menopause and ERT/HRT before they reach menopause. A discussion of the needs and concerns of a woman early in her premenopausal stage will help the healthcare provider identify her health priorities. Table 5 presents recommendations made by NAMS in its consensus opinion about ERT/HRT continuance.

Table 5. Counseling recommendations to improve ERT/HRT continuance

- Involve the woman in the decision-making process, and recognize that decision making involves making daily decisions. Decision making between the woman and her healthcare provider should be shared to optimize treatment planning and subsequent continuance.

- Explain the benefits and risks with clarity, personalizing information by translating population data to the personal risk profile.

- Determine the woman's preferences early in the decision-making process and use these preferences to modify a regimen to improve continuance.

- Provide educational information in words that the woman can understand.

- Help the woman systematize medication taking.

- Ensure adequate follow-up. Schedule regular contact through visits or phone calls.

- Set expectations that it may be necessary to try more than one regimen.

The North American Menopause Society. *Menopause* 1998.

Women should be informed that multiple therapeutic options, regimens, and dosages are available, and that it may take time to achieve the right one for them. Women may be most likely to discontinue medication at the time of initiating treatment, with changes in treatment, and after a long period of treatment when a change occurs in their life. The key is to maintain communication channels so that if a woman chooses to discontinue, she will call the clinician and provide an opportunity to discuss and revise the regimen to achieve the clinical goal.

A number of barriers to counseling regarding ERT/HRT continuance have been identified. These include a lack of available information concerning the risks and benefits (eg, a lack of clinical trial data or data that are conflicting). In addition, peri- and postmenopausal women bring a variety of beliefs and expectations that must be addressed. Decreased length of office visits is a trend in managed care, which may limit available clinician time for meeting educational and psychosocial needs. Creative approaches to education, including group support sessions, nurse counseling, printed material, suggested Web sites, and decision supports, are additional resources for ERT/HRT counseling.

Some clinicians are unfamiliar with the variety of ERT/HRT regimens and how to use them, if the initial one is unacceptable. Clinicians must continuously be informed about emerging data regarding medications, including complementary and alternative therapies, to address specific therapeutic goals.

Most data related to continuance are based on studies involving middle-class Caucasian women who live in the United States. Cultural experiences, education, and economics can affect women's health decisions. More research is needed among women who are not included within these demographics.

The most successful regimens are those that are simple, do not interfere with the woman's lifestyle, and are inexpensive. Delivering instructions verbally and in writing reinforces continuance counseling. Continuance rates are greater when women have participated in the decision-making process and they feel their expectations have been met, the practitioner listens and respects their concerns, and adequate information has been provided regarding their condition and therapeutic progress.

Bibliography

Anderson LA, Caplan LS, Buist DS, et al. Perceived barriers and recommendations concerning hormone replacement therapy counseling among primary care providers. *Menopause* 1999; 6:161-166.

Angus Reid Group. Attitudes towards menopause and hormone replacement therapy [press release]. Toronto, ON, Canada: Angus Reid Group, September 7, 2000. Accessible at http://www.angusreid.com/pdf/media/mr000907.pdf.

Berman RS, Epstein RS, Lydick EG. Risk factors associated with women's compliance with estrogen replacement therapy. *J Womens Health* 1997;6:219-226.

Berman RS. Patient compliance of women taking estrogen replacement therapy. *Drug Info J* 1997;31:71-83.

Cano A. Compliance to hormone replacement therapy in menopausal women controlled in a third level academic centre. *Maturitas* 1995;20:91-99.

Coulter A. Patient-centered decision making: empowering women to make informed choices. *Womens Health Issues* 2001;11:325-330.

Cramer JA. Partial medical compliance: the enigma in poor medical outcomes. *Am J Manag Care* 1995;1:45-52.

Cramer JA, Mattson RH, Prevey ML, Scheyer RD, Ouellette VL. How often is medication taken as prescribed? A novel assessment technique. *JAMA* 1989;261:3273-3277.

Ettinger B, Li DK, Klein R. Continuation of postmenopausal hormone replacement therapy: comparison of cyclic versus continuous combined schedules. *Menopause* 1996;3:185-189.

Ettinger B, Pressman A, Bradley C. Comparison of continuation of postmenopausal hormone replacement therapy: transdermal versus oral estrogen. *Menopause* 1998;5:152-156.

Ettinger B, Pressman A, Silver P. Effect of age on reasons for initiation and discontinuation of hormone replacement therapy. *Menopause* 1999;6:282-289.

Ettinger B, Woods NF, Barrett-Connor E, Pressman A. The North American Menopause Society 1998 Menopause Survey. Part II: Counseling about hormone replacement therapy: association with socioeconomic status and access to medical care. *Menopause* 2000;7:143-148.

Faulkner DL, Young C, Hutchins D, et al. Patient noncompliance with hormone replacement therapy: a nationwide estimate using a large prescription claims database. *Menopause* 1998;5:226-229.

Gass MLS, Rebar RW, Liu JH, Cedars MI. Characteristics of women who continue using hormone replacement therapy. *Menopause* 1997;4:19-23.

Kaufert P, Boggs PP, Ettinger B, Woods NF, Utian WH. The North American Menopause Society 1997 Menopause Survey. Women and menopause: beliefs, attitudes, and behaviors. *Menopause* 1998;5:197-202.

MacLaren A, Woods NF. Midlife women making hormone therapy decisions. *Womens Health Issues* 2001;11:216-230.

Motheral BR, Fairman KA. Patient education programs and continuance with estrogen replacement therapy: evaluation of the Women's Health Exchange. *Menopause* 1998;5:35-42.

Newton KM, LaCroix AZ, Leveille SG, et al. Women's beliefs and decisions about hormone replacement therapy. *J Womens Health* 1997;6:459-465.

The North American Menopause Society. Achieving long-term continuance of menopausal ERT/HRT: consensus opinion of The North American Menopause Society. *Menopause* 1998;5:69-76.

Reynolds RF, Obermeyer CM, Walker AM, Guilbert D. Side effects and sociobehavioral factors associated with the discontinuation of hormone therapy in a Massachusetts health maintenance organization. *Menopause* 2001;8:189-199.

Reynolds RF, Walker AM, Obermeyer CM, Rahman O, Guilbert D. Discontinuation of postmenopausal hormone therapy in a Massachusetts HMO. *J Clin Epidemiol* 2001;54:1056-1064.

Ryan PJ, Harrison R, Blake GM, Fogelman I. Compliance with hormone replacement therapy (HRT) after screening for postmenopausal osteoporosis. *Br J Obstet Gynaecol* 1992; 99:326-328.

Utian WH, Boggs PP. The North American Menopause Society 1998 menopause survey. Part I: Postmenopausal women's perceptions about menopause and midlife. *Menopause* 1999;6:122-128.

Vestergaard P, Herman AP, Gram J. Improving compliance with hormonal replacement therapy in primary osteoporosis prevention. *Maturitas* 1997;28:137-145.

Walsh JME, Brown JS, Rubin S, Kagawa M, Grady D. Postmenopausal hormone therapy: factors influencing women's decision making. *Menopause* 1997;4:39-45.

White VE, Bennett L, Raffin S, Emmett K, Coleman MJ. Use of unopposed estrogen in women with uteri: prevalence, clinical implications, and economic consequences. *Menopause* 2000; 7:123-128.

Woods N, Falk S, Saver B, et al. Deciding about using hormone replacement therapy for preventing diseases of advanced age: women's models and implications for health care and decision support. *Menopause* 1997;4:105-114.

Zhang P, Tho G, Anderson LA. Prevalence of and factors associated with hormone replacement therapy counseling: results from the 1994 National Health Interview Survey. *Am J Public Health* 1999; 89:1575-1577.

Q.07. Importance of listening and building trust

Clinicians have various responsibilities when caring for women in their practice (see Table 6). Actively listening to what each woman says about her unique menopause experience is important for the following reasons:

- to identify individual health beliefs,

- to determine the best management approach,

- to identify motivation to change behaviors and level of commitment,

- to build trust in the therapeutic relationship.

Table 6. Clinician responsibilities

- Develop satisfactory clinical relationships through communication and listening.

- Provide all the information necessary for an informed decision.

- Provide unbiased, factual, and comprehensive information on the risks and benefits of any therapeutic initiative.

- Elicit and include the woman's preferences in any recommendations.

- Periodically evaluate treatment continuance and adjust the regimen, as needed.

- Regardless of adherence to the treatment, the clinician still has ethical and legal responsibility. To fulfill this responsibility, the clinician must understand the woman's comprehension of the instructions and capacity to follow the instructions.

When counseling, the following suggestions can be kept in mind.

- Put the woman at ease by ensuring as much privacy as possible during the interview. Use a concerned, friendly demeanor.

- Maintain eye contact. This assures the woman that she is being listened to and enables the provider to observe her expression. Don't look at your watch, glance toward the hallway, or interrupt the woman in mid-sentence. Avoid taking phone calls during the interview.

- Encourage the woman to speak spontaneously through open-ended questions or reflective statements, and allow adequate time for her to respond. Listen carefully to the answer. Some research indicates that women who are listened to first and have their emotions acknowledged are more likely to understand the medical information.

- Avoid judgmental statements and questions, which may put the woman on the defensive and break down the lines of communication. Refrain from making social criticisms or allowing personal feelings of dislike or disapproval to interfere.

- Ask specific questions to clarify the woman's statements. Avoid closed-ended questions such as, "Do you understand the instructions?" Those types of questions usually elicit a one-word response.

- Consider each woman as an individual. Don't assume that each woman will be influenced by the same information or motivators.

- Be aware of body language, both the woman's and the clinician's.

- Ensure that a woman has personal control over her selection of treatment. Providing women with enough information for them to make an informed decision can help build a trusting relationship.

- Be sensitive to conversations about menopause, which may be viewed negatively by the woman. Consider forming menopause discussion groups and forums for women to articulate their feelings about menopause with other women facing the same situation.

- Supplement verbal counseling with published literature, written material, or video or audio tapes. Education that includes a variety of strategies and media are the most effective. For example, providing both written instructions and take-home reading materials can reinforce the message and allow the woman more time to absorb the information.

- Short words and sentences are easy to understand and facilitate learning. Avoid jargon and medical abbreviations that may be misunderstood.

- When explaining material, allow time for questions. Reasons should be given for important instructions. Explain why a medication should be taken 1 or 2 hours after a meal (eg, needs to be taken on an empty stomach for absorption). Women who understand the reasons for particular instructions are more likely to adhere to them.

- Engage the woman in the treatment decision. Avoid counseling as if there were only one "right way." Shared decision making empowers the woman to take an active role in her health care. It may also reduce the risk of litigation should something go wrong.

- Involve each woman in monitoring for adverse drug reactions and interactions. Knowing what to expect can enhance feelings of control over treatment and avoid potentially dangerous side effects.

- Schedule follow-up contacts either by phone or office visit. A woman who might not contact the provider with a question may be more apt to share her concerns if contacted by the office staff.

- Be attentive to financial factors associated with a treatment plan. A woman who will have difficulty paying for a medication is less likely to continue the treatment plan.

- Be aware of (and avoid) perfunctory listening. This kind of listening is half-hearted and indifferent and does not convey the message of understanding that is necessary for a woman to feel as if she has been heard. Practice listening that includes responding to the expressed feeling or opinion of the woman. She will feel validated and respected, and she will be more likely to discuss issues of importance that relate to her health and well-being.

Bibliography

Anderson LA, Caplan LS, Buist DS, et al. Perceived barriers and recommendations concerning hormone replacement therapy counseling among primary care providers. *Menopause* 1999; 6:161-166.

Boggs PP. Telling isn't teaching: tips for optimal clinician-patient communication. *Menopause Management* 1998;7(4):13,21.

Kaufert P, Boggs PP, Ettinger B, Woods NF, Utian WH. The North American Menopause Society 1997 Menopause Survey. Women and menopause: beliefs, attitudes, and behaviors. *Menopause* 1998;5:197-202.

Nichols MP. *The Lost Art of Listening.* New York, NY: The Guildford Press; 1995.

Utian WH, Boggs PP. The North American Menopause Society 1998 menopause survey. Part I: Postmenopausal women's perceptions about menopause and midlife. *Menopause* 1999;6:122-128.

Woods NF. Midlife women health care patterns and choices. In: Falik M, Collins K, eds. *Women's Health: The Commonwealth Fund Survey.* Baltimore, MD: Johns Hopkins Press; 1996:145-174.

Q.08. Lesbian health

Approximately 5% to 10% of women have their primary emotional and sexual relationships with women. Lesbian (gay, homosexual) women live in all communities and represent a diverse group in race, ethnicity, education, age, and sexual practice. They may be celibate or sexually active with women, men, or both. Lesbians cannot be described as a group. However, some counseling guidelines can be offered.

The prospect of sharing information with a clinician about sexual orientation and lifestyle keeps some lesbians from seeking health care as frequently as desirable or at all. In a survey conducted in the 1980s, lesbians (N = 1,921) were asked about their experiences with healthcare practitioners. Responses included many accounts of insensitivity and heterosexism and even homophobia. Fortunately, tolerance for diversity in sexual orientation has improved since that time, but problems still remain. Lesbians in the United States are reported to see their healthcare providers less frequently than do other women; in Canada, frequency is reported to be about equal.

Although it is unknown whether lesbian women are at higher risk for certain chronic diseases that affect women at midlife and beyond (eg, some cancers and cardiovascular disease), their higher incidence of some risk lifestyle factors suggest that this might be the case. The Women's Health Initiative (WHI), which includes the largest number of women (N = 500) to identify themselves as lesbians in the medical literature, has found that the incidence of risk factors such as alcohol consumption, smoking, and overweight is higher in lesbian women. A smaller study found similar results. Thus, lifestyle more than heredity appears to be problematic.

Lesbians underestimate their risk of developing cancer, particularly cervical cancers, perhaps from the infrequency of heterosexual intercourse (although most lesbians have had sexual intercourse at some point in their lives). One large survey shows a lower rate of Pap smears in lesbians and bisexuals compared with that of heterosexual women. However, abnormal Pap smears and cervical cancer have been found, even among lifelong lesbians, making Pap smears an important part of the appropriate evaluation of a lesbian woman's health.

Other cancer risks should be evaluated. Although data on cancer incidence in lesbians are limited, they may be at a higher risk for cancer mortality because they are less likely to be screened with Pap smears, mammograms, and breast examinations. Because lesbian women are less likely to become pregnant, they may have a higher risk for certain diseases associated with nulliparity and low/no use of oral contraceptives. In addition, high-risk lifestyle factors, such as obesity, smoking, and alcohol consumption, may increase cancer risk. Furthermore, many lesbians do not think they need an annual gynecologic exam because they may not currently have sexual relations with a man. One study (WHI), however, showed no difference in the rate of breast cancer among the lesbian and bisexual participants compared with heterosexual women.

Lesbian women and their partners are at risk for contracting sexually transmitted infections (STIs). STIs can often be passed between female partners through skin-to-skin contact and through unsafe use of sex toys. Screening for STIs should be a concern. Viral infections (eg, herpes, HPV) can be transmitted from woman to woman, although some uncertainty exists with regard to HIV. Current thinking is that there are lesbians at high risk for HIV and AIDS, but that risk is related to IV drug abuse and their heterosexual/ bisexual practices. Safer sex practices should be encouraged. There is evidence that lesbians who engage in high-risk behaviors are less likely than heterosexual women to limit risk by practicing safer sex.

Neither gonorrhea nor chlamydia infections have ever been reported in a woman who has only had sex with women, but the rate of bacterial vaginosis appears to be higher among lesbians. Lesbians need to be advised that trichomonas can be transmitted between female partners.

History taking. For the lesbian woman to receive appropriate health care, her sexual orientation and lifestyle must be known and understood by her healthcare provider.

Many healthcare providers assume that women are heterosexual. It is important to use language that is free of heterosexual assumptions (eg, asking method of birth control used). In addition, it is important not to assume that sexual relations are exclusively with other women.

In a recent Canadian survey, more than half (51%) of the women did not reveal their sexual orientation to their healthcare provider even though they believed that it was important to enhance quality care. The same survey found that only 32% of physicians asked about sexual orientation. Clinicians are encouraged to examine their biases. If they are uncomfortable with counseling lesbian women, they should refer the women to other providers who possess a nonjudgmental attitude.

Clinicians should be alert to the possibility of current or previous physical/sexual abuse; approximately 38% of lesbians are survivors of childhood sexual abuse. About 40% report sexual assault, similar to women in the general population. Lesbians are also targets for antigay verbal abuse, threats, and violence.

For tips on how lesbian and bisexual women can avoid sexually transmitted infections, see Section Q.10.

Clinical care. Healthcare providers are encouraged to refine their attitudes regarding sexual orientation so they can obtain an in-depth sexual history and provide clinical care for lesbian women without becoming awkward or uncomfortable (see Table 7). If appropriate care cannot be provided, referral to another clinician is advised.

Table 7. Suggestions when counseling lesbian women

- Use a questionnaire that includes a question about sexual orientation. One survey found that 97% of lesbians and gays revealed their sexual orientation through this procedure.

  Suggested questions could include:
  Are you in a relationship?
  Are you sexually active?
  Do you have a partner or partners?
  Is your partner a man or a woman?
  Have you ever been sexually active with a man, woman, or both?

- Instill trust that the information will be treated with respect and confidentiality.

- Use language free of heterosexual assumptions until sexual orientation is known (eg, avoid asking what type of birth control is used).

- Don't assume that sexual relations are exclusively with other women.

- Respect the role of the lesbian's partner in her life and health-related decisions, treating her as a spouse. Instead of asking for the spouse's name, ask, "Whom would you like to be involved in the discussion of your treatment/surgery?" Give her partner complete access if she is hospitalized; if needed, suggest obtaining a durable power of attorney or healthcare power of attorney. Be aware of insurance issues, especially when the partner is the only one working and the employer does not recognize the patient as family.

Bibliography

Bailey JV, Kavanagh J, Owen C, et al. Lesbians and cervical screening. *Br J Gen Pract* 2000;50:481-482.

Berger BJ, Kolton S, Zenilman JM, et al. Bacterial vaginosis in lesbians: a sexually transmitted disease. *Clin Infect Dis* 1995; 21:1402-1405.

Bradford J, Ryan C, Rothblum ED. National lesbian health care survey: implications for mental health. *J Consult Clin Psychol* 1994;62:228-242.

Carroll NM. Optimal gynecologic and obstetric care for lesbians. *Obstet Gynecol* 1999;93:611-613.

Christilaw JE, Davis V, Edwards C, et al. Society of Obstetricians and Gynaecologists of Canada clinical practice guidelines: lesbian health guidelines. *J SOGC* 2000;22:202-205.

Chu SY, Buehler JW, Fleming PL, et al. Epidemiology of reported cases of AIDS in lesbians, United States 1980-89. *Am J Public Health* 1990;80:1380-1381.

Cochran SD, Mays VM, Bowen D, et al. Cancer-related risk indicators and preventive screening behaviors among lesbians and bisexual women. *Am J Public Health* 2001;91:591-597.

Denenberg R. Report on lesbian health. *Womens Health Issues* 1995;5:81-91.

Diamond M. Homosexuality and bisexuality in different populations. *Arch Sex Behav* 1993;22:291-310.

Dibble SL, Roberts SA, Davids HR, Pail SM, Scanlon JL. A comparison of breast cancer risk factor distributions between lesbian and bisexual women. *MS JAMA Online* 1999. Accessible at http://www.ama-assn.org/sci-pubs/msjamaarticles/vol_282/no_13/cancer.htm.

Dibble SL, Roberts SA, Robertson PA, Paul SM. Risk factors for ovarian cancer: lesbian and heterosexual women. *Oncol Nurs Forum* 2002;29:E1-E7.

Fethers K, Marks C, Mindel A, Estcourt CS. Sexually transmitted infections and risk behaviours in women who have sex with women. *Sex Transm Infect* 2000;76:345-349.

Grushkin EP, Hart S, Gordon N, Ackerson L. Patterns of cigarette smoking and alcohol use among lesbians and bisexual women enrolled in a large health maintenance organization. *Am J Public Health* 2001;91:976-979.

Kennedy M, Moore J, Schuman P, et al. Sexual behavior of HIV-infected women reporting recent sexual contact with women [Letter]. *JAMA* 1998;280:29-30.

Koh AS. Use of preventive health behaviors by lesbian, bisexual, and heterosexual women: questionnaire survey. *West J Med* 2000;172:379-384.

Krieger N, Sidney S. Prevalence and health implications of anti-gay discrimination: a study of black and white women and men in the CARDIA cohort. Coronary Artery Risk Development in Young Adults. *Int J Health Serv* 1997;27:157-176.

Michael RT, Gagnon JH, Laumann EO, Kolata GB. *Sex in America: A Definitive Survey.* Boston, MA: Little, Brown and Company; 1994.

Moran N. Lesbian health care needs. *Can Fam Phys* 1996;42:879-884.

Price JH, Easton AN, Telljohann SK, Wallace PB. Perceptions of cervical cancer and Pap smear screening behavior by women's sexual orientation. *J Community Health* 1996;21:89-105.

Raiteri R, Fora R, Sinicco A. No HIV-1 transmission through lesbian sex [Letter]. *Lancet* 1994;344:270.

Skinner WF, Otis MD. Drug and alcohol use among lesbian and gay people in a southern U.S. sample: epidemiological, comparative, and methodological findings from the Trilogy Project. *J Homosex* 1996;30:59-92.

Smith EM, Johnson SR, Guenther SM. Health care attitudes and experiences during gynecologic care among lesbians and bisexuals. *Am J Public Health* 1985;75:1085-1087.

Stevens PE. Structural and interpersonal impact of heterosexual assumptions on lesbian health care clients. *Nurs Res* 1995;44:25-30.

Valanis BG, Bowen DJ, Bassford T, Whitlock E, Charney P, Carter RA. Sexual orientation and health: comparisons in the Women's Health Initiative sample. *Arch Fam Med* 2000;9:843-853.

White JC, Dull VT. Health risk factors and health-seeking behavior in lesbians. *J Womens Health* 1997;6:103-112.

Q.09. Sexual function

Continued sexual activity is a realistic and expected part of aging. Healthcare professionals need to be sensitive and informed about sexuality issues to better counsel women on how to recognize and adjust to the changes. Clinicians are encouraged to be aware of these issues and to avoid imposing their own or society's views as to what constitutes normal sexuality in older women.

Confidentiality is a special concern when discussing sexual function. Clinicians should assure those they counsel that all discussions between the woman and her provider are strictly confidential.

Menopause is associated with anatomic, physiologic, and psychologic changes that often influence sexual function. For some women, physical changes associated with aging combined with societal influences that associate sex with youth may translate into a poorer self-image, diminution of self-esteem, and a loss of sexual desire. Urogenital atrophy is a major contributor to a decline in sexual activity after menopause. Declining sexual function or lack of an available partner also contributes to less frequent sexual activity.

As women age, they need to be educated regarding the physical, emotional, and social changes that occur, with suggestions made regarding how to accommodate those changes — as well as those of their partners, whether heterosexual or homosexual. Because a variety of psychologic, sociocultural, interpersonal, and biologic factors can contribute to sexual dysfunction, it is often helpful to counsel both the woman and her partner about the aging process and changes in sexual function that may concomitantly occur.

Men may experience an overall decline in sexual interest as well as difficulty achieving an erection or ejaculating. Couples need to be aware that both men and women may need more time and stimulation to achieve orgasm. Women without sexual partners have similar counseling requirements. As they age, they also will need more time and stimulation to reach an orgasm.

Education and communication are key elements for counseling women regarding sexual matters, Practitioners need to ask peri- and postmenopausal women about their sexual function when taking their medical history. Clinicians who are uncomfortable asking these questions during a face-to-face interview may need to offer women an alternate method of support, either reading material or discussion with another provider. A face-to-face interview is essential if women are to express any concerns or problems related to sexual function.

A study by The Robert Wood Johnson Medical School found that only 3% of women with sexual problems initiated discussion about them with their physicians. However, when asked specifically about sexual function, 19% reported a problem. Survey data indicate that between one-third and one-half of menopausal women recruited from the general population complain of a problem in one of more aspects of sexual functioning.

A survey published in 1999 reinforced the importance of clinicians initiating a discussion about sexual health. This survey showed that 71% of patients believed that their physician would dismiss any mention of sexual concerns; 68% believed their physician would be embarrassed by any discussion regarding sexual problems; and 76% did not think there were any treatments available to help with sexual problems.

Many sexual problems can be successfully treated. Women should be evaluated for underlying physiologic factors that may contribute to sexual problems, including vasomotor symptoms, medication side-effects, lifestyle issues (eg, drug or alcohol abuse), or medical conditions such as diabetes or cardiovascular or thyroid disorders.

For disorders related to lack of sexual desire, clinicians should evaluate the woman for the presence of depression, fatigue, or relationship problems, including sexual dysfunction of her partner.

Women and their partners should be reminded that intercourse does not have to be the primary or only sexual activity. Removing intercourse as the goal for every sexual encounter is useful advice for all couples, regardless of age. More attention may be devoted to other satisfying sexual behaviors, including oral sex, massage, sensual baths, manual stimulation, and caressing. A woman without a partner can explore masturbation — a normal and healthy expression of sexuality. Using a vibrator or dildo may enhance sexual pleasure. Some women may benefit from a referral to a counselor or a sex therapist.

For a women undergoing a hysterectomy, both she and her partner need to be assured that losing the uterus does not mean losing her sexual desire and femininity. Following hysterectomy, some women may notice a change in sensation during intercourse and orgasm, but, in general, these changes do not interfere with sexual functioning or achieving orgasm. Many women report improved sex lives after a hysterectomy due to relief of pain or bleeding and the lack of need for birth control. A minority of women can experience significant change in sexual response if surgery is extensive.

Women facing chemotherapy or pelvic radiation therapy should also be counseled about the special effects that these therapies have on sexual function (see Table 8).

Table 8. Suggestions for sexual counseling

Educate couples regarding normal age-related changes in sexual function:

- Women: Diminished lubrication, need for increased time and stimulation for arousal, decreased orgasmic contractions, decreased breast fullness and nipple erection, heightened clitoral sensitivity

- Men: Decreased penile rigidity, need for increased time and stimulation for erection and orgasm, longer refractory time

Encourage couples to accommodate changes in sexual function:

- Try warm baths before genital sexual activity

- Extend foreplay time to accommodate longer sexual arousal time

- Use sexual fantasies, erotic clothing or materials (eg, movies, literature), vibrators

- Experiment with noncoital activities such as massage, oral stimulation

- Use masturbation as an alternative to intercourse

- Change the sexual routine, such as having sex in the morning when energy levels are higher

- Experiment with positions other than the standard "missionary" position

---

Bibliography

Andersen BL, Cyranowski JM. Women's sexuality: behaviors, responses and individual differences. *J Consult Clin Psychol* 1995;63:891-906.

Andrews WC. Approaches to taking a sexual history. *J Womens Health Gend Based Med* 2000;9(suppl 1):S21-S24.

Basson R, Berman J, Burnett A, et al. Report of the international consensus and development conference on female sexual dysfunction: definitions and classifications. *J Urol* 2000; 163:888-893.

Hallström T, Samuelsson S. Changes in women's sexual desire in middle life: the longitudinal study of women in Gothenburg. *Arch Sex Behav* 1990;19:259-268.

Laan E, Everaerd W, Van der Velde J, Geer JH. Determinants of subjective experience of sexual arousal in women: feedback from genital arousal and erotic stimulus content. *Psychophysiol* 1995; 32:444-451.

Laumann EO, Paik A, Rosen RC. Sexual dysfunction in the United States: prevalence and predictors [erratum in *JAMA* 1999;281:1117]. *JAMA* 1999;281:537-544.

Marwick C. Survey says patients expect little physician help on sex. *JAMA* 1999;281:2173-2174.

Q.10. Preventing STIs

Although postmenopausal women are protected against pregnancy, they are not protected against sexually transmitted infections (STIs), often called sexually transmitted diseases (STDs). The risk of STIs — including syphilis, gonorrhea, genital herpes, human papilloma virus (genital warts), hepatitis B, and human immunodeficiency virus (HIV) — is a lifelong concern for women who are not in a long-term, mutually monogamous relationship. Most STIs are more easily transmitted man-to-woman rather than woman-to-man. Women are twice as likely as men to contract gonorrhea, hepatitis B, and HIV, if exposed. Moreover, STIs are less likely to produce symptoms in women and are, therefore, more difficult to diagnose until serious problems develop. (See Section Q.08 for specific information about lesbian health.)

Sexually active postmenopausal women with atrophic vaginitis may be at increased risk for STIs because the delicate vaginal tissue is prone to small tears and cuts that can act as pathways for infection. Avoidance of an STI is essential (see Table 9).

Table 9. Safer sex guidelines for all women

- Choose sex partners selectively.

- Discuss sexual history with a partner; do not let embarrassment compromise health.

- Always insist that male partners use a latex condom for genital, oral, and anal sex, unless in a long-standing, mutually monogamous relationship. Never use petroleum-based oils as lubrication for condoms because they can damage the condom, potentially causing a leak.

- Keep medically fit and have an annual physical examination, including (when indicated) a Pap test as well as tests to identify STIs.

- If exposed to an STI, or after a confirmed diagnosis, urge any partner(s) to be examined and treated.

Although lesbian women tend to have fewer STIs than heterosexual women, STIs can be passed from woman to woman and preventive measures are needed (see Table 10). Many lesbian women also have sex with men, often gay men. Lesbian and bisexual women not in a long-term, mutually monogamous relationship are at increased risk.

Table 10. Preventing STIs in a woman-to-woman sexual relationship

• Prevent transfer of any body fluids, including menstrual blood and vaginal fluids, from cuts or other openings.

• During oral sex, cover the partner's vaginal area with a barrier impermeable to fluid to avoid contact with vaginal secretions.

• Use a latex barrier between vaginas during vulva-to-vulva sex.

• Avoid sharing sex toys. Either clean them in hot, soapy water or use a new condom before switching users.

Bibliography

Brook MG. Sexual transmission and prevention of the hepatitis viruses A-E and G. *Sex Transm Infect* 1998;74:395-398.

Cohen MS. HIV and sexually transmitted diseases: the physician's role in prevention. *Postgrad Med* 1995;98:52-58.

Division of STD Prevention. *Sexually Transmitted Disease Surveillance, 2000.* Atlanta, GA: Centers for Disease Control and Prevention; 2001. Accessible at http://www.cdc.gov/std/stats/.

Elias CJ, Coggins C. Female-controlled methods to prevent sexual transmission of HIV. *AIDS* 1996;10(suppl 3):S43-S51.

Holtgrave DR, Qualls NL, Curran JW, Valdiserri RO, Guinan ME, Parra WC. An overview of the effectiveness and efficacy of HIV prevention program. *Public Health Rep* 1995;110:134-146.

Reyes EM, Legg JJ. Prevention of HIV transmission. *Prim Care* 1997;24:469-477.

Stratton P, Alexander NJ. Prevention of sexually transmitted infections: physical and chemical barrier methods. *Infect Dis Clin North Am* 1993;7:841-859.

Q.11. Domestic violence

Domestic violence is a significant public health problem for women (and men, although to a lesser extent). Domestic violence includes threatened or actual physical, sexual, emotional, or psychological abuse by partners or acquaintances.

Domestic violence raises a distinct set of challenges for the clinician because of its social rather than biomedical cause. Clinicians will need to move beyond the traditional medical paradigm to confront their own responses to abused women and to work with community groups to prevent domestic violence.

Clinicians must be alert for signs of this problem and to integrate routine inquiry about domestic violence into their examination. Healthcare providers explore the possibility of domestic violence with their patients less frequently than is recommended because they often feel as if they have nothing to offer the patient or that uncovering domestic violence may create a great deal of work for them.

Recognizing domestic violence and treating the physical injuries is one step. Clinicians can play a role in preventing both new and continued domestic violence through universal screening, assessment, treatment, documentation, and education. However, there are few published reports that have assessed the effectiveness of training healthcare professionals to screen and counsel women for domestic violence.

Detecting abuse can be difficult, since women are often reluctant to discuss it. Some clinicians find direct questioning to be more revealing than a questionnaire. Suggestions include direct questions such as: Have you ever been hurt or frightened by your partner? Does your partner ever threaten you? Let the woman know that you are concerned, that she does not deserve to be hurt, and that there are resources to support her.

Direct questioning is appropriate only if the partner is not present, because a woman is unlikely to answer truthfully in front of the perpetrator. If the partner is present, look for ways to separate them. One option is to send the partner to another area to answer billing or insurance questions. If it is not possible to talk with the woman alone during the examination, try to call her at her work or when her partner is at work.

Display posters and print materials discussing domestic violence in the office, which indicate your willingness to discuss the issue. The materials also can educate the woman regarding her options for responding to domestic violence. She may not be aware of the community outreach groups and safe shelters in her area, or she may not know how to contact them. Post the telephone number of the local women's shelter or hotline in the bathroom stall of the office or clinic.

Healthcare providers should be prepared to provide effective counseling for the acute resolution of this problem. This includes legal and social alternatives and resources, and the possibility of long-term therapy.

Be aware of the legal options in your area regarding both victim rights and requirements of the healthcare provider. Document violence in the woman's medical record both for follow-up care and for legal purposes. Many states require practitioners to report cases of domestic violence to a government agency, particularly when a woman has an injury that appears to have been caused by a weapon.

Bibliography

Barkan SE, Gary LT. Woman abuse and pediatrics: expanding the web of detection. *J Am Med Womens Assoc* 1996;51:96-100.

Davidson LL, Grisso JA, Garcia-Moreno C, Garcia J, King VJ, Marchant S. Training programs for healthcare professionals in domestic violence. *J Womens Health Gend Based Med* 2001; 10:953-969.

Dutton MA, Mitchell B, Haywood Y. The emergency department as a violence prevention center. *J Am Med Womens Assoc* 1996; 51:92-95.

Hyman A. Domestic violence: legal issues for health care practitioners and institutions. *J Am Med Womens Assoc* 1996; 51:101-105.

Short LM, Cotton D, Hodgson CS. Evaluation of the module on domestic violence at the UCLA School of Medicine. *Acad Med* 1997;72(suppl 1):S75-S92.

Sugg NK, Inui T. Primary care physicians' response to domestic violence: opening Pandora's box. *JAMA* 1992;267:3157-3160.

Tilden VP, Schmidt TA, Limandri BJ, et al. Factors that influence clinician's assessment and management of family violence. *Am J Public Health* 1994;84:628-633.

Q.12. Alcohol/drug abuse

There are three major groups of substance abuse. First is the area of legal drugs, such as alcohol and nicotine. The second is illicit drugs such as marijuana and cocaine. The third is prescription drugs, which include opiates (eg, oxycodone HCl, marketed as Oxycontin, and hydrocodone bitartrate and acetaminophen, marketed as Vicodin), benzodiazepines (eg, alprazolam, marketed as Xanax, and diazepam, marketed as Valium), and psychostimulants (eg, dextroamphetamine sulfate, marketed as Dexedrine, and methylphenidate HCl, marketed as Ritalin).

The lifetime incidence of alcoholism among women is approximately 10%. The lifetime incidence of illicit drug dependence among women is 5% to 6%. The lifetime incidence of nicotine dependence is 22%.

Women have lower rates than men for lifetime incidence of both alcohol and illicit drug use, but the incidence of nicotine dependence is nearly equal to that of men. The exact statistic of women's incidence rate of dependence on prescription drugs is not available; however, it is recognized that this is the one area of substance dependence where women have a higher rate than men. This is particularly true with the benzodiazepines.

Identification of women with substance dependence requires a careful history or questioning of the women regarding this area. The clinician working with peri- and postmenopausal women should be knowledgeable and willing to make inquiries regarding substance use, as well as to evaluate for comorbid issues such as anxiety and depression.

The standard for normal drinking for the postmenopausal women is no more than one standard alcoholic drink per day, with a standard alcoholic drink being defined as one 12 oz beer, 1 oz of distilled spirits, or 5 oz of table wine. Levels of alcohol consumption greater than this have been associated with increased risk of breast cancer and osteoporosis. Alcohol used in combination with nicotine exacerbates both of these problems. Medical problems often associated with excessive alcohol use include cirrhosis, cardiac failure secondary to cardiomyopathy, accidents, and being victimized by physical, sexual, and emotional abuse. Women who have a problem with alcohol or who are in recovery should never be prescribed a benzodiazepine, as this drug can trigger their addiction.

Nicotine use is by itself a chronic dependency and responsible for many adverse health consequences. These problems include emphysema, lung cancer, heart disease, and osteoporosis. Smoking in the adult female should raise the suspicion of coexistent conditions.

Traditional markers for alcoholism include tolerance, withdrawal symptoms, loss of control over drinking with social decline, and impaired working skills. Some of these symptoms may be confused with menopausal symptoms. Physical markers for recognizing alcohol abuse include frequent gastrointestinal disturbances, difficulty controlling health problems such as hypertension or diabetes, and unexplained seizures. Abnormal laboratory results that are consistent with alcoholism are an elevated gamma-glutamyl transferase or elevated mean corpuscular volume.

Peri- and postmenopausal women are more likely to abuse prescription medications if they have another identified chemical dependency, such as alcohol and/or nicotine. The woman may be obtaining prescriptions for these medications from several different clinicians, none of whom are aware that the woman is obtaining prescriptions from others. These women have a history of repeated refill requests for reasons such as "lost prescription" or the alleged use of the prescription by family members or friends.

Women who are abusing mood-altering drugs may have many physical concerns that are consistent with menopause symptoms. These include mood changes, vasomotor instability, and insomnia. A primary psychiatric problem, such as a depressive or anxiety disorder, may also be part of the clinical picture.

In general, women are less likely to be involved with illicit drugs than are men, with one exception: younger women are more prone to cocaine dependence than are males. The clinician should be comfortable in asking questions concerning illicit drug use. However, the woman's response may vary from candid honesty to complete misrepresentation of her drug use.

In detecting problematic drug use, the clinician should look for preoccupation with a particular drug in conjunction with an entire lifestyle that appears centered around drug procurement and use. The clinician should assess adverse consequences of continued drug abuse (eg, physical, psychologic, spiritual, and social). Many women tend to minimize or deny their degree of abuse or the extent of adverse consequences. Such women will typically lack insight into the problems created by their drug use. They may be quite unaware of the impact of their addiction on family members, friends, and business associates.

Concern about use of alcohol or other drugs (including prescription medications) should be addressed in an immediate and direct fashion. If the clinician is uncomfortable dealing with these types of problems, there should be quick and easy access to another, more appropriate professional. This could include an addiction counselor or a physician or psychiatrist who is experienced in dealing with addictive disorders. It is possible that detoxification may be required. If so, clinicians should refer the woman to someone who is experienced in dealing with this type of problem.

Bibliography

Fiellin DA, Reid MC, O'Connor PG. Outpatient management of patients with alcohol problems. *Ann Intern Med* 2000;133:815-827.

Lieber CS. Medical disorders of alcoholism. *N Engl J Med* 1995; 333:1058-1065.

Miller NS, Belkin BM, Gold MS. Alcohol and drug dependence among the elderly: epidemiology, diagnosis, and treatment. *Compr Psychiatry* 1991;32:153-165.

Winger G, Hofmann FG, Moods JH, eds. *A Handbook on Drug and Alcohol Abuse: The Biomedical Aspects.* 3rd ed. Oxford University Press: Oxford, Eng; 1992.

Ustun B, Compton W, Mager D, et al. WHO Study on the reliability and validity of the alcohol and drug use disorder instruments: overview of methods and results [erratum in: *Drug Alcohol Depend* 1998;50:185-186]. *Drug Alcohol Depend* 1997;47:161-169.

Xie X, Rehm J, Single E, Robson L. *The Economic Costs of Alcohol, Tobacco and Illicit Drug Abuse in Ontario, 1992.* Addiction Research Foundation: Toronto, ON, Canada; 1998.